Handbook of Systemic Drug Treatment in Dermatology

The *Handbook of Systemic Drug Treatment in Dermatology* helps prescribers and patients make rational decisions about drug treatment while considering known risks and potential unwanted effects. Written for dermatologists, family practitioners, pharmacists and specialist nurses, this completely revised and updated third edition of a bestseller provides an accessible and concise aid to prescribing and monitoring systemic dermatologic therapy. For each drug or drug class, the book lists its classification, mode of action, formulations, dosages, suggested regimens, contraindications, important drug interactions, adverse effects, patient information and more. This third edition includes new classes of drugs as well as information on updated guidelines for prescribing and monitoring established drugs.

FROM REVIEWS OF PREVIOUS EDITIONS

'This updated edition includes new arrivals … Quite simply, it is indispensable! I have it with me in every clinic and often refer to it in discussions with pharmacists (who have been known to borrow my copy and forget to return it).'

Dermatology in Practice

'… an outstanding resource that helps to alleviate worrying by providing precise guidelines and advice in managing our most infirm patients who require these medications.'

SkinMed

Handbook of
Systemic Drug Treatment
in Dermatology
Third Edition

Edited by

Sarah H. Wakelin, BSc, MBBS, FRCP
Consultant Dermatologist and Honorary Senior Lecturer
Imperial College Healthcare NHS Trust
London, UK

Howard I. Maibach, MD
Professor of Dermatology
University of California School of Medicine
San Francisco, California, USA

Clive B. Archer, BSc, MBBS, MSc Med Ed, MD (Lond), PhD, FRCP
Consultant Dermatologist
St John's Institute of Dermatology
Guy's and St Thomas' Hospitals NHS Foundation Trust
Honorary Professor of Dermatology and Immunopharmacology
University of Central Lancashire (UCLan)
Honorary Senior Clinical Lecturer
King's College London (KCL), London, UK

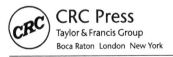
CRC Press
Taylor & Francis Group
Boca Raton London New York

CRC Press is an imprint of the
Taylor & Francis Group, an **informa** business

Third edition published 2023
by CRC Press

4 Park Square, Milton Park, Abingdon, Oxon, OX14 4RN

and by CRC Press

6000 Broken Sound Parkway NW, Suite 300, Boca Raton, FL 33487-2742

British Library Cataloguing-in-Publication Data
A catalogue record for this book is available from the British Library

---

Library of Congress Cataloging-in-Publication Data

Names: Wakelin, S. H. (Sarah H.), editor. | Maibach, Howard I., editor. |
Archer, Clive B., editor.
Title: Handbook of systemic drug treatment in dermatology / edited by Sarah
H. Wakelin, Howard I. Maibach, Clive B. Archer.
Description: Third edition. | Boca Raton : CRC Press, 2023. | Includes
bibliographical references and index.
Identifiers: LCCN 2022032357 (print) | LCCN 2022032358 (ebook) | ISBN
9780367860820 (hardback) | ISBN 9780367860813 (paperback) | ISBN
9781003016786 (ebook)
Subjects: MESH: Skin Diseases--drug therapy | Dermatologic
Agents--therapeutic use | Drug Interactions | Drug-Related Side Effects
and Adverse Reactions | Handbook
Classification: LCC RL801 (print) | LCC RL801 (ebook) | NLM WR 39 | DDC
616.5/061--dc23/eng/20221103
LC record available at https://lccn.loc.gov/2022032357

LC ebook record available at https://lccn.loc.gov/2022032358

ISBN: 978-0-367-86082-0 (hbk)
ISBN: 978-0-367-86081-3 (pbk)
ISBN: 978-1-003-01678-6 (ebk)

DOI: 10.1201/9781003016786

Typeset in Times
by KnowledgeWorks Global Ltd.

Contents

v

Preface

Since the second edition of this handbook in 2015, dermatological therapy has continued to advance at a pace. The prescriber can now offer patients a wide range of biologics for psoriasis and new biologics for eczema and urticaria. In addition, the licensing of Janus kinase (JAK) inhibitors for skin disease brings a completely new category of medication to the dermatologist's portfolio. Keeping up to date with new drugs and new treatment indications is a challenge in such a rapidly-changing field. The COVID-19 pandemic raised questions on our use of immunosuppressive drugs and the move to remote prescription and drug monitoring has altered the way we deliver care to our patients. Other societal changes include our ageing population especially those with frailty - now recognised as an emerging public health priority. Managing chronic disease in patients with complex multi-morbidities under time pressure in inadequately resourced and staffed systems, without inbuilt safety mechanisms is a recipe for disaster. This led the World Health Organisation (WHO) to launch its third global challenge, *Medication without harm*, in 2017, aiming to address the medication practices and errors that are a leading cause of injury and avoidable harm in health care systems across the world. Patients should be informed of the risks and benefits of therapy through detailed discussion supplemented with written information.

We hope that this third edition of the handbook will remain a practical and popular resource for prescribers and clinicians throughout their careers and help achieve the goal of safe prescribing. New drugs and updated guidelines are included which inevitably causes further gain in girth with age. At a time of potential information overload, our aim remains to provide an easily accessible and reliable 'how to' resource at the reader's fingertips that works when the internet connection fails and the computer crashes. While every effort has been made to ensure accuracy, prescribers are advised to check doses in up-to-date formularies and to consult the manufacturer's literature / summary of product characteristics.

The editors are very grateful to all contributors of this edition, and earlier editions. Last but not least we would like to thank Taylor & Francis, particularly Robert Peden for his support with this publication.

The Editors

Contributors

Elaine Agius
St John's Institute of Dermatology
Guy's and St Thomas' Hospitals NHS
    Foundation Trust
London, UK

Faisal R. Ali
Private Practice
London, UK

Iaisha Ali
The Harley Street Clinic
HCA Healthcare
London, UK

Mahreen Ameen
Royal Free Hospital
London, UK

Charles Archer
Oxford University Hospitals NHS
    Foundation Trust
Oxford, UK

Clive B. Archer
St John's Institute of Dermatology
Guy's and St Thomas' Hospitals NHS
    Foundation Trust
London, UK

Natalie R. Attard
St John's Institute of Dermatology
Guy's and St Thomas' Hospitals NHS
    Foundation Trust
London, UK

Susannah Baron
St John's Institute of Dermatology
Guy's and St Thomas' Hospitals NHS
    Foundation Trust
London, UK

Maria Bashyam
Wexham Park Hospital
Frimley Health NHS Foundation Trust
Slough, UK

John Berth-Jones
University Hospital
Coventry, UK

Leena Chularojanamontri
Faculty of Medicine Siriraj Hospital
Mahidol University
Bangkok, Thailand

Hannah Cookson
Royal Devon University Hospital
Devon, UK

Charles H. Earnshaw
Salford Royal Hospital
University of Manchester
Cancer Research UK
Manchester Institute
Manchester, UK

Charlotte L. Edwards
Chelsea and Westminster Hospital NHS
    Foundation Trust
London, UK

Michael P. Escudier
Faculty of Dentistry, Oral and Craniofacial
    Sciences
King's College London
London, UK

Hiva Fassihi
St John's Institute of Dermatology
Guy's and St Thomas' Hospitals NHS
    Foundation Trust
London, UK

Louise A. Fearfield
Chelsea and Westminster Hospital NHS
    Foundation Trust
London, UK

Steven R. Feldman
Wake Forest School of Medicine
Winston-Salem, North Carolina, USA

Rosanna Fox
Chelsea and Westminster Hospital NHS
    Foundation Trust
London, UK

L. Claire Fuller
Chelsea and Westminster Hospital NHS
    Foundation Trust
London, UK

Olga Golberg
Mid Essex Hospital Services NHS Foundation
    Trust
Chelmsford, UK

Mark Goodfield
University of Leeds
Leeds, UK

Clive Grattan
St John's Institute of Dermatology
Guy's and St Thomas' Hospitals NHS
    Foundation Trust
London, UK

Christopher E.M. Griffiths
Salford Royal Hospital
University of Manchester
NIHR Manchester Biomedical Research Centre
Manchester, UK

Richard W. Groves
St John's Institute of Dermatology
Guy's and St Thomas' Hospitals NHS
    Foundation Trust
London, UK

Karen Harman
University Hospitals of Leicester NHS Trust
Leicester, UK

Roderick J. Hay
King's College London
London, UK

Courtney E. Heron
Wake Forest School of Medicine
Winston-Salem, North Carolina, USA

Victoria J. Hogarth
Kingston Hospital
London, UK

Esther A. Hullah
Guy's and St Thomas' Hospitals NHS
    Foundation Trust
London, UK

Graham A. Johnston
University Hospitals of Leicester NHS Trust
Leicester, UK

Jonathan Kentley
Imperial College Healthcare NHS Trust
London, UK

Murtaza Khan
Mediclinic
Abu Dhabi, UAE

Shahid A. Khan
Imperial College Healthcare NHS Trust
London, UK

Brian Kirby
St Vincent's University Hospital
Dublin, Ireland

Joey E. Lai-Cheong
Private Practice
Windsor, UK

Alison M. Layton
University of York
York, UK

John T. Lear
The Alexandra Hospital
Manchester, UK

Hui Min Liew
Gleneagles Medical Centre
Singapore, Singapore

Antonia Lloyd-Lavery
Oxford University Hospitals NHS Foundation
    Trust
Oxford, UK

N. Farah Mahmood
University Hospitals of Leicester NHS Trust
Leicester, UK

Phil Mason
Oxford University Hospitals NHS Foundation
    Trust
University of Oxford
Oxford, UK

Simon Meggitt
Newcastle Hospitals NHS Foundation Trust
Newcastle upon Tyne, UK

Oonagh Molloy
St Vincent's University Hospital
Dublin, Ireland

Rachael Morris-Jones
St John's Institute of Dermatology
Guy's and St Thomas' Hospitals NHS
    Foundation Trust
London, UK

Alexander Nast
Charité – Universitätsmedizin Berlin
Berlin, Germany

Genevieve Osborne
Bristol Royal Infirmary
Bristol, UK

Gayathri K. Perera
Chelsea and Westminster Hospital NHS
    Foundation Trust
London, UK

Derrick Phillips
Imperial College Healthcare NHS Trust
London, UK

Andrew Pink
St John's Institute of Dermatology
Guy's and St Thomas' Hospitals NHS
    Foundation Trust
London, UK

Ellie Rashidghamat
St John's Institute of Dermatology
Guy's and St Thomas' Hospitals NHS
    Foundation Trust
London, UK

Chris Rutkowski
Department of Adult Allergy and St John's
    Institute of Dermatology
Guy's and St Thomas' Hospitals NHS
    Foundation Trust
London, UK

Robert P.E. Sarkany
St John's Institute of Dermatology
Guy's and St Thomas' Hospitals NHS
    Foundation Trust
London, UK

Julia J. Scarisbrick
University Hospital Birmingham
Birmingham, UK

Matthew Scorer
University Hospitals of Leicester NHS Trust
Leicester, UK

Alison Sears
St John's Institute of Dermatology
Guy's and St Thomas' Hospitals NHS
    Foundation Trust
London, UK

Jane Setterfield
Guy's and St Thomas' Hospitals NHS
    Foundation Trust
King's College London
London, UK

Manuraj Singh
St George's University Hospitals NHS
    Foundation Trust
London, UK

Sarita Singh
St John's Institute of Dermatology
Guy's and St Thomas' Hospitals NHS
    Foundation Trust
London, UK

Catherine Smith
St John's Institute of Dermatology
Guy's and St Thomas' Hospitals NHS
    Foundation Trust
London, UK

Lindsay C. Strowd
Wake Forest School of Medicine
Winston-Salem, North Carolina, USA

Thomas Tull
St John's Institute of Dermatology
Guy's and St Thomas' Hospitals NHS
    Foundation Trust
London, UK

Peter C.M. van de Kerkhof
Radboud University Nijmegen Medical Centre
Nijmegen, the Netherlands

Annette Wagner
Department of Adult Allergy and St John's
    Institute of Dermatology
Guy's and St Thomas' Hospitals NHS
    Foundation Trust
London, UK

Sarah H. Wakelin
Imperial College Healthcare NHS Trust
London, UK

Richard B. Warren
Salford Royal Hospital
University of Manchester
NIHR Manchester Biomedical Research Centre
Manchester, UK

Ricardo N. Werner
Charité – Universitätsmedizin Berlin
Berlin, Germany

Richard Woolf
St John's Institute of Dermatology
Guy's and St Thomas' Hospitals NHS
    Foundation Trust
London, UK

Shirin Zaheri
The Harley Street Clinic
HCA Healthcare
London, UK

List of Abbreviations

5-HT	5-hydroxytryptamine
ACE	angiotensin-converting enzyme
ACTH	adrenocorticotrophic hormone
AGEP	acute generalized exanthematous pustulosis
AIDS	acquired immunodeficiency syndrome
ALP	alkaline phosphatase
ALT	alanine aminotransferase
ANA	antinuclear antibodies (p)ANCA (perinuclear) antineutrophil cytoplasmic antibody
AST	aspartate aminotransferase
AV	atrioventricular
BAD	British Association of Dermatologists
BCC	basal cell carcinoma
BCG	bacillus Calmette–Guérin
Bd	twice daily, every 12 hours
BMD	bone mineral density
BMI	body mass index
BNF	British National Formulary
BP	blood pressure
BSA	body surface area
CBC	complete blood count (= FBC)
CBG	cortisol-binding globulin
CIN	cervical intraepithelial neoplasia
CK	creatine kinase
CKD	chronic kidney disease
CMV	cytomegalovirus
CNS	central nervous system
CS	glucocorticosteroids
CSM (UK)	Committee for Safety of Medicines
CTCL	cutaneous T-cell lymphoma
CXR	chest radiograph
CYP450	cytochrome P450
DCP	dexamethasone–cyclophosphamide pulse
DEXA	dual energy X-ray absorptiometry
DHT	dihydrotestosterone
DILI	drug-induced liver injury
DISH	diffuse idiopathic skeletal hyperostosis
DLE	discoid lupus erythematosus
DLQI	Dermatology Life Quality Index
DNA	deoxyribonucleic acid
DRESS	drug reaction (or rash) with eosinophilia and systemic symptoms
DVT	deep venous thrombosis
EBV	Epstein–Barr virus
ECG	electrocardiogram
ELISA	enzyme-linked immunosorbent assay
EMA	European Medicines Association
ENL	erythema nodosum leprosum

FBC	full blood count (= CBC)
FDA (USA)	Food and Drug Administration
FSH	follicle-stimulating hormone
G6PD	glucose-6-phosphate dehydrogenase
GAD-7	Generalised Anxiety Disorder Assessment-7
G-CSF	granulocyte colony-stimulating factor
(e)GFR	(estimated) glomerular filtration rate
GGT	gamma-glutamyl transferase
GI	gastrointestinal
GnRH	gonadotrophin releasing hormone
GSH	glutathione
HAART	highly active antiretroviral therapy
HBV	hepatitis B virus
HCV	hepatitis C virus
HDL	high-density lipoprotein
HIV	human immunodeficiency virus
HR	heart rate
HRT	hormone replacement therapy
HSV	herpes simplex virus
IBD	inflammatory bowel disease
IFN	interferon
Ig	immunoglobulin
IGRA	interferon-gamma release assay
IL	interleukin
i/m	intramuscular, intramuscularly
INR	international normalized ratio
ITP	idiopathic (immune) thrombocytopenic purpura
i/v	intravenous, intravenously
IVF	in vitro fertilization
KS	Kaposi's sarcoma
LDL	low-density lipoprotein
LE	lupus erythematosus
LFT	liver function test
LH	luteinizing hormone
MAOI	monoamine oxidase inhibitor
MCV	mean corpuscular volume
MF	mycosis fungoides
MHRA (UK)	Medicines and Healthcare Products Regulatory Agency
MI	myocardial infarction
MMR	mumps, measles, rubella
MPD	minimal phototoxic dose
MRI	magnetic resonance imaging
(CA/HA)-MRSA	(community-acquired/hospital-acquired) methicillin-resistant *Staphylococcus aureus*
MTX	methotrexate
NHL	non-Hodgkin's lymphoma
NICE (UK)	National Institute for Health and Care Excellence
nocte	at night
NMSC	non-melanoma skin cancer
NRTI	nucleoside reverse transcriptase inhibitor
NSAID	non-steroidal anti-inflammatory drug

NYHA	New York Heart Association
OCP	oral contraceptive pill
Od	once daily, every 24 hours
PIIINP	pro-collagen III peptides
PABA	para-aminobenzoic acid
PASI	Psoriasis Area and Severity Index
PE	pulmonary embolism
PGA	Physician's Global Assessment
PHQ-9	Patient Health Questionnaire-9
PML	progressive multifocal leukoencephalopathy
PPP	Pregnancy Prevention Programme
PSA	prostate-specific antigen
PT	prothrombin time
PTC	pseudotumour cerebri
PUVA	psoralen combined with ultraviolet A
PVL	Panton–Valentine leukocidin
Qds	four times daily, every 6 hours
RAR	retinoic acid receptor
RePUVA	PUVA with oral retinoid therapy
RNA	ribonucleic acid
RXR	retinoid X receptor
s/c	subcutaneous, subcutaneously
SCC	squamous cell carcinoma
SHBG	sex hormone-binding globulin
SLE	systemic lupus erythematosus
SPC	Summary of Product Characteristics
SSRI	selective serotonin reuptake inhibitor
STAT	signal transducer and activator of transcription
TB	tuberculosis
Tds	three times daily, every 8 hours
TEN	toxic epidermal necrolysis
TFT	thyroid function test
TGF-b	transforming growth factor-beta
TPMT	thiopurine methyltransferase
TSH	thyroid-stimulating hormone
U&E	urea and electrolytes
UVA	ultraviolet A
UVB	ultraviolet B
VTE	venous thromboembolism
VZIG	varicella/zoster immunoglobulin
VZV	varicella zoster virus
WBC	white blood cell count
WHO	World Health Organization

1 Acitretin

Peter C.M. van de Kerkhof

CLASSIFICATION AND MODE OF ACTION

By the 1960s, modifications of vitamin A (Figure 1.1) resulted in the discovery of the first-generation retinoids, all-trans-retinoic acid and 13-cis-retinoic acid. Further research led to development of the second generation of retinoids, the monoaromatic retinoids, etretinate and its metabolite, acitretin. Etretinate (which is no longer available) and acitretin are effective treatments for psoriasis and severe congenital disorders of keratinization.

A major problem with systemic retinoids is their teratogenicity, and separation of this from their therapeutic effects has never been achieved. Acitretin has a much shorter half-life than etretinate, but a long duration of pregnancy avoidance post-treatment is still advised, as acitretin can be converted to etretinate in the presence of alcohol, and the latter is stored in fat with a half-life of 120 days.

Acitretin is an established treatment for psoriasis and, despite development of biological agents (the biologics), it remains an important therapy due to its unique mode of action. It binds receptors belonging to the steroid–thyroid receptor superfamily. Subsequently, the ligand/receptor complex binds to specific gene regulatory regions to modulate gene expression. Acitretin has antiproliferative and anti-inflammatory properties. In the epidermis, acitretin reduces keratinocyte proliferation and normalises differentiation and cornification. It also inhibits production of vascular endothelial growth factor and inhibits intraepidermal neutrophil migration. Acitretin inhibits interleukin (IL)-6–driven induction of Th17 cells, which play a pivotal role in the pathogenesis of psoriasis and promote the differentiation of T-regulatory cells. Unlike other psoriasis therapies, acitretin lacks immunosuppressive effects, and this can be useful in patients with a history of internal malignancy, those with a history of skin cancer or severe sun damage, transplant recipients and those with underlying infections such as human immunodeficiency virus (HIV) infection. In addition, there is evidence that acitretin may be successfully combined with biologics.

INDICATIONS AND DERMATOLOGIC USES

The licensed indications for acitretin are as follows:

- Severe extensive psoriasis that cannot be managed by topical treatment or phototherapy.
- Palmoplantar pustular psoriasis.
- Severe Darier disease.
- Severe congenital ichthyosis.

Monotherapy is indicated for erythrodermic or pustular psoriasis, while combination therapy (with phototherapy) is often used for chronic plaque psoriasis. The efficacy of acitretin monotherapy in chronic plaque psoriasis is limited and dose-dependent, with approximately 70% of patients achieving a moderate or greater response. Various studies have reported partial clearance rates of 25–75% with daily doses of 30–40 mg. Lower doses (10 mg or 25 mg daily) have little therapeutic effect, whereas doses of 50 mg and 75 mg daily result in an improvement of at least 75% (PASI 75) in 25% of patients. Complete clearance is rare, and adherence at high dosage is often limited by side effects. In a more recent retrospective study, PASI 50, 75, 90 and 100 response was achieved by 53%, 48%, 28% and 14% of the patients, respectively, using acitretin at a daily dose of 25 mg.

DOI: 10.1201/9781003016786-1

1

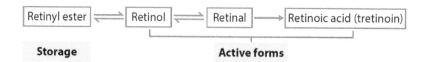

FIGURE 1.1   Simplified diagram to illustrate the three main active forms of vitamin A and a storage form.

The comparative efficacy of acitretin monotherapy in chronic plaque psoriasis is less than methotrexate and ciclosporin (cyclosporine). However, acitretin in combination with phototherapy (ultraviolet B [UVB] or psoralen combined with ultraviolet A [PUVA]) has an efficacy at least comparable with the other non-biologic systemic treatments. An additional advantage of combination treatment is that lower doses of acitretin and lower cumulative doses of UVA or UVB can be used. Topical therapy such as calcipotriol should be continued with acitretin, as it may enable increased efficacy at a lower dosage. There is also limited evidence for the effective combination of acitretin with etanercept and hydroxycarbamide (hydroxyurea).

As monotherapy, acitretin is highly effective in erythrodermic and pustular psoriasis. However, its efficacy in nail psoriasis and psoriatic arthritis is modest. Another potential therapeutic use of acitretin is the prophylaxis of non-melanoma skin cancer in organ transplant recipients. Acitretin may be considered a first-line systemic therapy for pityriasis rubra pilaris and lichen planus (especially the hyperkeratotic and erosive variants). Acitretin has similar efficacy to antimalarials in the treatment of cutaneous lupus erythematosus.

FORMULATIONS/PRESENTATION

Branded formulations exist with capsule sizes containing 10 mg and 25 mg of acitretin. In the United States, there are additional formulations containing 17.5 mg and 22.5 mg acitretin.

DOSAGES AND SUGGESTED REGIMENS

The recommended starting dose is 25–30 mg or 0.5 mg/kg once daily for chronic plaque psoriasis, with dose adjustment after 2–4 weeks according to clinical response and side effects. A lower starting dose of 0.25 mg/kg is advisable in erythrodermic psoriasis. For pustular psoriasis, the dose should be increased to the maximum maintenance dose of 75 mg or 1 mg/kg daily. An initial flare up of plaque psoriasis may occur, but improvement is usually evident by 4 weeks. Optimal response may take over 3 months.

Lower starting doses of 10 mg daily are indicated for Darier disease, with maintenance doses of 10–25 mg daily. Similar low doses can be used in conjunction with phototherapy.

With the availability of highly effective immunomodulatory/immunosuppressive treatments, it is important to have the availability of non-immunosuppressive treatments. In particular, in patients with malignancies and chronic infections, such as hepatitis, HIV and latent tuberculosis, acitretin may provide an adequate solution.

Acitretin should be taken with or after a fat-containing meal to maximize bioavailability.

BASELINE INVESTIGATIONS AND CONSIDERATIONS

- Pregnancy testing and enrollment in pregnancy prevention plan.
- Establishment of highly effective contraception in females of childbearing potential at risk of pregnancy.
- Full blood count (FBC) (complete blood count [CBC]).
- Liver function tests (LFTs).
- Serum urea, electrolytes and creatinine.
- Fasting lipids and glucose (consider testing HbA1c).
- Consider screening tests for mental illness (PHQ-9, GAD-7).

MONITORING

- Pregnancy testing (throughout and beyond treatment in females of childbearing potential).
- Fasting lipids and LFTs monthly for the first 2 months, then every 3–6 months.
- Fasting glucose if there is evidence of impaired glucose tolerance.
- Monitor for development of hyperostosis by history (twice yearly) and by skeletal X-ray if symptomatic.
- Growth charts for height and weight in those under 18 years.

CONTRAINDICATIONS AND CAUTIONS

The following are contraindications to systemic retinoid therapy:

- Pregnancy (see below).
- Lactation.
- Uncontrolled severe hyperlipidaemia.
- Hypersensitivity to retinoids or excipients.

Patients taking acitretin should not donate blood during treatment and for 3 years after stopping therapy. Extra caution should be taken when acitretin is prescribed in the following cases:

- Liver dysfunction.
- Severe renal dysfunction (elimination reduced).
- Hyperlipidaemia.
- Alcohol dependency.
- History of pancreatitis.
- Diabetes (glucose tolerance may be impaired).
- Obesity.
- Arteriosclerosis.
- Contact lens use.
- Serious disorders of the retina.
- History of or current mental health disorder.

IMPORTANT DRUG INTERACTIONS

- Ciclosporin (cyclosporine) metabolism: This may be inhibited by acitretin, as both drugs are metabolized by the same cytochrome P450 (CYP450) system, leading to a risk of ciclosporin toxicity.
- Glibenclamide: Acitretin enhances the hypoglycaemic effect of glibenclamide.
- Methotrexate and acitretin: These have been used successfully as combination therapy in those patients in whom all other psoriasis treatments have failed. However, severe hepatotoxicity has been reported, so careful monitoring is mandatory. As methotrexate itself causes hepatotoxicity, it is unclear what role acitretin plays in hepatotoxicity.
- Oral contraceptive pill (OCPs): There is an additive effect on the elevation of serum triglycerides and cholesterol, but there is no effect on the anti-ovulatory action of the combined OCPs.
- Phenytoin: Protein binding is reduced by acitretin, but the clinical significance of this is unknown.
- Tetracyclines: These should be avoided during acitretin therapy, as both drugs can cause benign intracranial hypertension; the risk may be increased if they are used concurrently.
- Vitamin A: Intake should not exceed the recommended dietary allowance (4,000–5,000 units/day), so supplements should be avoided.
- Alcohol: Alcohol promotes the esterification of acitretin to etretinate ('back metabolism'), which is far more slowly eliminated. This may prolong the risk of teratogenicity in females of childbearing potential.

ADVERSE EFFECTS AND THEIR MANAGEMENT

- Teratogenicity: This is the principal problem with all systemic retinoids. Both natural forms of vitamin A in high doses (but not its pro-vitamin, beta-carotene) and synthetic retinoids are highly teratogenic. Teratogenic effects include cardiac defects, microcephaly, spina bifida and limb defects. A retinoid pregnancy prevention program should be followed in all females of childbearing potential (see Chapter 22).
- Hyperlipidaemia: Hyperlipidaemia is a concern with long-term therapy. Triglycerides and cholesterol rise during acitretin treatment in about 30% of patients, with an increase in the low-density lipoprotein (LDL) to high-density lipoprotein (HDL) ratio (atherogenic index). This occurs particularly in patients with risk factors for hyperlipidaemia, i.e. excessive alcohol intake, diabetes mellitus, obesity or a family history of hyperlipidaemia. The elevation is dose-related and can be managed by dietary control, dose reduction or, in some circumstances, by lipid-lowering drugs. If the cholesterol cannot be maintained below 8.5 mmol/L and the triglyceride level below 3.0 mmol/L, treatment should be discontinued.
- Hepatitis: A transient modest rise in liver transaminases is common, but acute hepatitis and jaundice are rare. Elevation of liver enzymes above two to three times the upper limit of normal should lead to discontinuation of treatment. If the elevation of liver enzymes is less than twice the upper limit of normal, the patient can be managed by more frequent monitoring, e.g. every 2 weeks.
- Mucocutaneous: In view of the commonly occurring dryness or erosions of the skin and mucous membranes, topical emollients and lip salves should be used routinely. Scaling, dryness, skin thinning and erythema may also be seen, particularly on the face and palmoplantar skin. Rarer cutaneous manifestations include skin fragility, photosensitivity and development of excessive granulation tissue. Epistaxis may occur occasionally. Petrolatum can be smeared into the nostrils to alleviate dryness.
- Hair loss: Hair loss is dose-dependent and occurs in up to 75% of patients receiving acitretin, but only a minority are severely affected. Hair loss diminishes over time and is usually reversible within 6 months of discontinuation. Development of curly hair has been reported as a rare effect.
- Ocular adverse effects: These include sore eyes and decreased tolerance of contact lenses, which can be alleviated using eye drops ('artificial tears'). A decrease in night vision has occasionally been reported.
- Musculoskeletal adverse effects: These include arthralgia and myalgia, which are usually mild but may result in reduced exercise tolerance. Long-term (>2 years) treatment with second-generation retinoids has been associated with an increased risk of calcification of extraspinal tendons and ligaments, especially ankles, pelvis and knees, and diffuse idiopathic skeletal hyperostosis (DISH)–like changes in the spine. However, this is not clearly correlated with dose or duration. Routine monitoring with X-rays is therefore not justifiable in asymptomatic patients, but targeted radiography may be indicated for atypical musculoskeletal pain.
- Premature epiphyseal closure: This can occur in children. In view of the effect of retinoids on the growth plates, there is a potential risk of decreased growth. However, it is advisable to monitor growth at regular intervals in children who are treated with acitretin.
- Neurologic: Headache, drowsiness and benign intracranial hypertension have occasionally been reported. Subclinical dysfunction of sensory nerve fibres has been detected after 1 month of treatment. Taste disturbance may occur.
- Systemic: Non-specific symptoms such as nausea, malaise or sweating can sometimes occur.
- Psychiatric: Depression, insomnia, aggressive feelings, self-harm and suicidal ideation have been reported. It remains unclear if these are directly due to the drug/a retinoind class effect.

USE IN SPECIAL SITUATIONS

PREGNANCY

Acitretin is absolutely contraindicated in pregnancy, and females should not become pregnant for at least 3 years after stopping treatment. This duration is recommended by the British Association of Dermatologists (BAD). FDA and BNF recommend a 3-year time interval. Pregnancy must be excluded before starting therapy. Females of childbearing potential should have a negative pregnancy test not more than 2 weeks before starting acitretin.

Highly effective contraception must be used for 1 month before, during and for at least 3 years after cessation of treatment, even in those with a history of infertility. Precise recommendations will differ between countries.

Acitretin therapy should begin on the second or third day of the menstrual cycle.

The patient must be able to understand the risks of acitretin treatment, the consequences of a pregnancy and be able to comply with effective contraception. Information on how to obtain emergency contraception may be provided.

There is no evidence of impaired fertility or mutagenic risk in males who receive acitretin.

LACTATION

Acitretin is excreted in breast milk, and mothers taking this medication should not breastfeed.

CHILDREN

Acitretin may be used in carefully selected cases under expert supervision, e.g. in severe ichthyosis. The main concern in this age group is the risk of premature epiphyseal closure, though it is not clear if this is relevant with low-dose acitretin. Doses of 0.5–1.0 mg/kg/day may be used, up to a maximum of 35 mg/day, but the maintenance dose should be kept as low as possible. In female children approaching menarche, use of acitretin should be critically reviewed.

ESSENTIAL PATIENT INFORMATION

Patients should be warned of the possible side effects and given an up-to-date drug information leaflet as provided by the manufacturer.

Females should avoid pregnancy throughout treatment and for at least 3 years after stopping acitretin. Females of childbearing potential should sign an acknowledgement form regarding the risks associated with pregnancy.

Patients should not donate blood during or for at least 3 years after treatment. They should avoid tetracyclines, keratolytics, excessive sun exposure and ultraviolet lamps and supplements of vitamin A.

Wax epilation should be avoided due to the risk of increased skin fragility.

FURTHER READING

Chiricozzi A, Panduri S, Dini V, et al. Optimizing acitretin use in patients with plaque psoriasis. Dermatol Ther. 2017;30:e12453; https://doi.org/10.1111/dth.12453.

Griffiths CEM, Clark CM, Chalmers RJG, Li Wan Po A, Williams HC. A systematic review of treatments for severe psoriasis. Health Technol Assess. 2000;4(40):25–49.

Jessop S, Whitelaw DA, Delamere FM. Drugs for discoid lupus erythematosus. Cochrane Database Syst Rev. 2009;4:CD002954.

Kaushik SB, Lebwohl MG. Psoriasis: Which therapy for which patient: Focus on special populations and chronic infections. J Am Acad Dermatol. 2019;80:27–40.

Ormerod AD, Campalani E, Goodfield MJD. British Association of Dermatologists guidelines on the efficacy and use of acitretin in dermatology. Br J Dermatol. 2010;162:952–63.

2 Acne Antibiotics

Alexander Nast, Ricardo N. Werner and Natalie R. Attard

CLASSIFICATION AND MODE OF ACTION

Certain antibiotics are widely prescribed in the treatment of acne. They decrease the number and function of Cutibacterium acnes (formerly known as Propionibacterium acnes), a commensal lipophilic bacterium that colonizes the pilosebaceous duct. Additional non-antimicrobial actions may be of importance, including anti-inflammatory effects on neutrophils, impairment of matrix metalloproteinase activity and inhibition of pro-inflammatory cytokines such as IL-1α and TNFα. The relative contribution in clinical efficacy of the antibacterial and anti-inflammatory effects of antibiotics in acne are unknown. Tetracyclines and macrolides exert broad-spectrum antibacterial effects by inhibiting bacterial protein biosynthesis, while trimethoprim inhibits bacterial folic acid metabolism. They work by slowing the growth of bacteria rather than killing them. Concomitant treatment with topical benzoyl peroxide has a bactericidal effect, reducing the risk of antibiotic resistance.

INDICATIONS AND DERMATOLOGICAL USES

The use of systemic antibiotics for the treatment of acne is indicated in the following:

- Widespread mild-to-moderate papulopustular (inflammatory) acne.
- Severe papulopustular/moderate nodular acne.
- Severe nodular/conglobate acne (as an alternative to oral isotretinoin).

Topical antiacne therapy with a single fixed-dose formulation of combined benzoyl peroxide and retinoid (adapalene) or azelaic acid should be co-prescribed in all situations above.

FORMULATIONS/PRESENTATION

These include the following:

- Doxycycline: 40 mg (modified release), 50 mg and 100 mg capsules; 100 mg dispersible tablets.
- Lymecycline: 408 mg capsules.
- Minocycline: 50 mg and 100 mg tablets and capsules.
- Tetracycline and oxytetracycline: 250 mg tablets.
- Erythromycin: 250 mg and 500 mg tablets and capsules; 125 mg/5 mL suspensions (including sugar-free suspensions).
- Trimethoprim: 100 mg and 200 mg tablets; 50 mg/5 mL suspension.

Erythromycin is formulated as erythromycin base, estolate, ethyl succinate and stearate.

DOSAGES AND SUGGESTED REGIMENS

There is currently no clear evidence to guide the optimal duration of treatment. Antibiotics work relatively slowly in acne, and the initial duration of therapy is generally 3 months. If there is no improvement after this time, another drug should be considered. A further 3 months could be

DOI: 10.1201/9781003016786-2

prescribed if the acne has not completely cleared. Ideally, courses for longer than 6 months' duration should be avoided.

A clear explanation of the likely timelines of improvement, common side effects and the reason for additional topical treatment during the initial consultation is likely to improve patient adherence and outcome.

- First-choice treatment
  - Doxycycline: 100 mg once daily (or 50 mg–200 mg daily).
  - Lymecycline: 408 mg once daily.
- Second-choice treatment
  - Tetracycline and oxytetracycline: 500 mg twice daily.
- Third-choice treatment
  - Minocycline: 100 mg once daily.
  - Trimethoprim: 300 mg twice daily (unlicensed use).
- During pregnancy and lactation
  - Erythromycin: 500 mg twice daily (not erythromycin estolate).

Published trials show a trend towards superior efficacy for tetracyclines compared with macrolides. Although all tetracyclines appear to have comparable efficacy against inflammatory acne lesions, lymecycline and doxycycline are preferred due to their lack of interaction with milk and once-daily dosage. Due to the risk of irreversible pigmentation and other adverse effects with minocycline, it should not be used as a first-line therapy. Sarecycline is a new semi-synthetic tetracycline with a narrow antibacterial spectrum, developed for treatment of inflammatory acne. It was approved by the FDA in 2018 to treat non-nodular moderate-to-severe acne in patients 9 years and older.

Trimethoprim is unlicensed for the treatment of acne and therefore considered a third-choice antibiotic to be used under a specialist's recommendation. Erythromycin can be a useful treatment in pregnant or breastfeeding patients and when tetracyclines are contraindicated.

Once inflammatory lesions have resolved, maintenance topical treatment should be prescribed (retinoids and/or benzoyl peroxide or azelaic acid) and continued for a minimum of 6 months.

Failure to respond may be a consequence of the following:

- Poor patient adherence.
- C. acnes resistance.
- Inadequate dose or duration of therapy.
- Interactions impairing antibiotic absorption.

ANTIBIOTIC RESISTANCE

C. acnes resistance is increasing and widely reported globally. The clinical relevance of this is not clear, as acne antibiotics also exert anti-inflammatory effects. It is important to be aware of the principals of antibiotic stewardship when considering treatments for acne.

This is outlined in Figure 2.1.

Suspect resistance if:

- The patient has received many long-term sequential oral and/or topical antibiotics.
- Patient not improving.
- The patient relapses after the initial response to treatment despite continued therapy.

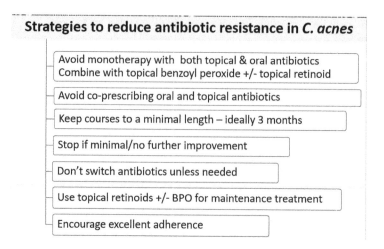

FIGURE 2.1   Consider adopting these strategies when treating acne to reduce the risk of antibiotic resistance.

MONITORING

- Routine monitoring is not required before or during treatment of acne with oral antibiotics.
- Baseline investigations and monitoring every 3 months for hepatotoxicity and lupus (ANA and LFTs) have been suggested for patients receiving minocycline.

CONTRAINDICATIONS

- Tetracyclines (doxycycline, minocycline, tetracycline and lymecycline)
  - Severe renal impairment (except doxycycline).
  - Children <12 years.
  - Pregnancy and lactation.
  - Systemic lupus erythematosus or family history of lupus (minocycline).
- Erythromycin
  - QT interval prolongation and combination with agents that can result in QT interval prolongation (risk of ventricular arrhythmias).
  - Hypokalaemia, hypomagnesaemia due to risk of QT interval prolongation.
  - Severe hepatic impairment, history of hepatitis caused by macrolides and cholestasis.
- Trimethoprim
  - Severe renal impairment.
  - Severe liver impairment.
  - Haematological disease (thrombopenia, granulocytopenia and megaloblastic anaemia).
  - Pregnancy and lactation.

CAUTIONS

- Tetracyclines
  - Hepatic impairment.
  - Renal impairment (dose reduction, consider determining drug serum level in long-term therapy – see Chapter 39).
  - Personal or close family history of lupus-like disorders (minocycline).
  - Myasthenia gravis, due to possible potentiation of neuromuscular blockade.
- Erythromycin
  - Hepatic impairment.
  - Severe renal impairment (risk of irreversible hearing loss).

- Trimethoprim
  - Hepatic impairment.
  - Renal impairment (dose reduction required).
  - Folic acid deficiency.
  - Risk of hyperkalaemia (risk may be increased).

IMPORTANT DRUG INTERACTIONS

Tetracyclines should not be prescribed with the following:

- Oral retinoids, due to a potential increased risk of benign intracranial hypertension (see Chapter 22).
- Penicillins, as the bactericidal action of penicillins may be reduced due to pharmacodynamic antagonism.

Care should be taken if tetracyclines are prescribed with the following:

- Digoxin, due to increased absorption and potential toxicity of digoxin.
- Oral anticoagulants, as tetracyclines may enhance anticoagulant effects due to a reduction in prothrombin activity.
- Salts of calcium, iron, strontium, bismuth, aluminium, zinc, magnesium, antacids and quinapril (contains magnesium), which may reduce absorption of tetracyclines and diminish their effectiveness.
- Oral hypoglycaemic agents, as the glucose-lowering effect of sulphonylureas may be increased.
- Ciclosporin (cyclosporine) and methotrexate, due to possible increased toxicity.
- Diuretics (lymecycline).

Erythromycin has numerous drug interactions due to its inhibitory effects on the cytochrome P450 (CYP450) 3A isoenzyme, and the cardiotoxicity of certain drugs may also be increased. It should not be prescribed with the following:

- Antipsychotic drugs, including droperidol, pimozide and sertindole.
- Ergot alkaloids (unlicensed use for headache), due to increased risk of ergotism.
- Mizolastine, due to QT prolongation.
- Simvastatin, lovastatin, due to increased risk of myopathy.

Care should be taken if erythromycin is prescribed with the following:

- Atorvastatin and pravastatin, as a lower dose should be used, and patients should be monitored carefully for signs of myopathy. Other statins which are not metabolized by CYP3A4 (rosuvastatin, fluvastatin) may carry less risk of myopathy.
- Ciclosporin metabolism, which may be inhibited with increased toxicity (see Chapter 13).
- Colchicine, due to increased risk of toxicity (see Chapter 14).
- Coumarin anticoagulants (e.g. warfarin), due to increased anticoagulant effects.
- Digoxin plasma concentrations, which are raised with risk of toxicity.
- Anticonvulsants (phenytoin, carbamazepine clozapine and valproic acid), due to decreased metabolic clearance and increased plasma levels.
- Theophylline, due to increased plasma theophylline, which may cause nausea, vomiting and seizures.
- Verapamil, due to increased risk of cardiotoxicity.

Trimethoprim should not be prescribed with the following:

- Cytotoxics (methotrexate, mercaptopurine and azathioprine), due to the increased risk of increased bone marrow toxicity.

Care should be taken if trimethoprim is prescribed with the following:

- Ciclosporin, due to possible increased nephrotoxicity.
- Coumarin anticoagulants, due to possible enhanced anticoagulant effect.
- Dapsone, as plasma concentrations of both drugs may increase.
- Pyrimethamine, due to possible blood dyscrasia.
- Oral hypoglycaemic agents, due to possible enhanced effects.
- Phenytoin, lamivudine, zidovudin, digoxin and procainamide, due to increased plasma level and potential toxicity.

Oral antibacterial drugs may inactivate oral typhoid and cholera vaccines. Vaccination with oral typhoid should be delayed for >72 hours and oral cholera vaccines should be delayed for >14 days after administration of antimicrobial agents.

SPECIAL POINT

The UK's Faculty of Sexual and Reproductive Health 2020 guidelines state that that most antibiotics do not affect combined hormonal contraceptives (with the exception of enzyme-inducing drugs such as rifampicin) unless they cause vomiting or severe diarrhoea (which can affect absorption and reduce contraceptive efficacy). The drug package information leaflet may contain contradictory advice, such as the need to use additional barrier contraception.

ADVERSE EFFECTS AND THEIR MANAGEMENT

Nonspecific effects of oral antibiotic therapy include the following:

- Gastrointestinal effects such as nausea, colic and diarrhoea may occur with all acne antibiotics but are particularly common with erythromycin, as it enhances gastroduodenal motility.
     Epigastric discomfort is common with doxycycline and may be improved by taking the medication after food (which may decrease absorption up to 20%).
- Vaginal candidiasis is a common side effect. Effective therapy is available without prescription.
- Severe cutaneous adverse drug reactions have been reported rarely with acne antibiotics. They include acute generalized exanthematous pustulosis, drug reaction with eosinophilia and systemic symptoms (DRESS) and Stevens-Johnson syndrome/toxic epidermal necrolysis. Milder rashes, urticaria and pruritus are not uncommon with trimethoprim.
- Hormonal contraceptive failure may occur if the user is affected by vomiting or diarrhoea. See Special Point.
- Clostridium difficile-associated diarrhoea (CDAD) and especially pseudomembranous colitis are very rare with oral acne antibiotics. They require prompt and specific treatment with metronidazole or vancomycin.

Specific drug side effects include the following:

- Hyperpigmentation with minocycline may affect various body sites including skin, nails, mucosae, eyes and bones ('black bones') due to the deposition of black metabolites of the drug. Blue/grey/muddy brown discoloration may be localized or diffuse. The risk is generally related to the duration of treatment, and pigmentation may persist after stopping therapy, especially on sun-exposed sites. Q-switched ruby laser therapy may help.

- Photosensitivity (phototoxicity) may occur with all tetracyclines but is especially common with doxycycline and demeclocycline. Phototoxicity ranges from mild sunburn to oedematous plaques, blisters and a lichenoid rash. It may be accompanied by photo-onycholysis, which can be delayed by several weeks. The triggering spectrum is mainly UVA1 (340–400 nm), so UV-protective products that cover this range should be used.
- Pseudotumor cerebri syndrome (benign intracranial hypertension) has been reported as a rare adverse effect of tetracyclines, especially with doxycycline. It usually occurs within 4 weeks of starting therapy. Symptoms include a severe headache, often pulsatile, which is worsened by coughing, straining and physical activity, visual disturbances, diplopia, pulsatile tinnitus, nausea and vomiting. It may result in permanent visual loss. If suspected, an ophthalmological or neurological examination for papilledema is required.
- Minocycline-induced lupus-like syndrome with hepatitis, polyarthralgia and positive antinuclear antibodies has been reported rarely (approximately 1 case per 10,000 person-years), especially with prolonged treatment. Perinuclear antineutrophil cytoplasmic antibodies (p-ANCAs) may also occur in some individuals. The risk of developing a lupus-like disorder has been estimated to be increased 2–5-fold during minocycline treatment, so the use of this drug should be avoided if possible.
- Oesophagitis may occur with all tetracyclines, especially doxycycline. Medication should be taken when upright and with plenty of water at least 30 minutes before going to bed to reduce the risk. Symptoms usually settle within a week of drug withdrawal.
- Tooth staining is a recognized adverse effect of all tetracyclines. This may affect the primary or secondary dentition and has been reported to develop in adults after prolonged therapy. It occurs due to the ability of this group of antibiotics to chelate calcium ions, leading to their incorporation into teeth, cartilage and bone.
- Drug-induced liver injury is a very rare adverse effect of tetracyclines (see Chapter 40). Cholestatic hepatitis has been reported as a hypersensitivity reaction to erythromycin, especially the estolate. The latency is usually short (1–3 weeks or <1 week on re-exposure). Eosinophilia and fever are common. Right upper quadrant pain and jaundice may be confused with cholecystitis. Abrupt severe liver injury with elevated liver enzymes may also occur.
- Idiosyncratic blood dyscrasias, including agranulocytosis, thrombocytopenia and anaemia, may occur with trimethoprim.

USE IN SPECIAL SITUATIONS

PREGNANCY AND PRE-CONCEPTION

Tetracyclines (formerly FDA Category D) are contraindicated. They cross the placenta and can have toxic effects on fetal development, particularly retardation of skeletal development. Embryotoxicity in early pregnancy has been noted in animals. Use of tetracyclines during the last half of pregnancy may cause permanent discoloration of the infant's teeth.

Erythromycin may be considered as a suitable oral therapy in severe disease in pregnancy. The estolate salt is contraindicated.

Trimethoprim should be avoided in pregnancy, as it is a folate antagonist.

Tetracycline and erythromycin have been shown to impair sperm motility in vitro. Tetracycline has been shown to achieve higher concentrations in prostatic and seminal fluid, so erythromycin may be the preferred option.

LACTATION

Tetracyclines should not be used, as they are excreted in breast milk and may cause permanent tooth discoloration and enamel hypoplasia in the developing infant.

Erythromycin is excreted in breast milk but can be considered in severe cases (strict indication).

Due to a relatively low rate of excretion in breast milk, trimethoprim can be considered in severe cases (strict indication).

CHILDREN

Tetracyclines are contraindicated in young children due to the risk of permanent tooth discoloration. The British National Formulary advises against their use in children under the age of 12 years due to the risk of permanent dental staining. Organizations in the United States recommend a lower age limit of 8 years.

Erythromycin is licensed for use in childhood and may be considered in severe infantile acne.

FURTHER READING

Nast A, Dréno B, Bettoli V et al. European evidence-based (S3) guideline for the treatment of acne – update 2016 – short version. J Eur Acad Dermatol Venereol. 2016 Aug;30(8):1261–8.

National Institute for Health and Care Excellence (NICE). Acne vulgaris: Management. 2021; https://www.nice.org.uk/guidance/ng198.

Simmons KB et al. Drug interactions between non-rifamycin antibiotics and hormonal contraception: A systematic review. Am J Obstet Gynecol. 2018 Jan;218:88.

Walsh TR, Efthimiou J, Dréno B. Systematic review of antibiotic resistance in acne: An increasing topical and oral threat. Lancet Infect Dis. 2016;16(3):e23–33.

Zaenglein AL, Pathy AL, Schlosser BJ et al. Guidelines of care for the management of acne vulgaris. J Am Acad Dermatol. 2016 May;74(5):945–73.

3 Alitretinoin

N. Farah Mahmood and Graham A. Johnston

CLASSIFICATION AND MODE OF ACTION

Alitretinoin (9-cis-retinoic acid) is an endogenously occurring retinoid which is structurally related to vitamin A. It acts as a pan-agonist at retinoid receptors, binding with high affinity to both retinoic acid receptors (RARs) and retinoid X receptors (RXRs). The latter are capable of binding to a range of different nuclear receptors to modulate gene expression (Figure 3.1). The precise mode of action of alitretinoin in chronic hand eczema remains unclear, but retinoids are known to affect multiple processes at a cellular level including proliferation, differentiation and apoptosis. They may also have anti-inflammatory and immunomodulatory effects, including suppression of nitric oxide and tumour necrosis factor (TNF)-alpha production, impairment of T-cell activation and down-regulation of chemokine synthesis (CXCL9 and CXCL10), thereby impairing the recruitment of inflammatory leukocytes. Alitretinoin has been shown to suppress the expression of co-stimulatory molecules on the surface of antigen-presenting cells, which may be of relevance to a therapeutic effect in contact dermatitis. In contrast to isotretinoin, alitretinoin has a minimal effect on sebum secretion.

Alitretinoin has a much shorter half-life (an average of 9 days) compared to acitretin and isotretinoin, and levels of the drug and its metabolites return to the normal range within 2–7 days of stopping established treatment.

INDICATIONS AND DERMATOLOGICAL USES

- The only licensed indication for alitretinoin in the UK is severe chronic hand eczema that is unresponsive to potent topical steroids in adults. Severe chronic hand eczema is defined by a clinical score – the Physician's Global Assessment (PGA) – and a Dermatology Life Quality Index (DLQI) score of at least 15.

A large, randomized placebo-controlled study (the Benefit of Alitretinoin in Chronic Hand [BACH] eczema study) demonstrated the efficacy of alitretinoin in adult patients with severe chronic hand eczema. This reported that almost half of all patients receiving a 30 mg daily dose of alitretinoin achieved a rating of 'clear' or 'almost clear' at the 24-week endpoint. A lower dose of 10 mg daily was less effective but still superior to placebo. Both hyperkeratotic disease and pompholyx/fingertip variants of hand eczema were reported to respond.

Smaller studies have reported benefits in palmoplantar psoriasis, chronic hyperkeratotic palmar psoriasis and chronic foot eczema. There are also reports of a benefit in Darier disease, Hailey–Hailey disease, pityriasis rubra pilaris, mycosis fungoides and palmoplantar keratoderma.

FORMULATIONS/PRESENTATION

- 10 mg and 30 mg alitretinoin in soft capsules (Toctino®).
- Capsules contain soya bean oil and sorbitol.

A topical formulation of alitretinoin is FDA approved in the United States for use in acquired immunodeficiency syndrome (AIDS)-associated Kaposi sarcoma.

DOI: 10.1201/9781003016786-3

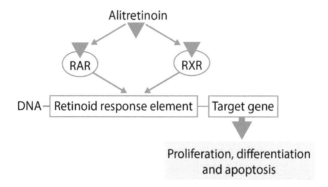

FIGURE 3.1   Schematic diagram of the retinoic acid receptor (RAR), retinoid X receptor (RXR) and binding to the retinoid response element in the promoter region of a gene.

SPECIAL POINT

Alitretinoin and acitretin are both prescribed by dermatologists and are 'soundalike' drugs. This raises the potential for prescribing and dispensing error with potentially serious consequences and litigation. Prescribing by brand may reduce this risk. Pharmacists who dispense alitretinoin should be alert to the potential for confusion.

DOSAGES AND SUGGESTED REGIMENS

The usual starting dose is 30 mg once daily. The capsule should be swallowed whole with or after a meal to maximize bioavailability. If side effects are not tolerated, the dose can be reduced to 10 mg daily. In patients with diabetes, hyperlipidaemia or risk factors for cardiovascular disease, a lower starting dose of 10 mg once daily is recommended. This can be increased if necessary to a maximum daily dose of 30 mg.

The onset of action is slow, but there is usually some improvement within the first month. UK NICE guidelines recommend that clinical response should be assessed at 12 weeks and treatment be discontinued if inadequate. For those who respond, the total duration of treatment is recommended to be 12–24 weeks. Treatment should be stopped once an adequate clinical response ('clear' or 'almost clear') has been achieved. At 24 weeks, around half of patients will be 'clear' or 'almost clear' of disease. A further response of 39–50% can be achieved if the course of treatment is extended by a further 12–24 weeks. Alitretinoin has been found to be well-tolerated up to 48 weeks. Relapse tends to occur slowly over several months; retreatment may be necessary.

BASELINE INVESTIGATIONS AND CONSIDERATIONS

Patch testing should be performed before starting alitretinoin to exclude a significant underlying contact allergy. This is an important consideration, as allergic contact dermatitis of the hands may be impossible to distinguish from an endogenous dermatitis on clinical grounds alone.

Patients with diabetes, a history of hyperlipidaemia or risk factors for cardiovascular disease should be identified and screened before starting treatment and closely monitored during treatment. Baseline investigations consist of:

- Pregnancy testing (and enrollment in a pregnancy prevention programme [PPP] for all females of childbearing potential).
- Full blood count (FBC) (complete blood count [CBC]).

- Urea, electrolytes and creatinine.
- Liver function tests (LFTs).
- Fasting lipids and glucose.
- Thyroid function tests (if clinically indicated).
- Consider screening tests for mental illness (PHQ-9, GAD-7).

SPECIAL POINT

Patients whose jobs may be impacted by visual disturbance such as drivers, airline pilots, military personnel and those who operate heavy machinery should discuss this medication before starting and check with current UK Civil Aviation Guidelines or local equivalent.

MONITORING

- A PPP should be followed in females of childbearing potential (see Chapter 22).
- Fasting lipids (cholesterol and triglycerides) should be monitored in order to detect hyperlipidaemia. In the absence of specific advice from the manufacturers, testing every 3–6 months is reasonable. Monthly monitoring may be indicated for those with diabetes, pre-existing hyperlipidaemia or risk factors for cardiovascular disease.
- Urea and electrolytes and LFT monitoring is reasonable, though not specifically advised by the manufacturer.
- Thyroid function should be monitored in those with pre-existing diseases. In normal individuals, low thyroid-stimulating hormone (TSH) levels may occur during treatment, but thyroid medication is not usually required.

CONTRAINDICATIONS AND CAUTIONS

The following are contraindications to systemic retinoid therapy including alitretinoin:

- Pregnancy (see below).
- Hypersensitivity to retinoids or excipients.

Alitretinoin capsules (Toctino) contain soya bean oil. While soya beans and peanuts are both legumes, each of these foods stand alone in terms of immunogenicity, and patients who are peanut allergic do not routinely need to avoid soya-containing products. Where the history is unclear, skin prick tests can be considered and, if negative, a test dose can be given under clinical supervision.

Blood donation should be avoided during treatment and for at least one month after stopping treatment.

Extra caution should be taken when alitretinoin is prescribed in the following:

- Liver dysfunction/cirrhosis (close monitoring is required; see Chapter 40).
- Renal impairment (alitretinoin metabolites are mainly excreted in the urine; see Chapter 39).
- Uncontrolled hypothyroidism.
- Uncontrolled hyperlipidaemia.
- Diabetes.
- Depression.
- Hypervitaminosis A.
- Disorders associated with ocular dryness.
- Concomitant treatment with tetracycline antibiotics.
- History of or current mental health disorder.

IMPORTANT DRUG INTERACTIONS

- Simvastatin: A slight reduction of simvastatin plasma levels was observed when co-administered with alitretinoin.
- Vitamin A: Supplements are contraindicated due to the risk of hypervitaminosis/retinoid toxicity.
- Tetracyclines: This is due to the increased risk of benign intracranial hypertension.

ADVERSE EFFECTS AND THEIR MANAGEMENT

- Teratogenicity: In females of childbearing potential, the PPP should be followed unless the individual has signed a disclaimer that she is not sexually active and at risk of pregnancy. The monitoring requirements are identical to those for oral isotretinoin (see Chapter 22). In the UK this includes the following:
  - Pregnancy testing before starting alitretinoin, at monthly intervals thereafter during treatment and at 5 weeks after the completion of treatment.
  - Females at risk of pregnancy must use adequate contraception for at least 1 month before starting treatment, during treatment and for at least 1 month after stopping treatment.
  - Females should be advised to use at least one method of highly effective contraception, and they should consider using two methods. The progesterone-only oral contraceptive pill (OCP) (mini-pill) or barrier contraception alone are not considered adequate but can be combined with other contraceptive methods. The effectiveness of hormonal contraceptives is not impaired by alitretinoin.
  - Females should be advised to discontinue treatment and to seek prompt medical attention if they become pregnant during treatment or within 1 month of stopping treatment.
- Hyperlipidaemia: Raised total cholesterol and triglycerides may occur during treatment. This effect is usually dose-related and reversible and usually responds to dosage reduction. If these measures fail and hyperlipidaemia is severe, treatment must be discontinued. Hypertriglyceridaemia is associated with an increased risk of pancreatitis, especially if levels exceed 9 mmol/L.
- Headache and flushing: These are the most common initial adverse effects and affect about half of all patients. They are a more frequent problem with alitretinoin than other systemic retinoids and tend to improve after several weeks of continued treatment. Simple analgesics and taking the medication shortly before sleep may be helpful.
- Benign intracranial hypertension (pseudotumour cerebri): This is a very rare adverse effect common to all retinoids, especially when taken with tetracyclines. Symptoms are severe headache, nausea and vomiting and visual disturbance. If untreated, there is a risk of permanent visual loss.
- Ocular adverse effects: These effects include blurred vision, conjunctivitis, photosensitivity, impaired night vision, cataracts, keratitis and eye irritation. If night vision is impaired patients should avoid driving and operating heavy machinery. Night vision changes can be permanent in extremely rare circumstances.
- Cutaneous adverse effects: These include flushing and pruritus, dryness, cheilitis, epistaxis, asteatotic eczema, vasculitis and alopecia. Cheilitis and alopecia are less common than with isotretinoin and acitretin, respectively. Photosensitivity can occur, so patients should be advised to avoid use of sunbeds and to protect their skin against excessive sun exposure. Use of a high-protection sunscreen of at least SPF 30 is advised. As skin fragility may occur,

hair removal using waxing, epilation, dermabrasion or laser treatment, as well as tattoos and piercings should be avoided during treatment and for 6 months afterwards.

- Musculoskeletal adverse effects: The effects common to oral retinoids include exercise-induced fatigue, myalgia and arthralgia. These may be associated with elevation of serum creatine kinase. Radiological changes with long-term retinoid therapy include hyperostosis and spondylitis (rare).
- Psychiatric disturbance including depression: This is a potential adverse effect (class effect) of all oral retinoids, especially isotretinoin (see Chapter 22). It is not yet clear if this applies to alitretinoin, which has generally been used in older patients with a different psychosocial profile from those with acne. Patients affected by mood change may be evaluated for depression and anxiety using PHQ-9 and GAD-7, respectively.

USE IN SPECIAL SITUATIONS

PREGNANCY AND PRE-CONCEPTION

Alitretinoin is a potent teratogen and absolutely contraindicated in pregnancy. Females should not become pregnant within 1 month of discontinuing treatment (see Chapter 22).

Very low amounts of alitretinoin have been detected in the semen of males taking alitretinoin. As with the other oral retinoids, isotretinoin and acitretin, these levels are too low to pose a teratogenic risk to the unborn baby of a female partner.

LACTATION

Alitretinoin is lipophilic and likely to be distributed to breast milk, so it is contraindicated in breast-feeding females.

CHILDREN

Alitretinoin is only licensed for use in those over 18 years. Clinical trials of high-dose 9-cis-retinoic acid in childhood malignancy reported benign intracranial hypertension as a frequent adverse effect, especially in younger children. There is insufficient evidence at present to support the use of alitretinoin in dermatological diseases in children.

ESSENTIAL PATIENT INFORMATION

- Patients should be informed of the likely side effects and the monitoring requirements.
- It should be explained that treatment will cease if there is an inadequate response at 3 months, after completion of a 6-month course or earlier if disease remission is achieved.
- Females should be fully informed of the requirements of the PPP.

FURTHER READING

Brown RG. Pharmacology of oral alitretinoin: A novel treatment for severe chronic hand eczema. Clin Exp Dermatol. 2011;36(Suppl. 2):1–34.

National Institute for Health and Care Excellence. NIoHaCE Final appraisal determination – Alitretinoin for the treatment of severe chronic hand eczema. Technology Appraisal Guidance (TA177). 2009. https://www.nice.org.uk/guidance/ta177.

Park HK, Kim EJ, Yo JY. Alitretinoin: Treatment for refractory palmoplantar keratoderma. Br J Dermatol. 2016;174(5):1143–4.

Patel AN, Wooton CI, Babakinjad P, English JS. Alitretinoin: The Nottingham experience. Clin Exp Dermatol. 2014;39:224–5.

Ruzicka T, Lynde CW, Jemec GBE, et al. Efficacy and safety of oral alitretinoin (9-*cis*-retinoic acid) in patients with severe chronic hand eczema refractory to topical corticosteroids: Results of a randomized, double-blind, placebo-controlled, multicentre trial. Br J Dermatol. 2008;158(4):808–17.

4 Antiandrogens

Shirin Zaheri and Iaisha Ali

CLASSIFICATION AND MODE OF ACTION

Antiandrogens are a group of drugs that block the action of androgens by two broad mechanisms:

- Competitive inhibition of binding of androgens (testosterone and dihydrotestosterone [DHT]) to the androgen receptor (androgen receptor antagonists).
- Inhibition of the enzyme 5α-reductase that converts testosterone to DHT.

Androgen receptor antagonists include drugs, such as the steroidal antiandrogens, spironolactone and cyproterone acetate, which also have direct inhibitory effects on androgen synthesis, and the non-steroidal or 'pure' antiandrogens, which are flutamide, bicalutamide, enzalutamide, darolutamide and apalutamide.

Flutamide is a potent antiandrogen. Its mechanism of action is inhibiting androgen uptake and nuclear binding of androgens in target tissues. Bicalutamide is a more potent antiandrogen with similar mechanisms of action. Bicalutamide was first developed for the treatment of prostate cancer, but at modified doses, bicalutamide has been found to be effective in the treatment of females with hirsutism. Enzalutamide, darolutamide and apalutamide and nilutamide have not been used for dermatological indications to date but are indicated for the treatment of prostate cancer.

Spironolactone is an aldosterone antagonist and acts as a potassium sparing diuretic. It inhibits the action of aldosterone on the distal renal tubule, increasing sodium and water excretion and reducing potassium excretion. Spironolactone is also a potent antagonist of the androgen receptor as well as an inhibitor of androgen production; hence, it is used to treat androgen-related skin disease in females, namely hirsutism, androgenic alopecia and acne.

Drospirenone is a spironolactone analogue with antimineralocorticoid activity. It also counteracts the oestrogen-stimulated activity of the renin–angiotensin–aldosterone system and has also been shown to possess mild antiandrogen activity. It is used in combination with oestrogen for hormonal oral contraception and hormone replacement therapy.

Cyproterone acetate is a synthetic derivative of 17-hydroxyprogesterone and acts primarily as an androgen receptor antagonist. It also has a weak progesterone agonist and glucocorticoid actions and inhibits androgen synthesis. Cyproterone acetate was the first antiandrogen in clinical use, and it was introduced in 1964. A low-dose combined preparation containing 2 mg of cyproterone acetate and 50 μg of ethinyloestradiol was first marketed in the UK in 1977, and it was subsequently reformulated with a lower oestrogen dose (Dianette®) to reduce oestrogen-related side effects (oedema, melasma and nausea).

5α-reductase inhibitors specifically prevent the conversion of testosterone to its more potent metabolite, DHT. In males with male pattern hair loss, the balding scalp contains miniaturized hair follicles and increased amounts of DHT. Administration of 5α-reductase inhibitors decreases scalp DHT concentrations and inhibits the process responsible for miniaturization of scalp follicles. Males with a genetic deficiency of type 2 5α-reductase do not suffer from male pattern hair loss. The enzyme 5α-reductase exists as two isoenzymes; type 1 is the dominant form in non-genital skin, including the scalp and the sebaceous glands, while type 2 is the dominant form in genital skin, the prostate and hair follicles of the scalp, where miniaturization takes place. Finasteride selectively inhibits the type 2 isoenzyme, whereas dutasteride inhibits both type 1 and type 2 5α-reductase. Although dutasteride reduces serum DHT levels more than finasteride, both drugs

DOI: 10.1201/9781003016786-4

have similar efficacy in the treatment of symptomatic benign prostatic hyperplasia, where they reduce prostate volume and have similar adverse event profiles.

Other drugs with antiandrogenic effects include the corticosteroids, prednisolone and dexamethasone, which inhibit adrenal androgen secretion, particularly when given as a nocturnal dose (see Chapter 15). Metformin, an insulin-sensitizing agent, has been suggested to have direct antiandrogen actions on ovarian steroid synthesis, as well as improving insulin sensitivity and reducing insulin levels, which leads to a reduction in circulating free androgens. Cimetidine has weak antiandrogenic effects due to competitive inhibition of DHT at peripheral androgen receptors. Gonadotrophin-releasing hormone (GnRH) agonists inhibit pituitary gonadotrophin release and are the most effective inhibitors of testosterone, while oral contraceptive pills (OCPs) inhibit ovarian androgen secretion. These agents have been reported to be useful in the treatment of skin conditions.

INDICATIONS AND DERMATOLOGICAL USES

Dermatological uses include the following (licensed indication*):

- Finasteride: Androgenetic alopecia (in males*).
- Dutasteride: Androgenetic alopecia.
- Flutamide: Hirsutism, female pattern hair loss.
- Bicalutamide: Hirsutism.
- Spironolactone: Female pattern hair loss, acne and hirsutism.
- Drospirenone: Acne.
- Cyproterone acetate as co-cyprindiol (Dianette): Acne (recalcitrant/severe*) and/or hirsutism (moderate*) in females. The combined preparation also functions as a hormonal contraceptive but is not licensed specifically for this purpose. It is not available in the United States.
- Cyproterone acetate (high dose): Female hair loss and hirsutism.

Other licensed uses are:

- Finasteride and dutasteride: Benign prostatic hyperplasia.
- Flutamide and bicalutamide: Metastatic prostate cancer.
- Spironolactone: Oedematous conditions, including congestive heart failure, nephrotic syndrome, cirrhosis with ascites, malignant ascites and primary aldosteronism.
- Drospirenone: OCPs.
- Cyproterone acetate (high dose): Male hypersexuality and advanced prostate cancer.

FORMULATIONS/PRESENTATION

- Finasteride: 1 mg and 5 mg tablets. The 1 mg dose is indicated for males with androgenetic alopecia.
- Dutasteride: 0.5 mg soft capsules.
- Flutamide: 125 mg tablets.
- Bicalutamide: 25 mg tablets.
- Spironolactone: Tablets containing 25 mg, 50 mg and 100 mg of spironolactone. Oral suspensions ranging from 5 to 100 mg/5 mL are available on special order.
- Drospirenone: Combined preparation of 3 mg drospirenone and 30 μg ethinyloestradiol as oral contraception (Yasmin®) and 0.5 mg of drospirenone and 1 mg of oestradiol (Angeliq®) as hormone replacement therapy in post-menopausal females.
- Cyproterone acetate: Scored tablets containing 50 mg and 100 mg of cyproterone acetate. A combined preparation, co-cyprindiol, containing cyproterone acetate 2 mg and ethinyloestradiol 35 μg is available as sugar-coated tablets (Dianette).

DOSAGES AND SUGGESTED REGIMENS

FINASTERIDE

The recommended dose for male androgenic alopecia is 1 mg daily. A higher daily dose (5 mg) is used for the treatment of benign prostatic hyperplasia but does not increase efficacy in hair loss.

DUTASTERIDE

The recommended dose for benign prostatic hyperplasia is 0.5 mg daily, and this dose has also been found to be effective in male androgenic alopecia. A placebo-controlled study reported that this dose had superior effects to finasteride on hair growth and hair count. Capsules should be swallowed whole, not chewed or opened, as contact with the contents may cause irritation of the oropharyngeal mucosa.

The onset of effect of these agents in male androgenic alopecia is slow, and it usually takes 6 months to stabilize hair loss. Treatment arrests the progression of disease, but regrowth is partial at best, and continued treatment is required to sustain benefit. If treatment is stopped, the beneficial effects begin to reverse by 6 months and return to baseline by 9–12 months. At the recommended dose, finasteride has been shown to improve the anagen (growing phase) follicle count in males with vertex baldness while those given placebo lost anagen hair. The majority of males continue to benefit from long-term treatment (up to 10 years). The most common adverse effect is sexual dysfunction and can carry a 1.57-fold risk of sexual dysfunction. Efficacy in females with androgenic alopecia is controversial. No adjustment in dosage is necessary in renal impairment or in older people. Finasteride has a much shorter half-life than dutasteride.

FLUTAMIDE

Low doses of 125–250 mg daily are effective for hirsutism. Doses of up to 750 mg have been used (i.e. the recommended dose for prostate cancer). Treatment may be given with a combined OCP and in a reverse sequential regimen as below.

BICALUTAMIDE

Low doses of 25 mg daily for treatment of hirsutism.

SPIRONOLACTONE

A low starting dose of 25–50 mg daily is recommended to reduce side effects, followed by dose increases up to 200 mg daily. Low maintenance doses of 50–100 mg daily may be effective in acne, with higher doses used to treat hair loss and hidradenitis suppurativa. (Doses of up to 400 mg daily are used in oedema and ascites.) Medication should be taken with food to aid absorption.

DROSPIRENONE

The combined OCP preparation Yasmin is taken once daily for 21 days, followed by a 7-day tablet-free interval.

CYPROTERONE ACETATE

For the treatment of hirsutism and female pattern hair loss, 50 mg daily is usually sufficient, although up to 100 mg/d may be used. Side effects are dose-dependent, so the lowest effective dose should be given. To prevent pregnancy and minimize menstrual irregularities, it should be taken daily with the first 10 pills of a combined OCP, i.e. a reverse sequential regimen. Co-cyprindol is taken once daily for 21 days, followed by a 7-day tablet-free interval when a withdrawal bleed should occur.

Following a finding of an increased risk of meningioma with cyproterone acetate, the European Medicines Agency's safety committee recommended in 2020 that daily doses of 10 mg and above should only be used for androgen-dependent conditions such as hirsutism, alopecia and acne if lower doses and other treatment options have failed. Once a therapeutic response has been achieved, the dose should be gradually reduced to the lowest effective dose. Available data do not indicate a risk for low-dose cyproterone medicines containing 1 or 2 milligrams cyproterone in combination with ethinylestradiol or oestradiol valerate; however, as a precaution, they should not be used in people who have or have had a meningioma.

Patients must be monitored for symptoms of meningioma (see below). If a patient is diagnosed with meningioma, treatment with cyproterone medicines must be stopped permanently.

BASELINE INVESTIGATIONS, CONSIDERATIONS AND MONITORING

- Females who are overweight or obese (body mass index [BMI] ≥30) should be advised to lose weight, as this may improve androgen-related symptoms.
- In females with severe/progressive hirsutism or acne (especially if associated with menstrual disturbance), undertake blood tests for androgen profile, serum cortisol and pelvic ultrasound scan.
- Pregnancy should be excluded before starting oral antiandrogen therapy.
- Ensure adequate contraception in females of childbearing potential.

FINASTERIDE/DUTASTERIDE

- Serum prostate specific antigen (PSA).
- Prostate evaluation by urologist for older males.
- Monitoring: Check PSA values regularly and refer to individual's baseline value. PSA usually falls with treatment. Any increase in PSA level may indicate the presence of prostate cancer and needs further evaluation even if within the normal range. PSA levels should return to baseline within 6 months of discontinuing treatment.
- Assessment for depression/suicidal ideation. Rare reports of depression and suicidal thoughts have been addressed by the Medicines and Healthcare Regulatory Agency (MHRA). Guidance is to advise patients to stop finasteride immediately and inform a healthcare professional if they develop depression.

FLUTAMIDE/BICALUTAMIDE

- Baseline: Full blood count (FBC) (complete blood count [CBC]), urea and electrolytes and liver function tests (LFTs).
- Monitoring: LFTs monthly for first four months, then three times monthly. Discontinue if alanine aminotransferase (ALT) increases to twice the upper limit of normal. Monitor methaemoglobin levels in patients susceptible to the effects of hypoxia. Monitor for respiratory symptoms during the first few weeks of treatment as cases of interstitial pneumonitis are reported.

SPIRONOLACTONE

- Baseline: BP, weight and BMI.
- Urea and electrolytes.
- Monitoring: Urea and electrolytes if at risk of hyperkalaemia/hyponatraemia. Discontinue if hyperkalaemia occurs.

DROSPIRENONE (YASMIN)

- Baseline: BP, weight and BMI.
- Check patient suitability for a combined OCP.

- The risk of venous thromboembolism (VTE) should be assessed (personal or close family history). The risk of VTE may be greater in females taking drospirenone compared to the risk associated with low dose combined OCPs (see below).
- Start treatment on the first day of the menstrual period.
- Monitoring: As for OCPs includes review after 3 months, then every 6–12 months, with measurement of BP and assessment of new risk factors.

CYPROTERONE ACETATE AS CO-PYRINDIOL (DIANETTE)

- Baseline: BP, weight and BMI.
- Check patient suitability for a combined OCP.
- Neurological history and examination and monitoring for symptoms of meningioma, including vision change, hearing loss or tinnitus, anosmia, headaches, memory loss, seizures or weakness in the arms and legs.
- The risk of VTE should be assessed (personal or close family history), as VTE occurs more frequently in females taking co-cyprindiol than in those taking low-dose combined OCPs (see below).
- Start treatment on the first day of the menstrual period.
- Monitoring: As for OCPs (see Drospirenone).

CYPROTERONE ACETATE (HIGH DOSE)

- Baseline tests as above.
- Regular laboratory monitoring (FBC, urea and electrolytes, glucose and LFTs).

CONTRAINDICATIONS

All antiandrogens are contraindicated in pregnancy (see Pregnancy and Preconception).

- Flutamide/bicalutamide
  - Severe hepatic disease.
- Spironolactone
  - Hyperkalaemia and severe renal impairment.
  - Postural hypotension.
  - Addison disease.
- Drospirenone (Yasmin)
  - Contraindications to a combined OCP.
  - Renal or liver impairment.
  - Adrenal insufficiency.
- Cyproterone acetate as co-pyrindiol (Dianette)
  - History of meningioma.
  - Contraindications for a combined OCP, including personal or close family history of VTE.
- Cyproterone acetate (high dose)
  - Meningioma or past history of meningioma.
  - Severe depression.

CAUTIONS

- Finasteride/dutasteride
  - Although the overall risk of prostate cancer is decreased, there is an increased risk of high-grade disease, and PSA tests are more difficult to interpret.

- Flutamide/bicalutamide
  - Cardiac disease.
  - Hepatic impairment – closer monitoring needed.
  - Renal impairment.
- Spironolactone
  - Use with caution in older people (over 65).
  - Renal impairment, diabetes mellitus and increased risk of hyperkalaemia (see below).
  - Porphyria.
  - Patients suffering from menstrual abnormalities or breast enlargement.
- Drospirenone
  - As for a combined OCP, including diabetes, hypertension, age over 35 years, obesity and those at risk of thromboembolic disease, depression. All combined OCPs are associated with an increased risk of VTE; the size of this risk is related to the dose of oestrogen and the progestogen. The risk of a VTE is highest during the first year of treatment or when switching/restarting after a pill-free period of at least 1 month. Epidemiological studies have shown that the incidence of VTE for combined OCPs containing 30–35 µg ethinyloestradiol and drospirenone, cyproterone acetate, gestodene and desogestrel are similar and about 50–80% higher than for combined OCPs with levonorgestrel.
  - Increased risk of hyperkalaemia (in renal impairment, hepatic impairment and adrenal insufficiency).
- Cyproterone acetate as co-pyrindiol (Dianette)
  - As for a combined OCP (see above).

IMPORTANT DRUG INTERACTIONS

- Finasteride and dutasteride: Combination therapy with an alpha blocker, especially tamsulosin, may precipitate cardiac failure.
- Dutasteride: Verapamil, diltiazem, isoniazid, and macrolide antibiotics—These can increase dutasteride serum concentrations.
- Flutamide: Corticosteroids delay its metabolism and may increase plasma concentrations of flutamide. Avoid concomitant administration of potentially hepatotoxic drugs or excessive alcohol consumption. Concomitant administration with theophylline increases theophylline plasma concentration. It also enhances the anticoagulant effect of warfarin.
- Bicalutamide: This drug inhibits cytochrome P450 (CYP450) 3A4 and should be used with caution with other drugs which are metabolized by this enzyme system, e.g. ciclosporin, cimetidine and calcium channel blockers. It also enhances the anticoagulant effect of warfarin.
- Spironolactone: Due to the drug's diuretic actions, there is an increased risk of hyponatraemia with chlorpropamide and hyperkalaemia with potassium-sparing diuretics, ciclosporin, trimethoprim, non-steroidal anti-inflammatory drugs (NSAIDs) and tacrolimus. The nephrotoxicity of drugs such as NSAIDS may be increased and excretion of digoxin and lithium reduced, so closer therapeutic monitoring is required.
- Drospirenone: This may worsen hyperkalaemia (see Spironolactone). Drug interactions are also relevant to the oestrogenic component in Yasmin, and agents that induce CYP3A4 may increase metabolism of oestrogen and cause loss of efficacy (see formulary for full prescribing information).
- Cyproterone acetate: Oral antidiabetic drug or insulin requirements may change. Drug interactions are also relevant to the oestrogenic component in Dianette as for Yasmin (see above and consult full prescribing information).

ADVERSE EFFECTS AND THEIR MANAGEMENT

FINASTERIDE/DUTASTERIDE

- Infertility: There have been sporadic reports of infertility and/or poor seminal quality, but in some cases patients had additional risk factors for infertility. Normalization or improvement of seminal quality has been reported after discontinuation of finasteride.
- Sexual adverse effects: In a placebo-controlled trial, a slight increase in the incidence of sexual adverse effects, such as decreased libido, impotence and ejaculatory dysfunction was reported with finasteride. These adverse effects gradually disappeared during prolonged treatment. However, persistence of decreased libido and erectile dysfunction after discontinuation has been reported in post-marketing data. The risk of sexual dysfunction is slightly greater in males taking dutasteride compared with finasteride.
- Breast cancer: This has been reported in males taking finasteride and dutasteride. Physicians should advise patients to report any changes in their breast tissue, such as lumps, pain, gynaecomastia or nipple discharge.
- Cutaneous adverse effects: These include rash and pruritus, urticaria, localized oedema, angioedema, alopecia (primarily body hair loss) and hypertrichosis.

FLUTAMIDE/BICALUTAMIDE

- Hepatotoxicity ranges from mild transaminitis and jaundice to hepatic necrosis and encephalopathy. It may be less frequent with bicalutamide than flutamide. Careful monitoring is required with early discontinuation if LFTs are deranged.
- Sexual adverse effects are common with non-steroidal antiandrogens, including loss of libido, gynaecomastia, breast tenderness and galactorrhoea. Dry skin, pruritus and flushing may occur.
- Gastrointestinal adverse effects are common and include nausea and dyspepsia.
- Haematological adverse effects include anaemia and, very rarely, methemoglobinemia (flutamide).
- Cutaneous adverse effects including photosensitivity and a systemic lupus erythematosus-like syndrome have been described.
- Bicalutamide appears to have fewer side effects than flutamide at the higher doses used in the treatment of prostate cancer.

SPIRONOLACTONE

- Hyperkalaemia is dose-related and more common in people over 65 and those with renal impairment or cardiac impairment. It may lead to arrhythmia and cardiovascular collapse. Review other medication (see Important Drug Interactions) and discontinue if necessary.
- Non-specific side effects such as fatigue, headache and dizziness are common.
- Gastrointestinal adverse effects include gastritis and an increased risk of gastroduodenal bleeding (dose-related).
- Sexual adverse effects include gynaecomastia, breast tenderness, loss of libido and alteration in voice pitch. These are usually reversible on discontinuation, but in rare instances breast enlargement and voice change may persist. Menstrual irregularities are common with doses above 100 mg daily and may be improved by combination with an OCP or cyclical therapy (days 4–21 of menstrual cycle).

- Cutaneous adverse effects include pruritus, alopecia, immediate-type hypersensitivity and severe cutaneous adverse reactions (Drug Reaction with Eosinophilia and Systemic Symptoms [DRESS] and Stevens–Johnson syndrome).
- Other adverse effects include osteomalacia, agranulocytosis, eosinophilia, thrombocytopenia and hyponatraemia.
- Carcinogenicity has not been established in large epidemiological studies, though isolated reports have raised concerns, especially when long-term treatment is considered in young females.

DROSPIRENONE (YASMIN)

- Combined oral contraceptive adverse events: Arterial and venous thromboembolism, hypertension, weight gain, depression, headache and melasma.
- Hyperkalaemia: A potential adverse effect due to the drug's potassium sparing diuretic actions, but large studies in healthy female users have not shown this metabolic abnormality.

CYPROTERONE ACETATE AS CO-PYRINDIOL (DIANETTE)

- Combined oral contraceptive adverse effects (see above).

CYPROTERONE ACETATE (HIGH DOSE)

- Neurological adverse effects include meningiomas (at doses of 10 mg daily and above) and depression. Overall, the risk of meningioma is small and estimated at between 1 to 10 in 10,000 people. The risk increases with increasing cumulative doses. Symptoms include changes in vision, hearing loss or tinnitus, loss of smell, headaches, memory loss, seizures or weakness in arms and legs. Treatment must be discontinued permanently if the patient develops a meningioma.
- Cardiovascular adverse effects include arterial and venous thromboembolism.
- Hepatotoxic adverse effects include hepatitis, jaundice and liver tumours (benign and malignant).
- Sexual adverse effects include decreased libido, erectile dysfunction, reversible inhibition of spermatogenesis, gynaecomastia, galactorrhoea and hot flushes.
- Metabolic adverse effects include changes in body habitus (central obesity).
- Other adverse effects include anaemia, osteoporosis, fatigue and lassitude.

USE IN SPECIAL SITUATIONS

PREGNANCY AND PRE-CONCEPTION

Antiandrogens are contraindicated during pregnancy due to the risk of feminization of the male fetus. Small amounts of finasteride/dutasteride have been detected in the semen of males taking this medication. It is not known whether a male fetus may be adversely affected by in utero exposure to the semen of a male treated with finasteride or dutasteride, but condom use is advised. Likewise, it is advised that crushed or broken tablets should not be handled during pregnancy.

Bicalutamide, cyproterone acetate, drospirenone, dutasteride and finasteride were FDA Category X, indicating potent teratogenicity. Flutamide was FDA Category D, and spironolactone was FDA Category C.

Finasteride/dutasteride have been reported to adversely affect sperm counts and quality in healthy males and an impairment of male fertility cannot be excluded. Flutamide and bicalutamide have both been shown to adversely affect male fertility.

Antiandrogens are contraindicated during breastfeeding. Canrenone, the principal metabolite of spironolactone, has been detected at low levels in breast milk, so an alternative method of infant feeding should be instituted.

Cyproterone acetate and drospirenone (Yasmin) may lead to a reduction in the volume of milk produced and to a change in its composition. Minute amounts of these active substances are excreted with the milk. These amounts may affect the child, particularly in the first 6 weeks post-partum.

CHILDREN

Antiandrogen therapy is not relevant in paediatric dermatology, as the skin disorders they are used to treat do not occur before puberty. Use of spironolactone in adolescent girls ≥12 has been reported.

ESSENTIAL PATIENT INFORMATION

- Females should be advised of the need to avoid pregnancy during antiandrogen therapy.
- There should be counselling for the risks and benefits of combined hormonal contraception for Yasmin and Dianette.

FURTHER READING

Arowojolu AO, Gallo MF, Lopez LM, et al. Combined oral contraceptive pills for treatment of acne. Cochrane Database Syst Rev. 2012;7:CD000425.

Azarchi S, Bienenfeld A, Lo Sicco K, et al. Androgens in women: Hormone-modulating therapies for skin disease. J Am Acad Dermatol. 2019 Jun;80(6):1509–21.

Blume-Peytavi U, Hahn S. Medical treatment of hirsuitism. Dermatol Therapy. 2008;21:329–39.

Brown J, Farquhar C, Lee O, et al. Spironolactone versus placebo or in combination with steroids for hirsuitism and/or acne. Cochrane Database Syst Rev. 2009;2:CD000194.

Champeaux-Depond C, Weller J, Froelich S, et al. Cyproterone acetate and meningioma: A nationwide population based study. J Neurooncol. 2021 Jan;151(2):331–8.

European Medicines Agency (EMA). Cyproterone-containing medicinal products. 2020; https://www.ema.europa.eu/en/medicines/human/referrals/cyproterone-containing-medicinal-products#key-facts-section.

Vargas-Mora P, Morgado-Carrasco D. Use of spironolactone in dermatology: Acne, hidradenitis supurativa, female alopecia and hirsutism. Actas Dermosifiliogr. 2020;155:639–649.

5 Antibiotics Commonly Used for Skin Infections

Hui Min Liew, Victoria J. Hogarth and Roderick J. Hay

Antibiotics are drugs with therapeutic activity against living organisms, the term usually reserved for drugs active against bacteria. They are commonly described as either bacteriostatic or bactericidal, depending on whether, at any given concentration, they inhibit or kill the bacteria. Site of infection, strain of organism and drug molecular structure and concentration are all important in determining this characteristic. This chapter is concerned with the antibiotics most commonly used in dermatology, including broad- and narrow-spectrum drugs. One of the problems dominating antibiotic usage is the rising prevalence of resistance among bacteria, either because of intrinsic drug resistance or acquired resistance due to mutation or transfer of plasmid-based resistance genes.

PENICILLINS

CLASSIFICATION AND MODE OF ACTION

Penicillins are bactericidal because they inhibit bacterial cell wall synthesis leading to death of the microorganism. The basic structure of a penicillin consists of a thiazolidine ring, a β-lactam ring and a variable side chain. They are usually divided into penicillinase-sensitive (e.g. benzylpenicillin/penicillin G and phenoxymethylpenicillin/penicillin V) or penicillinase-resistant penicillins (e.g. methicillin, flucloxacillin), broad-spectrum penicillins, antipseudomonal penicillins and mecillinams. All penicillins are readily and actively secreted by the renal tubules, and most are eliminated, almost completely unchanged, in the urine.

INDICATIONS AND DERMATOLOGICAL USES

- Penicillins are first-line drugs for infections by Staphylococcus aureus, Streptococcus pyogenes group A, Treponema pallidum and suspected meningococcal septicaemia, as well as yaws, actinomycosis and diphtheria. Most S. aureus strains are resistant to benzylpenicillin because they produce penicillinases.
- Flucloxacillin is resistant to degradation by this enzyme and therefore is effective against penicillin-resistant staphylococci. Penicillin V (also known as phenoxymethylpenicillin) has similar antibacterial properties to benzylpenicillin, but it is less active and produces variable plasma concentrations.

In dermatology, flucloxacillin is indicated for pyodermas such as extensive impetigo, early furunculosis, erysipelas and cellulitis. If the patient is acutely unwell, IV penicillins, e.g. piperacillin, should be considered. Oral penicillin V has a role in prophylaxis against recurrent streptococcal cellulitis in patients with lymphoedema.

Infection with S. aureus strains resistant to methicillin (MRSA) and to flucloxacillin has become a serious concern, as it is endemic in many hospitals and is also becoming a problem in the community setting. The hospital-acquired strains (HA-MRSAs) show multiple drug resistance, whereas

DOI: 10.1201/9781003016786-5

community-acquired strains (CA-MRSAs) usually show resistance to a smaller range of penicillins, e.g. methicillin. Treatment of MRSA is guided by the sensitivity of the infecting strain and local hospital eradication policy regime.

Strains of CA-MRSA, unlike HA-MRSA, usually carry a gene encoding the Panton–Valentine leukocidin (PVL) toxin. This is a virulence determinant and is associated with multiple skin and soft tissue infections, such as abscesses. PVL-positive strains may also occur without methicillin resistance, but even then flucloxacillin is usually ineffective and may increase PVL production. In such cases, two antibiotics are advised, e.g. rifampicin and clarithromycin, in consultation with local infections teams.

FORMULATIONS/PRESENTATION

- Penicillin V: Tablets (250 mg); oral solution (125 mg/5 mL or 250 mg/5 mL).
- Benzylpenicillin sodium powder: 600 mg vials.
- Flucloxacillin: Capsules (250 mg or 500 mg); oral solution (125 mg/5 mL or 250 mg/5 mL); injection either IM, slow IV or IV infusion (250 mg or 500 mg vial).

DOSAGES AND SUGGESTED REGIMENS

Penicillin V

In adults, 500 mg every 6 hours can be increased up to 1 g every 6 hours in severe infections. In children up to 1 year, 62.5 mg every 6 hours; 1–6 years, 125 mg every 6 hours; 6–12 years, 250 mg every 6 hours. If the infection is severe, the dose can be increased up to 12.5 mg/kg every 6 hours.

Benzylpenicillin

In adults, 0.6–1.2 g every 6 hours, by IM injection, slow IV injection or infusion. Increased dosages (by IV route only) and frequency of injection may be indicted in severe infection. In children 1 month–18 years, 25 mg/kg every 6 hours (see children's formulary for further information in severe infections).

Flucloxacillin

In adults, 250–500 mg every 6 hours, at least 30 minutes before food or 2 hours after food, or by IM injection, usually for 5–7 days. By slow IV injection or by IV infusion, 0.25–2 g every 6 hours. In children 1 month–2 years, 62.5–125 mg every 6 hours; 2–10 years, 125–250 mg every 6 hours.

For these short half-life penicillins, high peaks are much less important than duration of exposure, so for parenteral administration, continuous IV infusion may optimize therapy.

BASELINE INVESTIGATIONS AND CONSIDERATIONS

No investigations are required. Patients should be asked about previous hypersensitivity reactions to β-lactam antibiotics (see Special Point: Immediate Hypersensitivity).

MONITORING

Monitoring is not necessary unless the patient is on a prolonged course of flucloxacillin or is known to have renal or hepatic impairment.

CONTRAINDICATIONS

Penicillins are contraindicated in patients with known penicillin or β-lactam antibiotic hypersensitivity (see Special Point: Immediate Hypersensitivity).

CAUTIONS

- Chronic renal impairment: Reduce the dose of flucloxacillin if the estimated glomerular filtration rate (eGFR) is less than 10 mL/min/1.73 m^2 (see Chapter 39).
- Hepatic impairment (flucloxacillin).
- Patients over the age of 65 and those with serious underlying disease (increased risk of hepatitis with flucloxacillin).

IMPORTANT DRUG INTERACTIONS

There are few significant drug interactions. The following should be noted:

- Neomycin reduces the absorption of penicillin V.
- Coumarin oral anticoagulant actions (and INR) can be altered by penicillins, in particular the broad-spectrum penicillins; close monitoring is required.
- Methotrexate excretion may be reduced by penicillins, increasing the risk of toxicity.
- Oral typhoid vaccine may be inactivated by penicillins, as with other antibiotics.

ADVERSE EFFECTS AND THEIR MANAGEMENT

- Minor gastrointestinal (GI) upset and diarrhoea are common problems, while antibiotic-associated colitis is very rare. The penicillin must be stopped immediately and treatment given with oral vancomycin or metronidazole.
- Hypersensitivity reactions vary according to the underlying immunological mechanism. Immediate drug withdrawal is usually needed, and treatment may be required (e.g. anaphylaxis therapy, corticosteroids). If further treatment with the antibiotic is essential, drug desensitization may be considered.
- Immediate-type hypersensitivity reactions with urticaria, angioedema and anaphylaxis may follow parenteral or oral therapy. Serum sickness-type hypersensitivity reactions with fever, arthralgia and rashes can occur.
- Drug rashes are usually morbilliform ('measles-like'), but a range of drug eruptions can occur, including Stevens–Johnson syndrome, acute generalized exanthematous pustulosis and toxic epidermal necrolysis.
- Hepatitis and cholestatic jaundice are very rare idiosyncratic adverse effects, especially with flucloxacillin. The onset may be delayed for up to 2 months post-treatment and may persist for months. Risk factors include age over 55 years and duration of therapy over 2 weeks.
- Other very rare reactions include interstitial nephritis, haemolytic anaemia, leukopenia, thrombocytopenia and coagulation disorders.

USE IN SPECIAL SITUATIONS

Pregnancy

Penicillins are not known to be harmful in pregnancy and were formerly classified as FDA Category B.

LACTATION

Penicillins are not known to be harmful in lactation. Trace amounts of penicillins are excreted in human breast milk.

CHILDREN

It is safe to use penicillins in children when clinically indicated. The dosing is according to age and weight.

OLDER PEOPLE

Penicillin V is not known to cause any problems in older people, but careful note should be made of concurrent drugs to avoid interactions.

SPECIAL POINT: IMMEDIATE HYPERSENSITIVITY

Patients with IgE (immediate-type) hypersensitivity to penicillins may be reactive to the β-lactam ring that is common to all β-lactams (including cephalosporins, carbapenems and monobactams) or the R-group side chain that distinguishes different penicillins from one another. Although a 5–10% cross-reactivity rate with cephalosporins in penicillin-allergic patients with IgE-mediated reactions was reported in early studies, most penicillin-allergic patients can tolerate third- and fourth-generation cephalosporins, because the R-group side chain (rather than the β-lactam ring) appears to play the dominant role in cephalosporin allergy.

The use of in vivo skin tests (skin prick tests and intradermal tests) is well-validated for β-lactam antibiotics. Commercial reagents are available in many countries. In vitro diagnostic immunoassays are generally more expensive and less sensitive. Finally, drug provocation testing may be required to exclude cross-reactivity.

ESSENTIAL PATIENT INFORMATION

Patients should be informed about the side effect profile of penicillins.

ERYTHROMYCIN AND CLARITHROMYCIN

CLASSIFICATION AND MODE OF ACTION

Macrolides, including erythromycin and clarithromycin, are antibiotics whose structure is based on a large macrocyclic lactone ring. They act by inhibiting protein synthesis through binding to ribosomes and are mainly bacteriostatic.

INDICATIONS AND DERMATOLOGICAL USES

- Erythromycin is the most widely used macrolide. It is active mainly against Gram-positive organisms such as staphylococci and streptococci. Staphylococci and streptococci may become erythromycin-resistant, including as many as 50% of staphylococcus strains. However, erythromycin may be active against many penicillin-resistant staphylococci. Uses include staphylococcal and streptococcal pyodermas, especially in penicillin-allergic patients, erythrasma and acne. Macrolides may be more effective than penicillins for the treatment of cellulitis. Macrolides may also be used for atypical mycobacterial infections and for Lyme disease and syphilis.

- Clarithromycin is an erythromycin derivative with slightly greater activity and greater tissue concentrations. Although not widely used in dermatology, it is licensed for treatment of skin infections and is also used for the treatment of atypical mycobacterial infections.

FORMULATIONS/PRESENTATION

- Erythromycin: 250 mg, 500 mg tablets and capsules, 125 mg/5 mL suspensions (including sugar-free suspensions).
- Clarithromycin: 250 mg, 500 mg tablets, 125 mg/5 mL suspension, granules 250 mg/sachet.

DOSAGES AND SUGGESTED REGIMENS

- Erythromycin: Adults and children over 8 years: 250–500 mg every 6 hours or 0.5–1 g every 12 hours; up to 4 g daily in divided doses in severe infections. Younger children: 1 month–2 years: 125 mg every 6 hours; 2–8 years: 250 mg every 6 hours. Doses are doubled for severe infections. Lyme disease: 500 mg 4 times daily for 14–21 days. By IV infusion: Adult and child severe infections, 50 mg/kg daily by continuous infusion or in divided doses every 6 hours, mild infections (oral treatment not possible), 25 mg/kg daily.
- Clarithromycin: Adults and children over 12 years: 250 mg every 12 hours for 7 days, increased in severe infection up to 500 mg every 12 hours for up to 14 days. By IV infusion into a larger proximal vein: 500 mg twice daily. For younger children (1 month–12 years), the dosage depends on body weight: <8 kg: 7.5 mg/kg twice daily; 8–11 kg: 62.5 mg twice daily; 12–19 kg: 125 mg twice daily; 20–29 kg, 187.5 mg twice daily; 30–40 mg, 250 mg twice daily.

BASELINE INVESTIGATIONS AND CONSIDERATIONS

No routine investigations/monitoring are required in the absence of renal impairment.

CONTRAINDICATIONS

- Erythromycin or clarithromycin hypersensitivity.
- Severe hepatic impairment, history of hepatitis caused by macrolides and cholestasis.
- Clarithromycin, which is contraindicated in patients with prolonged QT intervals, ventricular dysrhythmias and hypokalaemia.

CAUTIONS

ERYTHROMYCIN

- Maximum dose of 1.5 g daily in severe renal impairment (risk of hearing loss).
- Avoid in acute porphyria.
- Risk of hypertrophic pyloric stenosis in neonates under 2 weeks.
- Predisposition to QT interval prolongation; therefore, caution with concomitant use of drugs that prolong QT interval and electrolyte disturbances.

CLARITHROMYCIN

- Caution is advised in hepatic impairment, as clarithromycin is mainly excreted by the liver.
- The dosage should be reduced in moderate-to-severe renal impairment.

IMPORTANT DRUG INTERACTIONS

Macrolide antibiotics have numerous drug interactions due to inhibitory effects on the cytochrome P450 (CYP450) 3A4 isoenzyme and it may, for instance, enhance the cardiotoxicity of certain drugs. Prescribers are advised to consult an updated drug formulary.

Macrolides should not be prescribed with the following:

- Antipsychotic drugs, including droperidol, pimozide and sertindole.
- Cisapride (no longer widely available), due to the risk of ventricular dysrhythmias.
- Ergot alkaloids (unlicensed use for headache), due to increased risk of ergotism.
- Mizolastine, due to QT prolongation.
- Simvastatin and lovastatin, due to increased risk of myopathy.

Care should be taken if erythromycin or clarithromycin are prescribed with the following:

- Atorvastatin and pravastatin, in which a lower dose should be used and patients monitored carefully for signs of myopathy (muscle pain and weakness). Other statins that are not metabolized by CYP3A4 (rosuvastatin, fluvastatin) may carry less risk of myopathy. Measurement of serum creatine kinase (CK) is helpful, as modest elevations (up to 5 times above the upper limit of normal) are common and usually related to exercise. A rise in CK of more than 10 times above the upper limit of normal can indicate significant myopathy and a risk of rhabdomyolysis, which is a medical emergency.
- Calcium channel blockers, in which the risk of hypotension or shock is increased with erythromycin and clarithromycin. In older patients at risk, azithromycin is the macrolide of choice.
  - Chloroquine and hydroxychloroquine; co-administration of systemic macrolide antibiotics may be associated with an increased risk of cardiovascular events (including angina or chest pain and heart failure) and cardiovascular mortality.
- Ciclosporin (cyclosporine), since metabolism may be inhibited, with increased toxicity (see Chapter 13).
- Colchicine. There may be increased risk of colchicine toxicity (see Chapter 14).
- Coumarin anticoagulants (e.g. warfarin). There may be increased anticoagulant effects with risk of serious haemorrhage. Close monitoring of INR is essential.
- Digoxin plasma concentrations are raised with risk of toxicity.
- Methyl prednisolone metabolism may be inhibited.
- Oral contraceptives, in which there may be a short-term impairment in the contraceptive effects of oestrogen-containing pills due to alteration of gut flora.
- Oral hypoglycaemic agents/insulin, in which the concomitant use of macrolides and certain oral hypoglycaemic agents and/or insulin can result in significant hypoglycaemia. Careful monitoring of glucose is recommended.
- Phenytoin, carbamazepine, clozapine and valproate may be subject to decreased metabolic clearance and increased plasma levels.
- Theophylline, due to increased plasma theophylline, may cause nausea, vomiting and seizures.
- Verapamil may increase the risk of cardiotoxicity.

ADVERSE EFFECTS AND THEIR MANAGEMENT

Erythromycin

- Cholestatic hepatitis can occur with erythromycin estolate.
- GI effects, such as nausea and colicky pains, are common, with occasional vomiting and diarrhoea. Symptoms may be improved by giving a lower dose (250 mg four times daily).

- Hypersensitivity reactions are rare. They include Stevens–Johnson syndrome and toxic epidermal necrolysis.
- Reversible hearing loss and tinnitus have been reported after large IV doses and in renal impairment.
- Other effects include pancreatitis, cardiac effects and myasthenia-like syndrome/exacerbation of myasthenia gravis.

CLARITHROMYCIN

The adverse reaction profile is similar to that of erythromycin:

- Hepatitis and cases of fatal hepatic failure have been reported. Advise patients to stop treatment and contact their doctor if signs and symptoms of hepatic disease develop.
- Tooth and tongue discolouration, smell and taste disturbances, stomatitis and glossitis.
- Arthralgia, myalgia and headache are less common.
- Dizziness, insomnia, nightmares, anxiety, confusion, psychosis, paraesthesia, convulsions, hypoglycaemia, renal failure, intestinal nephritis, leukopenia and thrombocytopenia have been reported very rarely.

Patients who are hypersensitive to clindamycin may also be hypersensitive to clarithromycin, so caution is required if they are prescribed clarithromycin.

USE IN SPECIAL SITUATIONS

PREGNANCY

Erythromycin crosses the placenta but is not known to be harmful in pregnancy. The manufacturers advise avoiding clarithromycin in pregnancy unless the potential benefit outweighs the risk.

LACTATION

Only small amounts of erythromycin are found in breast milk, and this is not known to be harmful. The manufacturers advise avoiding clarithromycin in lactation unless the potential benefit outweighs the risk.

CHILDREN

Both drugs are available in paediatric formulations. Remember the risk of pyloric stenosis in neonates.

OLDER PEOPLE

Consider underlying renal impairment, which may affect drug dosage for clarithromycin.

CLINDAMYCIN

INDICATIONS AND DERMATOLOGICAL USES

Clindamycin is a lincosamide antibiotic with activity against Gram-positive cocci and many anaerobes. It has a bacteriostatic effect by inhibiting bacterial ribosomal translocation. It can be used as an alternative to macrolides for erysipelas or cellulitis and for infections associated with MRSA. It is also used in the treatment of diabetic foot. Topical clindamycin is licensed for use in acne and bacterial vaginosis.

FORMULATIONS/PRESENTATION

Capsules (75 mg, 150 mg), IM and IV preparations, lotions/gels (acne vulgaris) and cream (bacterial vaginosis).

DOSAGES AND SUGGESTED REGIMENS

The usual adult oral dose is 150–300 mg every 6 hours and up to 450 mg every 6 hours in severe infection. The recommended dose of clindamycin in children is 3–6 mg/kg every 6 hours.

A regimen of 300 mg clindamycin twice daily and 300 mg rifampicin (see below) twice daily for 10 weeks has been reported to be effective in the treatment of hidradenitis suppurativa (HS).

Deep IM or IV infusion in 2–4 divided doses/day may be used as an alternative to oral therapy or in severe infection. Injections containing benzyl alcohol should be avoided in neonates.

BASELINE INVESTIGATIONS AND CONSIDERATIONS

Liver function tests (LFTs) and renal indices in neonates and infants being treated for greater than 10 days.

MONITORING

LFTs and renal indices weekly for prolonged therapy (>10 days) in neonates and infants.

CONTRAINDICATIONS AND CAUTIONS

- Diarrhoea and colitis.
- Acute porphyria.

IMPORTANT DRUG INTERACTIONS

- Erythromycin should not be prescribed concurrently, as its antibacterial actions may be impaired by clindamycin.
- Neuromuscular blocking agent effects may be enhanced, and the effects of cholinesterase inhibitors may be prolonged.
- The oral typhoid vaccine is inactivated by antibacterials.

ADVERSE EFFECTS AND THEIR MANAGEMENT

- Clostridium difficile-associated diarrhoea (CDAD) is the most frequent cause of pseudo-membranous colitis, which is the most serious common adverse effect of clindamycin. Although CDAD can occur with almost all antibiotics (including β-lactams), it is classically linked to clindamycin use. Symptoms may develop several weeks after ceasing therapy. The drug should be discontinued immediately if marked diarrhoea or colitis develops (severe abdominal pains with passage of blood and mucus). If allowed to progress, it may lead to toxic megacolon, peritonitis and fatal septicaemic shock.

The disease is likely to follow a more severe course in older or debilitated patients. Diagnosis can be confirmed by colonoscopic demonstration of pseudomembranous colitis and culture of the stool for C. difficile or assay of the stool specimen for C. difficile toxin. Treatment is usually with oral vancomycin 125–500 mg 4 times a day for 7–10 days. Hypertoxin-producing strains of C. difficile can be refractory to antimicrobial therapy and may require a colectomy. Probiotics taken for the duration of antibiotic treatment and the following 2 weeks may have a protective effect. CDAD must be considered in all patients who present with diarrhoea following antibiotic use.

Other adverse effects include the following:

- Jaundice and hepatitis.
- Taste disturbance, oesophagitis and oesophageal ulceration.
- Hypersensitivity reactions, including urticaria, and anaphylactoid reactions.
- Dermatological effects; generalized mild-to-moderate morbilliform-like skin rashes are the most frequently reported rashes. Rare cases of erythema multiforme, Stevens–Johnson syndrome, pruritus, vaginitis, exfoliative or vesiculobullous dermatitis and toxic epidermal necrolysis have been reported.
- Induration, pain and abscess formation after IM injection; thrombophlebitis after IV injection.
- Haematological adverse effects, including eosinophilia, neutropenia and thrombocytopenia.

USE IN SPECIAL SITUATIONS

PREGNANCY

Clindamycin is not known to be harmful in pregnancy.

LACTATION

It is excreted in breast milk, but the amount is probably too small to be significant.

CHILDREN

Licensed for children aged above 1 month in the UK. A syrup formulation containing 75 mg clindamycin/5 mL may be obtained from outside the UK.

OLDER PEOPLE

Clindamycin should be used with caution in frail, older patients due to their increased susceptibility to complications of CDAD.

ESSENTIAL PATIENT INFORMATION

Patients should be fully informed about the risk of diarrhoea and colitis and advised to discontinue the drug immediately and to contact a doctor if symptoms develop. Capsules should be swallowed with a glass of water.

RIFAMPICIN

Rifampicin is a complex, synthetically modified antibiotic of the rifamycin group and has a concentration-dependent, prolonged postantibiotic effect. It is bactericidal and very effective against Mycobacterium tuberculosis, M. leprae, many atypical mycobacteria and Gram-positive cocci such as S. aureus.

INDICATIONS AND DERMATOLOGICAL USES

Rifampicin is always used in combination with other antimicrobials, such as clarithromycin or clindamycin, to prevent the rapid emergence of resistant strains. It is licensed for use in the following infections:

- Tuberculosis, for all forms of disease in combination with other drugs.
- Atypical mycobacterial infections.

- Leprosy, in combination with at least one other active antileprosy drug. It has also been recommended as a single dose for post-exposure prophylaxis of contacts of patients with leprosy.
- Brucellosis.
- Legionnaires' disease.
- Serious staphylococcal infections.

Dermatological uses include PVL-positive S. aureus. Benefit has also been reported in recalcitrant pustular/follicular diseases, including hidradenitis suppurativa (HS) and folliculitis decalvans/tufted folliculitis.

Rifampicin is also used in asymptomatic carriers to eliminate Neisseria meningitidis and Haemophilus influenzae.

FORMULATIONS/PRESENTATION

Rifampicin is available as 150 mg and 300 mg capsules and a 100 mg/5 mL syrup.

DOSAGES AND SUGGESTED REGIMENS

In adults, it is usual to prescribe 450–600 mg/d as a single dose before breakfast. Concomitant antacid administration may reduce absorption, so rifampicin should be given at least 1 hour before the ingestion of antacids.

BASELINE INVESTIGATIONS AND CONSIDERATIONS

LFTs may be checked at baseline, but monitoring is generally not necessary during treatment. Rifampicin may inhibit standard microbiological assays for serum folate and vitamin B12, so alternative assay methods should be considered.

CONTRAINDICATIONS

Severe liver impairment or jaundice.

CAUTIONS

- Liver impairment: A reduced dose is indicated due to impaired elimination with regular monitoring of liver enzymes every 2–4 weeks during therapy.
- Alcohol dependence: Regular monitoring of liver enzymes is advised.

IMPORTANT DRUG INTERACTIONS

Rifampicin is a potent inducer of certain CYP450 enzymes. Concurrent administration of rifampicin with other drugs that are also metabolized through these pathways may accelerate the metabolism and reduce the activity of these other drugs with loss of therapeutic effectiveness. The number of potential interactions is large and includes the following:

- Antiarrhythmics, calcium channel blockers and cardiac glycosides (digoxin).
- Oestrogens, progestogens in hormonal contraceptives and hormone antagonists (antioestrogens, e.g. tamoxifen). Advise patients to use alternative, non-hormonal methods of birth control during rifampicin therapy.
- Antipsychotics, anxiolytics, barbiturates and anticonvulsants (phenytoin).

- Anticoagulants (e.g. coumarins).
- Azole antifungals.
- Antiretrovirals (e.g. saquinavir, indinavir, efavirenz, amprenavir, nelfinavir, atazanavir, lopinavir and nevirapine). When rifampicin is given concomitantly with the combination saquinavir/ritonavir, the potential for hepatotoxicity is increased. Therefore, concomitant use of this drug combination is contraindicated.
- Antibacterials (e.g. clarithromycin, dapsone, doxycycline and fluoroquinolones).
- Corticosteroids.
- Oral hypoglycaemic agents for diabetes. Diabetes may become more difficult to control.
- Immunosuppressive agents (e.g. ciclosporin [cyclosporine], sirolimus and tacrolimus).
- Thyroid hormone (levothyroxine).
- Statins metabolized by CYP3A4 (e.g. simvastatin).
- Theophylline.

ADVERSE EFFECTS AND THEIR MANAGEMENT

Rifampicin is generally regarded as a relatively safe drug, but the following adverse reactions have been described:

- Cutaneous adverse effects that are mild and self-limiting consist of flushing and pruritus with or without a rash. Urticaria and more serious cutaneous adverse drug reactions are uncommon. Exfoliate dermatitis, bullous dermatoses, erythema multiforme/Stevens–Johnson syndrome and vasculitis have been reported rarely.
- Gastrointestinal adverse effects are common and consist of anorexia, nausea, vomiting, abdominal discomfort and diarrhoea.
- Hepatitis is usually characterized by transiently elevated transaminases. Hyperbilirubinemia can occur in the early days of treatment due to competition between rifampicin and bilirubin for hepatic excretion.
- Thrombocytopenia with or without purpura may occur and is in association with intermittent therapy. Eosinophilia, leukopenia and agranulocytosis have also been reported.
- A flu-like syndrome consisting of episodes of fever, chills, headache, dizziness and bone pain has mainly been reported with intermittent or irregular therapy and may represent drug hypersensitivity. Anaphylaxis has also been described.
- Red-orange discolouration of the urine, sweat, sputum and tears is common and may lead to permanent staining of soft contact lenses.

USE IN SPECIAL SITUATIONS

Pregnancy

Animal data indicate that there is a potential risk to the fetus, but there is no confirmatory information in humans. Caution is therefore advised, but depending on the condition under treatment, the benefits may outweigh any risk.

Lactation

Rifampicin is excreted in breast milk at low concentrations. The amounts are considered too small to be harmful.

Children

Rifampicin is used in special situations, such as tuberculosis in childhood.

ESSENTIAL PATIENT INFORMATION

- The drug should be stopped immediately if purpura develops and should not be given again.
- Patients should be advised how to recognize signs of liver disorders, and to stop treatment immediately and seek advice if symptoms such as persistent nausea, vomiting, malaise, jaundice or bruising develop.

FLUOROQUINOLONES

The fluoroquinolones or 4-quinolones are antibiotics whose principal use in dermatology is the treatment of Gram-negative infections. Their mode of action is by inhibition of DNA synthesis. Generally, only one of these agents, ciprofloxacin, is used in dermatology. Other fluroquinolones include norfloxacin and ofloxacin.

INDICATIONS AND DERMATOLOGICAL USES

Ciprofloxacin is used in the treatment of lower respiratory tract, GI, urinary tract and genital tract infections. In dermatology, it is used for Gram-negative infections of the skin and soft tissue and Gram-negative folliculitis.

FORMULATIONS/PRESENTATION

Ciprofloxacin is available in 100 mg, 250 mg, 500 mg and 750 mg tablets, a strawberry-flavoured suspension of 250 mg/5 mL and powder for IV infusion. Topical liquid formulations are available for eye and ear infections.

DOSAGES AND SUGGESTED REGIMENS

For most skin infections, the usual dose is 250–750 mg twice daily for 7–14 days, depending on severity. For unresponsive cellulitis, the higher dose of 750 mg twice daily is used. Ciprofloxacin is well-absorbed after oral administration and rarely needs to be given parenterally.

MONITORING

Routine monitoring is not required.

CONTRAINDICATIONS

Patients with known hypersensitivity to quinolones.

CAUTIONS

- Lower dosages are used in patients with renal impairment (see Chapter 39).
- Use with caution in patients with cardiac disease due to possible QT interval prolongation.

IMPORTANT DRUG INTERACTIONS

- Drugs causing QT interval prolongation.

- Ciprofloxacin inhibits the enzyme CYP1A2 and thus may cause increased serum concentration of concomitantly administered drugs metabolized by this enzyme (e.g. theophylline, clozapine, olanzapine, ropinirole, tizanidine and duloxetine). Co-administration of ciprofloxacin and tizanidine (a muscle relaxant) is contraindicated.
- Methotrexate excretion may be inhibited, leading to toxicity.

ADVERSE EFFECTS AND THEIR MANAGEMENT

- Hypersensitivity and anaphylactic reactions have been described.
- Phototoxicity may occur, so avoid excess sunlight or artificial ultraviolet (UV) exposure.
- QT interval prolongation may occur in patients with cardiac disorders, electrolyte imbalance (hypokalaemia and hypomagnesaemia) and drug therapy (see above).
- Tendonitis and tendon rupture (especially the Achilles tendon) may occur even within the first 48 hours of treatment. Inflammation and rupture can also occur up to several months after therapy. The risk is increased in older patients and those receiving corticosteroids. The drug should be discontinued at any sign of tendonitis and care taken to rest the affected limb.
- Seizure threshold may be lowered in predisposed patients with CNS disorders. Polyneuropathy, depression and psychosis have been reported.
- Haemolytic reactions may occur in patients with glucose-6-phosphate dehydrogenase (G6PD) deficiency.
- Hepatitis ranges from mildly abnormal LFTs to hepatic necrosis and life-threatening hepatic failure.

USE IN SPECIAL SITUATIONS

PREGNANCY

Effects on immature cartilage have been observed in animal studies, so avoid if possible in pregnancy.

LACTATION

Ciprofloxacin is excreted in breast milk and should not be used in lactation due to the potential risk of joint damage.

CHILDREN

Ciprofloxacin is associated with an increased risk of musculoskeletal disorders in children and is therefore not recommended except in severe infections.

OLDER PEOPLE

Older patients and females may be more sensitive to QT-prolonging medications. Therefore, caution should be taken when using ciprofloxacin in these populations.

ESSENTIAL PATIENT INFORMATION

Advise patients about signs and symptoms of tendonitis and hepatitis.

FURTHER READING

Carter EL. Antibiotics in cutaneous medicine: An update. Semin Cutan Med Surg. 2003;22:197–211.

Kilburn SA, Featherstone P, Higgins B, Brindle R. Interventions for cellulitis and erysipelas. Cochrane Database Syst Rev. 2010;6:CD004299.

Rayner C, Munckhof WJ. Antibiotics currently used in the treatment of infections caused by *Staphylococcus aureus*. Intern Med J. 2005;35(Suppl. 2):S3–16.

Shaker M, McWilliams S, Greenhawt M. Update on penicillin allergy delabelling. Curr Opin. Pediatrics. 2020;32:321–27.

Sousa-Pinto B, Tarrio I, Blumenthal KG, et al. Accuracy of penicillin allergy diagnostic tests: A systematic review and meta-analysis. J Allergy Clin Immunol. 2021 Jan;147(1):296–308. doi: 10.1016/j.jaci.2020.04.058.

Turner NA, Sharma-Kuinkel BK, Maskarinec SA, et al. Methicillin-resistant *Staphylococcus aureus*: An overview of basic and clinical research. Nat Rev Microbiol. 2019;17:203–18.

6 Antifungals

Rachael Morris-Jones

CLASSIFICATION AND MODE OF ACTION

Systemic antifungal drugs are highly effective in treating superficial dermatomycoses acquired in temperate climates. Unfortunately, tropical and deep fungal infections often remain recalcitrant to treatment despite high-dose prolonged therapy with newer agents. Topical treatment is often adequate for localized superficial yeast and dermatophyte infection, but nail and scalp infections usually require systemic therapy to enable adequate delivery of the drug to the infected hair shafts and nail plates.

Fungi are broadly divided into moulds and yeasts. A mould is made up of multinucleate filaments called hyphae, which can be divided by septae and grow continuously from their apical tip. Yeasts are unicellular and usually oval in shape. They mainly replicate by budding. Some fungi, including Candida and dimorphic species (such as Aspergillus), are able to switch between producing hyphae and yeast forms depending on the environment. Hyphal forms are usually necessary for invasion of cells and tissue, whereas yeast forms appear to be important for dissemination to distant sites.

The plasma membrane of fungal cells contains ergosterol rather than cholesterol as in mammalian cells and the majority of antifungal drugs exert their selective effects by interfering with the enzymatic pathway of ergosterol biosynthesis (see Table 6.1). However, some of these enzymes are also involved with cholesterol metabolism. The majority of antifungal drugs are fungistatic (inhibiting fungal cell growth) at concentrations achievable at sites of infection. Only a minority have the advantage of being fungicidal (killing fungal cells), which enables more effective clearance of fungal infections with a shorter course of treatment and less evolution of drug resistance.

The main categories of antifungal drugs are listed in Table 6.1, which summarizes their classification and mechanism of action (see also Figure 6.1). The systemic antifungal drugs used in dermatology (terbinafine, azoles and griseofulvin) are discussed in more detail.

Patients at risk from superficial fungal infections include children (tinea capitis), older people (onychomycosis), the immunosuppressed, animal handlers (zoophilic tinea corporis), athletes (tinea pedis, tinea cruris) and those with diabetes (candidiasis). Human immunodeficiency virus (HIV) infection may predispose individuals to more severe and more frequent infections, particularly onychomycosis, which may fail to respond to conventional doses of antifungals.

AZOLE ANTIFUNGAL DRUGS

CLASSIFICATION AND MODE OF ACTION

Azole antifungals are a synthetic group of fungistatic agents with a broad spectrum of activity. They are based on a 5-member ring structure and classified into two groups: Imidazoles and triazoles. They bind to the iron atom in the haem component of lanosterol-14 demethylase (or CYP51A1, P45014DM), a cytochrome P450 enzyme that converts lanosterol to ergosterol, a major fungal wall component. This leads to arrested fungal growth. Triazoles have a higher specificity of binding than imidazoles, leading to increased potency. Overexpression of CYP51A1 or impairment of energy-dependent facilitated diffusion of azoles into fungal cells are mechanisms underlying drug resistance. Most imidazole antifungal drugs are only formulated for topical use (clotrimazole, miconazole and econazole) to treat the skin and nails. Ketoconazole was the exception, but it is no longer recommended for systemic use due to the risk of hepatotoxicity. Triazoles (itraconazole,

DOI: 10.1201/9781003016786-6

TABLE 6.1

Classification and Mechanism of Action of Antifungal Drugs

Group	Examples	Mode of Action	Main Indications
Azoles	Clotrimazole	Inhibit C-14 sterol demethylase via cytochrome P450 leading to a reduction in ergosterol	Tinea infections
Imidazoles	Econazole		*Candida* skin infections
	Ketoconazole		Vaginal candidiasis
	Miconazole		
	Tioconazole		Onychomycosis
	Itraconazole		Oropharyngeal candidiasis
Triazoles	Fluconazole		Vaginal candidiasis
			Sporotrichosis
			Tinea skin infections
			Onychomycosis
	Voriconazole		*Fusarium, Mycetoma,* chromoblastomycosis
	Posaconazole		Coccidioidomycosis
			Scedosporium, Candida
Allylamines	Terbinafine	Inhibit squalene epoxidase causing squalene accumulation	Tinea infections
	Naftifine		
Echinocandins	Caspofungin	Inhibit (1-3)-β-D-glucan synthase, a component of fungal cell wall	Invasive aspergillosis
	Micafungin		Invasive candidiasis
	Anidulafungin		
Morpholines	Amorolfine	Inhibits 14 reductase epoxidase causing squalene accumulation	Dermatophyte onychomycosis
Polyenes	Amphotericin B	Binds to ergosterol in fungal cell walls and disrupts membrane structure	Invasive candidiasis
	(Nystatin)		Invasive aspergillosis
	(Natamycin)		Cryptococcosis
			Sporotrichosis
Others	Griseofulvin	Disrupts microtubule function in nuclear division	Tinea infections
			Onychomycosis
	Flucytosine (5-fluorocytosine)	Inhibits DNA and RNA synthesis	Cryptococcosis
			Invasive candidiasis

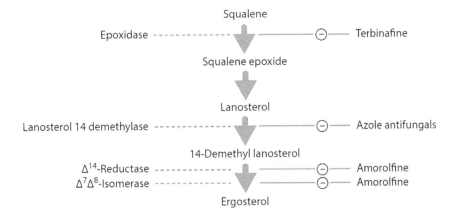

FIGURE 6.1   Points of action of antifungal drugs in the pathway of ergosterol biosynthesis.

fluconazole, voriconazole and posaconazole) are used systemically and have a higher specificity against fungal cytochrome P450 (CYP450) than imidazoles and less human toxicity. Fluconazole has good activity against fungal yeast forms, but it lacks activity against moulds, whereas itraconazole has a wider spectrum of action, but less reliable bioavailability. Voriconazole and posaconazole are used for invasive fungal infections. The adverse effects of voriconazole include hepatitis, hair loss, nail changes, visual disturbance, phototoxicity and squamous cell carcinoma.

The widespread therapeutic and prophylactic use of azole antifungal drugs has led to an increase in the rate of drug resistance. This can relate to the ability of some fungal species to switch from yeast to hyphal forms in the presence of azole drugs.

ITRACONAZOLE

Itraconazole is highly lipophilic and well-absorbed with a prolonged half-life. The therapeutic effect in the skin is achieved by passive diffusion into basal keratinocytes, a high rate of excretion in sebum and, to a lesser degree, excretion in sweat. Extensive tissue (protein) binding in skin and hair has been demonstrated, so the active drug persists for several weeks after stopping therapy.

INDICATIONS AND DERMATOLOGICAL USES

The licensed dermatological indications for itraconazole are:

- Dermatophytosis caused by tinea species (tinea corporis, tinea pedis, etc.).
- Onychomycosis caused by dermatophytes and/or yeast.
- Pityriasis versicolor.
- Vulvovaginal and oropharyngeal candidiasis.

Itraconazole has a broad spectrum of antifungal action and is also widely used to treat systemic fungal infections (e.g. aspergillosis, candidiasis, cryptococcosis and histoplasmosis), deep mycoses (e.g. sporotrichosis, chromoblastomycosis, paracoccidiodomycosis and histoplasmosis) and for prophylaxis of fungal infection in patients with neutropenia and HIV.

It is effective in both a continuous and pulsed regimen for fungal nail infections. Candida onychomycosis responds very well to pulsed itraconazole; however, non-dermatophyte moulds causing onychomycosis (such as Scytalidium) do not respond. When onychomycosis is treated with systemic drugs, the causative organism should therefore be identified and host factors such as comorbidities and concurrent medication carefully considered, as well as the extent and severity of disease.

FORMULATIONS/PRESENTATION

- 100 mg capsules (a super bioavailable 65 mg formulation, SUBA® itraconazole, has been approved by the FDA for systemic fungal infection – see Table 6.2).
- Oral solution (10 mg/mL), which is suitable for children and HIV/immunosuppressed patients with oral or oesophageal candidiasis. (Higher bioavailability than standard capsules.)
- IV infusion for systemic fungal infections.

DOSAGES AND SUGGESTED REGIMENS

See Table 6.2. Itraconazole capsules should be taken immediately after a meal to maximize absorption. Absorption is inconsistent and impaired by any drug or factors that reduce gastric acidity. Increasing stomach acidity with cranberry juice or non-diet cola can enhance absorption. The treatment regimen and dosage vary according to indication. In the treatment of fungal nail disease, improvement may be slow and full benefit not apparent until after treatment has been completed. The oral solution bioavailability is not affected by the gastric pH and should be taken on an empty stomach.

TABLE 6.2

Indications and Dosage Regimens of Itraconazole for Skin Disease

Indication	Dose
Vulvovaginal candidiasis	200 mg twice daily for 1 day
Pityriasis versicolor	200 mg once daily for 7 days
Tinea corporis, tinea cruris	100 mg once daily for 15 days or 200 mg once daily for 7 days
Tinea pedis, tinea manuum	100 mg once daily for 30 days or 200 mg twice daily for 7 days
Tinea capitis in younger children (unlicensed)	3–5 mg/kg/d up to 200 mg daily for 2–6 weeks or pulsed regimen (see Use in Special Situations – Children)
Oropharyngeal candidiasis	100 mg once daily for 15 days
Onychomycosis (dermatophyte or *Candida*)	200 mg once daily for 3 months or a pulsed regimen of 200 mg twice daily for 7 days a month, i.e. subsequent courses repeated after 21-day intervals; 2 pulses for fingernails, 3 pulses for toenails
Super bioavailable capsule formulation (SUBA)	Itraconazole is licensed to treat blastomycosis, histoplasmosis and aspergillosis (130–260 mg daily); it should be taken with food

BASELINE INVESTIGATIONS AND CONSIDERATIONS

- Mycology should confirm a fungal infection before starting treatment for suspected onychomycosis.
- Liver function tests (LFTs) should be performed in patients with a history of liver disease.
- There should be pregnancy testing and effective contraception should be ensured in females of childbearing potential.

MONITORING

LFTs in patients with pre-existing liver disease, those taking continuous treatment over a month or if receiving other hepatotoxic drugs.

CONTRAINDICATIONS

- Hypersensitivity to itraconazole or related azoles.
- Acute porphyria.
- Pregnancy.

CAUTIONS

Use itraconazole only after careful consideration and with caution:

- Liver disease: Use at reduced dosage if the benefit outweighs risk of hepatotoxicity. LFTs should be monitored.
- Cardiac failure: Itraconazole has been associated with congestive cardiac failure after high doses and long treatment courses. Caution is advised in patients at high risk of heart failure, i.e. older people and those with cardiac disease. Baseline echocardiography may be indicated.

IMPORTANT DRUG INTERACTIONS

As itraconazole is mainly metabolized by CYP3A4, potent inhibitors of this enzyme may increase its bioavailability. Examples include: Ritonavir, indinavir, clarithromycin and erythromycin. Enzyme inducers and medications that reduce gastric acidity and absorption of itraconazole may reduce its bioavailability, such as rifampicin, lansoprazole, omeprazole, pantoprazole and raniti-dine. Itraconazole may also inhibit the metabolism of many other drugs metabolized by CYP450 3A4 and lead to an increased risk of toxicity.

Multiple drugs are contraindicated with itraconazole, including mizolastine, triazolam, oral mid-azolam, quetiapine, pimozide, dofetilide, dabigatran, ticagrelor, quinidine, and statins metabolized by CYP3A4 (atorvastatin, lovastatin and simvastatin).

Caution is advised with the following drugs:

- Calcium channel blockers, which is due to pharmacological interactions and additive negative inotropic effects which may precipitate cardiac failure.
- Cardiac glycosides (digoxin).
- Ciclosporin, tacrolimus and sirolimus metabolism are inhibited. Reduced dosage and monitoring of drug levels may be required.
- Colchicine is contraindicated in those with renal or hepatic impairment.
- Coumarin anticoagulants' and non-vitamin K oral anticoagulants' (NOACs) effect may be enhanced.
- Inhaled corticosteroids, because metabolism may be impaired with long-term itraconazole, leading to iatrogenic Cushing syndrome.
- HIV protease inhibitors such as ritonavir, indinavir and saquinavir.

ADVERSE EFFECTS AND THEIR MANAGEMENT

- Gastrointestinal: Nausea and abdominal pain are the most common side effects and are generally mild. Side effects are dose-dependent; therefore, the dose can be reduced.
- Hepatitis: This is very uncommon (<1/10,000) but potentially serious. The risk is increased in pre-existing liver disease, with prolonged therapy (>1 month) and high dosage. Patients should be advised of the signs and symptoms of hepatitis (see below) and treatment stopped immediately. In most cases, LFTs normalize after withdrawal of treatment.
- Dermatological: Pruritus, acute generalized exanthematous pustulosis, urticaria, Stevens–Johnson syndrome and photoallergic reactions have been reported. Adverse cutaneous reactions are more common in immunosuppressed patients.
- Cardiovascular: See Cautions.
- Headache, dizziness, hypersensitivity reactions, thrombocytopenia and decreased libido can also occur.

USE IN SPECIAL SITUATIONS

PREGNANCY AND PRE-CONCEPTION

Itraconazole is embryotoxic and teratogenic in animals, so it is contraindicated in pregnancy except for life-threatening infections. Effective contraception must be used during treatment and until the next menstrual period following treatment cessation. It may cause menstrual irregularities.

LACTATION

Small amounts of itraconazole are excreted in human breast milk, so it should not be taken during lactation.

CHILDREN

Itraconazole is unlicensed in children under the age of 12 years, but it has been proven to be safe, effective and well-tolerated. It is commonly prescribed for tinea capitis due to Trichophyton species.

Its efficacy is comparable to griseofulvin and terbinafine, with high complete cure rates when given for 2–3 weeks. Itraconazole is superior to terbinafine for the treatment of Microsporum species, but griseofulvin remains the treatment of choice in many countries due to its lower cost. The duration of treatment is 2–6 weeks, and dosage is based on weight and formulation, up to a maximum of 200 mg daily. The dose for capsules is 5 mg/kg/d and for oral solution is 3 mg/kg/d.

For tinea capitis, treatment can be given continuously for 2–6 weeks or as a pulsed regimen of 1 week of itraconazole, then 2 weeks off between each pulse, for up to 3 pulses in total. The schedule for pulsed treatment for onychomycosis is the same as in adults with a dose of 5 mg/kg.

OLDER PEOPLE

Care should be taken in those at risk of cardiac failure and those taking drugs which may interact with itraconazole. The prevalence of onychomycosis in older people is high, but generally morbidity is low; therefore, the risks/benefits of treating onychomycosis with any oral antifungal should be carefully considered before embarking on potentially lengthy courses of treatment.

SPECIAL POINT

Itraconazole has been shown to suppress tumour growth by inhibiting the Hedgehog signalling pathway and angiogenesis and is currently undergoing trials in various malignant diseases. Its inhibitory effects are similar to vismodegib (see Chapter 37) and may underlie its teratogenic effects.

ESSENTIAL PATIENT INFORMATION

Females of childbearing potential should avoid pregnancy and use effective contraception.

Patients should be informed of the signs and symptoms of liver dysfunction, e.g. anorexia, nausea, vomiting, fatigue, abdominal pain or dark urine, and should be advised to discontinue treatment and seek medical advice if affected.

FLUCONAZOLE

Fluconazole is very well-absorbed after oral administration and does not undergo first-pass metabolism, so serum concentrations are identical, whether administered orally or parentally. Unlike itraconazole, it is highly water-soluble, and absorption is not affected by food intake or gastric acidity. It is distributed widely throughout the body and appears to be eliminated from the skin more slowly than from the plasma. Most of the drug is excreted unchanged in the urine.

INDICATIONS AND DERMATOLOGICAL USES

- Genital candidiasis and oropharyngeal candidiasis.
- Systemic candidiasis, including candidemia and disseminated candidiasis.
- Superficial mycoses: Tinea pedis, tinea corporis, tinea cruris, pityriasis versicolor and dermal candidiasis.

Other uses include:

- Tinea capitis in children (off-label).
- Recalcitrant toenail onychomycosis (off-label).
- Prophylaxis or treatment of systemic mycoses such as cryptococcosis and candidosis in HIV infection, treatment of histoplasmosis and coccidiomycosis and prevention of fungal infections in immunocompromised patients.

FORMULATIONS/PRESENTATION

- Capsules containing 50 mg, 150 mg and 200 mg fluconazole. A 150 mg single-capsule pack is available from pharmacies without prescription for the treatment of vaginal candidiasis.
- Oral suspension: 50 mg/5 mL, 35 mL oral suspension, 200 mg/5 mL, 35 mL oral suspension.
- IV infusion (infuse slowly over 1–2 hours).

DOSAGES AND SUGGESTED REGIMENS

- Genital candidiasis: 150 mg as single oral dose.
- Oropharyngeal/oesophageal candidiasis: 50 mg daily (100 mg maximum daily in recalcitrant infection) given for 7–14 days.
- Chronic atrophic candidiasis associated with dentures: 50 mg daily for 14 days.
- Oesophageal and mucocutaneous candidiasis: 50 mg for 14–30 days. In unusually difficult cases of mucosal candidal infections, the dose may be increased to 100 mg daily.
- Tinea pedis, tinea corporis, tinea cruris, pityriasis versicolor and dermal candidiasis: 50 mg daily for 2–4 weeks (up to 6 weeks in tinea pedis).

Other reported regimens (unlicensed) include pulse dosing of 150 mg fluconazole once weekly for tinea corporis and tinea cruris, and 300 mg once weekly for 6–9 months for onychomycosis. However, fluconazole is not licensed for the treatment of nail disease and has lower efficacy than other licensed drugs, so it should only be considered when these are contraindicated or not tolerated.

SPECIAL POINT

Resistant strains of Candida may emerge during prolonged treatment with fluconazole. C. krusei, C. glabrata, C. auris and certain strains of C. albicans are also primarily resistant to this drug.

BASELINE INVESTIGATIONS AND CONSIDERATIONS/MONITORING

- Baseline: Full blood count (FBC) (complete blood count [CBC]), renal indices and liver function tests (LFTs) in those with underlying illnesses. Pregnancy test.
- During therapy: Repeat LFTs after 6 weeks of treatment.

CONTRAINDICATIONS

- Fluconazole should not be used in patients with known hypersensitivity to it or related azoles.
- Pregnancy.

CAUTIONS

Dose reduction required in renal impairment, as fluconazole is mostly excreted unchanged by the kidneys.

IMPORTANT DRUG INTERACTIONS

Fluconazole inhibits the 2C9, 3A4 and 2C19 isoforms of CYP450, which leads to multiple potential interactions:

- Rifampicin: Modest reduction in fluconazole levels due to CYP450 induction by rifampicin.
- Phenytoin: Levels may be increased, so monitoring is required.

- Ciclosporin: Levels may be increased, so monitoring is required.
- Warfarin: Activity may be enhanced.

It should also be avoided with drugs that may prolong the QT interval, including erythromycin and hydroxychloroquine, especially in the presence of hypokalaemia.

- Hydrochlorothiazide may increase levels of fluconazole.

ADVERSE EFFECTS AND THEIR MANAGEMENT

The adverse effect profile of fluconazole is similar to itraconazole (see above), but fluconazole is less frequently associated with hepatotoxicity. Adverse events usually occur with treatment duration of over 1 week, but most are reversible when the drug is discontinued.

Fixed drug eruption is a recognised adverse effect of fluconazole and may be underreported. Other azole antifungals may be tolerated. Patch tests on lesional skin can confirm the diagnosis.

USE IN SPECIAL SITUATIONS

PREGNANCY

Fluconazole is contraindicated in pregnancy, as it has been associated with birth defects in the children born to mothers taking high-dose long-term treatment. Pregnancy should be excluded before starting therapy, and females of childbearing potential should use adequate contraception.

LACTATION

Fluconazole is excreted in breast milk at similar levels to plasma and should not be used during lactation.

CHILDREN

Fluconazole is licensed for use in children, including neonates, in the treatment of mucosal candidiasis, invasive Candida infections and cryptococcal infections, but not for superficial skin infection. Clearance is faster than in adults, so higher doses are needed (up to 12 mg/kg/d for severe infection). Fluconazole has been reported to be effective in childhood tinea capitis at doses of 6 mg/kg/day for 3–6 weeks with comparable efficacy to griseofulvin and the advantage of a shorter treatment duration.

VORICONAZOLE

INDICATIONS AND DERMATOLOGICAL USES

Aspergillus (including extrapulmonary and disseminated infection), disseminated Candida infections (including/wounds and chronic mucocutaneous candidiasis), Coccidioidomycosis, Scedosporium fusarium, Talaromyces marneffei, resistant dermatophyte infections (such as terbinafine-resistant Trichophyton interdigitale (mentagrophytes) and Paecilomyces lilacinus.

FORMULATIONS AND PRESENTATIONS

Oral tablets and oral suspension, and lyophilized powder to form a solution for intravenous infusion.

DOSAGES AND SUGGESTED REGIMENS

- Oral administration: If less than 40 kg, then 100 mg every 12 hours; and if greater than 40 kg, 200–300 mg every 12 hours (or 3–4 mg/kg every 12 hours). For severe infections, the dose can be increased to 400 mg every 12 hours.
- IV initially: 6 mg/kg every 12 hours for 2 doses, then maintenance with 4 mg/kg every 12 hours.

BASELINE INVESTIGATIONS AND MONITORING

- LFTs (aspartate transaminase [AST] and alanine transaminase [ALT] levels), urea and electrolytes, plasma calcium and magnesium levels.
- Electrocardiogram (ECG). Voriconazole may prolong the QT interval, so in those with underlying cardiac conditions, a baseline ECG should be obtained.
- Liver toxicity usually occurs within the first 10 days of treatment, so in at-risk individuals, check liver function tests and electrolytes after 1 week. The dose should be reduced in patients with liver impairment.
- With prolonged use, there is an increased risk of skin malignancies, particularly squamous cell carcinoma. Patients with sun-damaged skin should be advised to use high-SPF sunscreen and protective clothing and seek advice about any new skin lesions.

CONTRAINDICATIONS AND CAUTIONS

Voriconazole should be avoided in patients with acute porphyrias. Caution should be taken using voriconazole in patients with symptomatic arrhythmias, prolonged QT interval, cardiomyopathy, bradycardia, electrolyte disturbances and those at risk of pancreatitis.

IMPORTANT DRUG INTERACTIONS

Voriconazole interacts with several drugs due to inhibition of the cytochrome P450 enzyme. Some combinations can be prescribed but may require additional monitoring.

It should be avoided with multiple drugs, including carbamazepine, ergotamine, everolimus, phenobarbital and long-acting barbiturates, pimozide, quinidine, rifampicin, ritonavir and St John's wort.

Drugs that require additional monitoring or dose adjustment include ciclosporin, tacrolimus sirolimus, coumarin anticoagulants, opioid analgesics, oral contraceptives, benzodiazepines, efavirenz, NSAIDs, statins, omeprazole, sulphonylureas, methadone, phenytoin and rifabutin.

ADVERSE EFFECTS AND THEIR MANAGEMENT

- Hypertension and rashes can occur in approximately 10% of children who take voriconazole and 2% and 5% of adults, respectively.
- Hyperkalaemia is more common in adults (17%) and hypokalaemia in children (11%).
- Gastrointestinal upset can occur in up to 20% of patients.
- Abnormal liver function tests affect about a quarter of patients (raised AST/ALP or bilirubin).
- Transient visual disturbance is common and usually occurs shortly after dosage. It includes enhanced/altered light and colour perception and photophobia. This is due to selective reversible dysfunction of the retinal ON-bipolar cells in both rod and cone pathways.
- Increased serum creatinine in about 20% of adults and <5% of children.
- Epistaxis and fever can occur in up to a quarter of children.
- Rare cases of malignancy (melanoma and squamous cell carcinoma) have been reported. Phototoxicity may be a precursor. The risk is duration-dependent, and malignancies tend to be more aggressive and multifocal.

The drug should be stopped, or dose reduced according to the severity of the adverse effect.

USE IN SPECIAL SITUATIONS

PREGNANCY AND LACTATION

Voriconazole should not be taken during pregnancy or breastfeeding.

CHILDREN

Oral suspension of voriconazole should be given either one hour before or one hour after food. The suspension should be shaken for at least 10 seconds before use; it should not be mixed with other medications or flavouring liquids. Most of the studies in children that are based on the oral suspension indicate that in children, higher doses (mg/kg) may be required compared to adults, especially those <15 years and weighing <50 kg. Most children are treated with IV voriconazole first and only switch to oral once significant clinic improvement has been seen.

OLDER PEOPLE

No special considerations are required; however, in the obese patient, use ideal body weight to calculate drug doses.

SPECIAL POINT

Drug trough levels can be monitored if there are concerns about lack of efficacy or toxicity or for prolonged treatment in disseminated infection. Levels should be checked after 5–7 days of consistent voriconazole therapy, when the drug has reached a steady state. Serum samples should be taken immediately before the next dose. The safe and effective trough level is between 2–6 mg/L.

KETOCONAZOLE

Ketoconazole was the first broad-spectrum imidazole for oral use in the treatment of systemic mycoses. However, in 2013, the European Medicines Association (EMA) issued advice against the use of oral ketoconazole for treatment of fungal infections due to the risk of severe, progressive and potentially fatal liver damage and the availability of safer alternatives. Females over the age of 40 years on long-term therapy appeared to be at highest risk. Although the estimated incidence of severe hepatotoxicity was less than 1 in 10,000, in view of this serious hazard and availability of safer drugs, the EMA advised that its use was no longer justified. Topical ketoconazole is still available in cream and shampoo formulations for the treatment of seborrheic dermatitis and pityriasis versicolor.

TERBINAFINE

CLASSIFICATION AND MODE OF ACTION

Terbinafine is a synthetic allylamine which is highly effective against a broad spectrum of dermatophyte infections. It inhibits the biosynthesis of fungal ergosterol at the point of squalene epoxidase. (See Figure 6.1.) This leads to accumulation of the intermediate squalene, which appears to be fungicidal, and deficiency of the end product, ergosterol, which is fungistatic. Ergosterol is an integral component of fungal cell membranes, and squalene is thought to interfere with fungal membrane function and cell wall synthesis. Although the biosynthesis of cholesterol relies on the activity of squalene epoxidase, terbinafine has a much lower binding affinity for the mammalian enzyme and therefore demonstrates selective toxicity to fungal systems.

Terbinafine is well-absorbed after oral dosage (especially after a high-fat meal/with acidic food) and reaches peak plasma concentrations within about 2 hours. Primary metabolism occurs in the liver and involves at least seven CYP450 enzymes. Inactive metabolites are slowly eliminated, mainly in the urine. The polyfunctional nature of terbinafine as a substrate reduces potential drug interactions. Terbinafine inhibits CYP2D6, and the activity of this enzyme may not return to normal for months following cessation of a prolonged course of treatment.

Terbinafine is preferentially taken up into fat and reaches high concentrations in the sebum, skin and nails. It is delivered to the stratum corneum primarily by sebum and to a lesser extent by diffusion through the dermo-epidermis. During the first 2 weeks of therapy, concentrations within the stratum corneum increase to 75 times greater than plasma concentrations. It is also incorporated into the hair matrix. The long terminal half-life of 200–400 hours may reflect its slow elimination from tissues, such as skin and adipose. The clinical efficacy of terbinafine is related to high drug levels at the site of infection and sustained fungicidal activity following discontinuation of therapy.

INDICATIONS AND DERMATOLOGICAL USES

The licensed indications of terbinafine are dermatophyte infections of the skin and nails where oral therapy is appropriate (site, severity, etc.).

Terbinafine is the most active anti-dermatophyte agent. It is the treatment of choice for dermatophyte onychomycosis, with superior long-term results in toenail disease to griseofulvin, fluconazole and itraconazole. Clinical trials have shown greater or equal efficacy compared with other antifungals, with the benefit of a shorter treatment period. It is also highly effective in treating chronic dermatophyte infections on the hands, feet and body.

Terbinafine is also an effective treatment for tinea capitis, though not licensed in the UK for treating children. It is however, licensed for this complaint in the United States and many parts of Europe. The most common causative agents for tinea capitis vary from one part of the world to another. In urban settings in Europe and the United States, the main dermatophyte fungi causing tinea capitis are Trichophyton species, which cause an endothrix pattern of infection where arthrospores are most abundant within the hair shaft (see Figure 6.2).

Oral terbinafine is usually ineffective at treating superficial yeast infections, such as candidosis and pityriasis versicolor.

FORMULATIONS/PRESENTATION

- Scored tablets containing terbinafine hydrochloride equivalent to 250 mg terbinafine.
- Topical formulation (terbinafine hydrochloride 1%) cream/gel/spray.

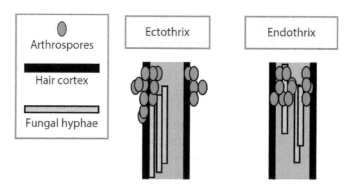

FIGURE 6.2   Different arthrosporic distribution in ectothrix and endothrix fungal hair infection.

DOSAGES AND SUGGESTED REGIMENS

The usual adult dose is 250 mg once daily. The duration of treatment depends on the site and severity of the infection. It is usually 2–6 weeks in tinea pedis, 2–4 weeks in tinea cruris, 4 weeks in tinea corporis and 6 weeks–3 months in nail infections (occasionally longer in toenail infections). Additional topical or surgical treatment to infected nails may improve cure rates. The maximum clinical effect in nail infections may not be seen for several months after cessation of treatment until the healthy nail has grown.

Although unlicensed in children in the UK, studies have confirmed good cure rates in tinea capitis.

- Child over 1 year, body weight 10–20 kg: 62.5 mg once daily.
- Child body weight 20–40 kg: 125 mg once daily.
- Child body weight over 40 kg: 250 mg once daily.

The duration of treatment for tinea capitis depends on the causative organism. Trichophyton species show good response rates within 4 weeks of treatment. Microsporum infection requires prolonged therapy of 6 weeks or more. The difference in clinical response may be related to the ectothrix infection pattern of Microsporum spp. as opposed to the endothrix pattern associated with the genus Trichophyton, with a consequent decreased accessibility of antimycotics to the fungal spores on the surface of the hair shaft in the former.

Treatment of onychomycosis in patients with HIV infection may require higher-dose therapy, e.g. 500 mg daily. Additional use of a topical antifungal preparation and avulsion of a diseased nail may improve cure rates in severe toenail onychomycosis.

BASELINE INVESTIGATIONS AND CONSIDERATIONS

Mycological confirmation of infection and causative organism should ideally be obtained before starting treatment, especially when prolonged treatment is likely (onychomycosis).

MONITORING

A baseline LFT is advised, but in young, fit, healthy children/adults, this is not routinely necessary for normal-dose short courses of treatment, such as up to 4 weeks. In patients who have previous or current liver dysfunction or relevant comorbidities, it is advised to check LFTs at baseline, then every 4–6 weeks during treatment.

Consider also checking the FBC in patients who are immunosuppressed if on treatment for more than 6 weeks.

CONTRAINDICATIONS

- Terbinafine hypersensitivity.
- Severe renal or liver impairment.

CAUTIONS

- Psoriasis: Exacerbation has been reported very rarely.
- Systemic and cutaneous lupus erythematosus: These conditions may be exacerbated or induced.
- Hepatic impairment: Hepatic clearance of terbinafine is reduced in liver disease, and as it may also cause hepatotoxicity, its use should be avoided in liver disease.

- Renal impairment: Reduce dosage by 50% if estimated glomerular filtration rate (eGFR) is <50 mL/min/1.73 m^2 and no suitable alternative is available.

IMPORTANT DRUG INTERACTIONS

- CYP450 enzyme inducers (e.g. rifampicin) and inhibitors (e.g. cimetidine) may accelerate or reduce terbinafine metabolism, respectively, and its dosage may need adjustment.
- CYP2D6-mediated drug metabolism is inhibited by terbinafine. Patients taking drugs metabolized by this enzyme (H1-antihistamines, SSRIs, MAOIs type B) may require closer monitoring.
- Oral contraceptive metabolism in not usually affected, but there have been sporadic reports of menstrual disturbances/breakthrough bleeding.
- Warfarin efficacy may be reduced so closer monitoring is indicated.

ADVERSE EFFECTS AND THEIR MANAGEMENT

- Gastrointestinal effects are mild and common (>2%). They include anorexia, nausea and diarrhoea. Symptoms may settle with continued treatment.
- Loss of taste/a metallic taste is not uncommon, and although usually reversible, permanent taste loss has been reported.
- Serious hepatotoxicity is very rare and is estimated to occur in 1 in 50,000–120,000 pre-scriptions. It may present with hepatitis or cholestasis. Clinical features include nausea, anorexia, fatigue, vomiting, dark urine and pale stools. Mild asymptomatic biochemical abnormalities are commoner. Elevated serum aminotransferases occur in less than 1% of patients and may resolve without discontinuation of treatment. Abnormalities requiring interruption of treatment occur in about 0.3% for courses of treatment between 2–6 weeks' duration and 0.44% for treatment courses longer than 8 weeks. Acute hepatotoxicity is thought to be a hypersensitivity reaction and is associated in Europeans with HLA-A*33:01 heterozygosity, which is found in less than 1% of the population. Treatment should be dis-continued immediately if signs of liver dysfunction develop. Liver injury usually recovers within 6 months of stopping the drug.
- Dermatological: Includes pruritus, urticaria, hair loss, photosensitivity, induction or exac-erbation of subacute cutaneous or systemic lupus erythematosus, exacerbation of psoria-sis and serious cutaneous adverse reactions (acute generalized exanthematous pustulosis, Stevens–Johnson syndrome and toxic epidermal necrolysis). Treatment should be discon-tinued immediately if a progressive rash develops.
- Psychiatric adverse effects have been reported very rarely.
- Blood disorders (including leukopenia and thrombocytopenia) have been reported very rarely.
- Other nonspecific adverse effects include headache and flu-like symptoms, occasionally with arthralgia or myalgia.

USE IN SPECIAL SITUATIONS

Pregnancy and Pre-Conception

Although there is no evidence of harm, the use of terbinafine is not recommended in pregnancy unless potential benefit outweighs risk.

Avoid as terbinafine is excreted in milk with a high ratio of drug in milk:plasma of 7:1 after oral administration.

CHILDREN

Although not licensed for use in children in the UK, terbinafine has been shown to be well-tolerated and effective in this age group. The drug may have a higher clearance and shorter half-life in this age group. It has been licensed by the FDA for use in children from the age of 4 years in the United States. For dosages in tinea capitis, see page 53.

ESSENTIAL PATIENT INFORMATION

Patients should be advised to seek prompt medical attention if they develop a new or worsening rash or signs and symptoms of liver dysfunction (e.g. jaundice, right upper abdominal pain, nausea, fatigue, vomiting, dark urine or pale stools). They should be advised to report any alteration in taste or smell or depressive symptoms.

SPECIAL POINT

Dermatophyte resistance to terbinafine is emerging as a global problem. Originally reported in India and presenting as treatment-unresponsive tinea cruris and corporis, this has now been reported in other regions including Europe.

GRISEOFULVIN

CLASSIFICATION AND MODE OF ACTION

Griseofulvin was first obtained from the mould Penicillium griseofulvum in 1939 and has been used as an oral therapy for superficial fungal infection since the 1960s. It has fungistatic actions and is most effective against dermatophytes that cause tinea (ringworm) infections. It is deposited in newly formed keratin in the skin and hair and is thought to act by inhibiting the formation of fungal microtubules. Griseofulvin may also have anti-inflammatory and immunomodulatory effects.

GI absorption varies considerably between individuals, mainly because the drug is insoluble in the upper GI tract. Absorption is improved if griseofulvin is taken after a fatty meal. Bioavailability is also improved by a reduction in particle size ('ultramicrosize'). It is metabolized in the liver and excreted in the urine, faeces and sweat.

The duration of treatment depends on the length of time required for the infected keratin to be shed, which may be several months. Effective delivery to the skin depends upon eccrine sweating and can be impaired in disease where the sweat ducts are obstructed.

INDICATIONS AND DERMATOLOGICAL USES

- Superficial dermatophyte infections (nail, skin, hair) where topical therapy has failed or is inappropriate (severe or widespread disease). Griseofulvin has specific activity against dermatophytes. It is a long-established treatment for infections of the scalp and nails and has been used safely in children for many years, being available as both tablet and suspension preparations. However, it has a bitter taste, and prolonged treatment may be required. For nail infection, newer, more effective antifungal drugs are preferred. Griseofulvin is licensed to treat tinea capitis in children and is still widely used in this context, but newer drugs (itraconazole and terbinafine) appear to be equally effective with shorter treatment durations. Griseofulvin is not effective against Candida, Pityrosporum, Scopulariopsis or Scytalidium spp.

- There have been anecdotal reports of benefit from griseofulvin treatment in a range of dermatological conditions, including lichen planus and eosinophilic fasciitis, and recent research has highlighted a potential anti-tumour effect.

FORMULATIONS/PRESENTATION

- Microsize tablets containing 125 mg and 500 mg griseofulvin.
- Ultramicrosize tablets containing 125 mg and 250 mg griseofulvin.
- A peppermint-flavoured oral suspension containing 125 mg/5 mL griseofulvin is useful for treating children.

DOSAGES AND SUGGESTED REGIMENS

The usual adult dose (microsize preparation) is 500 mg/d in a single or divided dose taken after meals. Where the ultramicrosize preparation is available, the dose is 375 mg/d. For children, see Use in Special Situations.

BASELINE INVESTIGATIONS AND CONSIDERATIONS

No routine investigations are needed for short courses (up to 6 weeks).

MONITORING

During therapy: FBC and LFTs after 3 months.

CONTRAINDICATIONS

- Hypersensitivity to griseofulvin or any component of the formulation.
- Severe liver disease.
- Porphyrias, particularly acute intermittent; avoid if possible in variegate and porphyria cutanea tarda.
- Systemic lupus erythematosus (SLE).
- Pregnancy.

CAUTIONS

- Hepatic impairment.
- Penicillin allergy: Hypersensitivity cross-reaction between penicillins and griseofulvin is possible.
- Photosensivity: Avoid exposure to intense sunlight to prevent photosensitivity reactions.

IMPORTANT DRUG INTERACTIONS

- Griseofulvin may decrease the blood level of drugs metabolized by CYP3A4, and adjustment of their dosage may be required.
- Coumarin anticoagulant activity (warfarin) is decreased, so closer monitoring is required.
- Oral contraception: Metabolism is increased, and contraceptive failure may occur, so additional precautions are required during griseofulvin treatment and for 1 month afterward.
- Ciclosporin: Serum levels are decreased by griseofulvin.

ADVERSE EFFECTS AND THEIR MANAGEMENT

The most common side effects of griseofulvin are listed below. Serious reactions are extremely rare.

- Headache: This is a common adverse reaction and is due to a reduction in vascular tone. It usually improves with continued treatment. Nausea, diarrhoea and vomiting are frequent side effects. These may be helped by dividing the dose.
- Dermatologic: These are rare and include urticaria, photosensitivity, erythema multiforme and toxic epidermal necrolysis. A dermatophytide (id or 'ide') reaction is occasionally seen after starting oral antifungal medication including griseofulvin. This usually presents with widespread follicular papules, especially on the face, and may be mistaken for a drug rash.
- Neuropsychiatric: Confusion, drowsiness, impaired concentration and peripheral neuropathy have been reported. The sedative effects of alcohol may be enhanced.
- SLE: This may be exacerbated or precipitated.
- Alcohol: Toxic effects are enhanced by griseofulvin and alcohol ingestion may precipitate a disulfiram-like reaction.

USE IN SPECIAL SITUATIONS

PREGNANCY AND PRE-CONCEPTION

Griseofulvin disrupts the mitotic spindle and is capable of inducing aneuploidy (abnormal segregation of chromosomes following cell division) and causing embryo toxicity. It was formerly classified as FDA Category C. Rare cases of conjoined twins have been reported following griseofulvin therapy in early pregnancy. The drug should not be taken during pregnancy and pregnancy must be avoided within 1 month of discontinuation. Men should not father children within 6 months of treatment.

LACTATION

Griseofulvin should be avoided in lactation as its safety is not established.

CHILDREN

Griseofulvin is the only licensed treatment for superficial fungal infections, including tinea capitis in children under the age of 12 years. In children, the recommended dose is 10 mg/kg/d (maximum 500 mg daily). The duration of treatment varies from 2–4 weeks in tinea corporis and 2–4 months in tinea unguium. The recommended duration of griseofulvin treatment for tinea capitis is 6–12 weeks. To avoid treatment failure, however, the dose may need to be increased to 20 mg/kg/d (maximum 1 g daily) for the same period of time. This is particularly advisable in patients with endothrix infection (see Table 6.3).

Griseofulvin is ineffective in at least one-third of children with tinea capitis, most likely due to inadequate dosing, poor adherence and insufficient treatment duration. Adjunctive therapy with an antifungal shampoo (ketoconazole or selenium sulphide) is recommended for the first 2 weeks to minimize transmission to others. Prolonged treatment is required to clear kerion (12–16 weeks), but the routine additional use of systemic corticosteroids confers no benefit and is not recommended.

SPECIAL POINT

Children with tinea capitis may continue on treatment to shed fungal spores for several months and do not need to be excluded from school. Children in contact with tinea capitis should be examined

TABLE 6.3

Oral Antifungal Agents for Tinea Capitis in Children

Agent	Dose
Griseofulvin[a]	10–20 mg/kg/d for 6–12 weeks
Terbinafine (for Trichophyton tonsurans)	<20 kg: 62.5 mg/kg
	20–40 kg: 125 mg/kg
	>40 kg: 250 mg – all daily for 1 month
Itraconazole	3–5 mg/kg/d (max 100 mg/d) for 2–6 weeks
	Or weekly pulses of 5 mg/kg/d every 4 weeks for 2–3 months
Fluconazole	3–6 mg/kg/d for 3–6 weeks

[a] Licensed in the UK for treatment of tinea capitis in children.

very carefully for signs of infection (which may be as little as a few broken hairs) and given oral antifungals if infection is confirmed. Asymptomatic carriers do not routinely need oral antifungals but should be given an antifungal shampoo at least twice weekly.

ESSENTIAL PATIENT INFORMATION

- Patients should be advised to avoid alcohol.
- Patients should avoid driving or operating machinery if affected by drowsiness.
- Patients should be advised about contraceptive and family planning precautions and the reduced effectiveness of oral contraceptives.

AMPHOTERICIN B AND LIPID-BASED FORMULATIONS

Amphotericin B (AmB) is a polyene antifungal drug with a broad spectrum of activity against yeast and mould fungi. It binds to ergosterol in the cell wall of the fungus, leading to holes which allow the contents to seep out. Due to toxicity, it is mainly used for life-threatening disseminated infections. It has very poor oral absorption (about 5%), so it is almost exclusively given parenterally. Liposomal formulations of AmB were developed in the 1990s using small, unilamellar vesicles of 60–80 nm in size (composed of hydrogenated soy phosphatidylcholine and distearoyl phosphatidylglycerol, stabilized by cholesterol). They are associated with reduced toxicity and similar efficacy to conventional AmB (as deoxycholate complex) and are generally preferred. They include AmB lipid complex (ABLC), liposomal AmB (L-AmB) and pegylated-liposomal AmB. Conventional AmB (as deoxycholate complex) is still also available.

INDICATIONS AND DERMATOLOGICAL USES

Amphotericin B (AmB) has activity against most Candida and Aspergillus species, Mucorales and all endemic mycoses, and most hyaline and brown-black moulds. It is also used to treat extensive cutaneous, mucocutaneous and visceral Leishmania.

FORMULATIONS AND PRESENTATIONS

- Powders for infusion and suspensions.

AmB is usually given intravenously but can administered intrathecally into the vitreous chamber of the eye, bladder and peritoneum, and a nebulised formulation is available to treat respiratory infections.

SPECIAL POINT

Conventional formulations of AmB and the different liposomal formulations are not interchangeable, and the formulation must be specifically prescribed to avoid potentially fatal medication errors.

Topical formulations of AmB are under development for the treatment of cutaneous fungal infections and cutaneous leishmaniasis.

DOSAGES AND SUGGESTED REGIMENS

- An initial test dose is usually followed by the remaining infusion given over several hours. The manufacturer's precise instructions should be followed according to the formulation.
- AmB doses range from 250 mcg/kg/day to 1.5 mg/kg/day (or alternate days). The maximum dose must not be exceeded due to potentially fatal cardiac toxicity.
- Liposomal formulations are given at a dose of 3–5 mg/kg/day for most indications, with up to 10 mg/kg/day for fungal meningitis.

BASELINE INVESTIGATIONS AND MONITORING

Renal indices, LFTs, FBC and electrolytes, including potassium and magnesium levels, should be measured at baseline and then daily (for daily infusions) or weekly depending on the frequency of the infusions and the results of the tests.

CONTRAINDICATIONS AND CAUTIONS

- Hypersensitivity to AmB.

IMPORTANT DRUG INTERACTIONS

- Nephrotoxic drugs should be avoided.
- Drugs that cause hypokalaemia should be avoided and not co-administered.
- Digoxin and muscle relaxant drug toxicity is increased by AmB-induced hypokalaemia.
- Micafungin (an echinocandin antifungal) may increase AmB toxicity.

ADVERSE EFFECTS AND THEIR MANAGEMENT

- Infusion reactions are the most common adverse effects with all forms of AmB with headache, fever, chills, shortness of breath, arrhythmias, nausea, vomiting, muscle cramps, weakness and increased/decreased urination. Slowing the infusion and use of antipyretics or hydrocortisone may ameliorate if ongoing medication is essential.
- Renal impairment affects about 10% of patients. Renal function usually improves on interruption of the treatment but may rarely be permanent.
- Electrolyte imbalances affect about 10% of patients and include hypokalaemia, hypomagnesaemia and, more rarely, hyperkalaemia and hypocalcaemia.
- Arrhythmias have been associated with rapid IV infusions. It may lead to cardiorespiratory arrest.
- Gastrointestinal upset affects about 10% of patients.
- Hepatitis occurs in about 10% of patients.
- Cutaneous adverse effects include urticaria, maculopapular rash, pruritus, exfoliation and, rarely, Stevens–Johnson syndrome and toxic epidermal necrolysis.

USE IN SPECIAL SITUATIONS

PREGNANCY AND LACTATION

AmB is not for use during pregnancy unless potential benefits outweigh the risks, though it is not known to be harmful in pregnancy. There is no information available on safety of AmB while breastfeeding.

CHILDREN

There is little data on the safety and efficacy of AmB in children; however, there are reported case series showing it is generally effective and well-tolerated. In this age group, the safety and efficacy of conventional AmB may be similar or better than that of LAmB. Dosages and regimens vary according to age and infectious agent.

OLDER PEOPLE

Case series of LAmB use in patients greater than 65 years of age show it is well-tolerated and effective, even if baseline creatinine levels are slightly elevated.

FURTHER READING

Ahmen M, Lear JT, Madan V, et al. British Association of Dermatologists guidelines for the management of onychomycosis. Br J Dermatol. 2014;171:937–58.

Bell-Syer SE, Khan SM, Torgerson DJ. Oral treatments for fungal skin infections of the foot. (Review). Cochrane Database Syst Rev. 2012;10:CD003584. doi: 10.1002/14651858.CD003584.pub2.

Fuller LC, Barton RC, Mohd Mustapa MF, et al. British Association of Dermatologists guidelines for the management of tinea capitis 2014. Br J Dermatol. 2014;171(3):454–63.

Groll AH, Rijnders BJA, Walsh TJ, et al. Clinical pharmacokinetics pharmacodynamics, safety and efficacy of liposomal amphotericin B. Clin Infect Dis. 2019;66(S4):S260–74.

Levine MT, Chandrasekar PH. Adverse effects of voriconazole: Over a decade of use. Clin Transplant. 2016;30:1377–86.

Moriarty B, Hay R, Morris-Jones R. The diagnosis and management of tinea. (Clinical Review). BMJ. 2012;435:37–42.

7 Antimalarials

Thomas Tull and Mark Goodfield

CLASSIFICATION AND MODE OF ACTION

Antimalarials are the first choice of oral therapy for all patients with cutaneous lupus erythematosus (LE), as well as the majority with systemic forms of the disease. They have been widely used since their introduction in 1894, particularly since the 1950s.

Hydroxychloroquine, mepacrine and chloroquine are all effective in the management of systemic lupus erythematosus (SLE), various forms of cutaneous lupus and rheumatoid arthritis, and are also used in a variety of other cutaneous disorders. They are safe when used appropriately and generally well-tolerated; they are probably under-prescribed.

Chloroquine and hydroxychloroquine are 4-aminoquinolones, while mepacrine (quinacrine), a 9-aminoacridine, has an extra benzene ring but is otherwise structurally similar. This structural change leads to a different side effect profile. The mode of action of antimalarials in dermatological disease is still uncertain, although recent research has led to a clearer understanding of their mode of action. Antimalarials inhibit toll-like receptors, particularly TLR9 and TLR7, thus reducing levels of tumour necrosis factor alpha (TNF-α) and type I interferons, which are important mediators of inflammation in lupus. Hydroxychloroquine also inhibits lysosomal degradation of endocytosed material or cellular components processed via the autophagy pathway. It can therefore prevent antigen processing and presentation via MHC class II molecules.

The antimalarials outlined above are well-absorbed orally and bind particularly to pigmented tissues, including the retina. They are metabolized by the liver and excreted renally, with a prolonged half-life of 40–50 days. There is a great inter-individual variability in blood levels between patients taking similar drug doses, and the onset of therapeutic effect varies between drugs.

INDICATIONS AND DERMATOLOGICAL USES

- All forms of cutaneous LE, including discoid lupus erythematosus (DLE) and subacute LE.
- SLE with disease symptoms, including arthralgia, myalgia, fatigue, rashes and alopecia.
- Other rheumatic diseases, including rheumatoid arthritis and juvenile chronic arthritis.

Hydroxychloroquine and chloroquine are both licensed in the UK for treatment of DLE and SLE, as well as 'skin conditions aggravated by sunlight.' Mepacrine is currently unlicensed for use in skin and connective tissue disorders.

Several randomized, controlled trials provide evidence that antimalarials are useful in suppressing disease activity in SLE, particularly skin manifestations and fatigue. Fewer studies demonstrate efficacy in cutaneous lupus specifically. Discontinuing hydroxychloroquine in stable SLE may lead to increased disease activity. The drugs may also reduce the risk of thrombotic episodes in patients with antiphospholipid antibody syndrome and reduce serum lipids.

In addition to cutaneous lupus, other evidence-based dermatological indications for antimalarials include:

- Polymorphic light eruption.
- Cutaneous sarcoidosis.
- Porphyria cutanea tarda.

DOI: 10.1201/9781003016786-7

Quinolone antimalarials have also been found to be useful in a number of other inflammatory dermatoses, including benign cutaneous lymphocytic infiltration (Jessner), reticular erythematous mucinosis syndrome, dermatomyositis, urticarial vasculitis, lichen planus and frontal fibrosing alopecia.

FORMULATIONS/PRESENTATION

- Hydroxychloroquine is available as 200 mg or 300 mg tablets.
- In the UK, chloroquine is dispensed as 250 mg tablets of chloroquine phosphate (containing 150 mg chloroquine base).
- Chloroquine phosphate syrup is available at a concentration of 80 mg/5 mL (containing 50 mg/5 mL chloroquine base).
- Chloroquine sulphate as 250 mg and 500 mg tablets are the most readily available forms in the United States.
- Mepacrine hydrochloride is available as 100 mg scored tablets.

DOSAGES AND SUGGESTED REGIMENS

There is little evidence of comparative efficacy of different antimalarials in skin disease, but hydroxychloroquine is used in preference to chloroquine due to its safety profile. Most patients will need repeated courses of therapy, or even continuous treatment, to deal with flares and adequately suppress disease. Cigarette smoking seems to impair the efficacy of antimalarials, but the mechanism remains unclear. Combinations of antimalarials, particularly hydroxychloroquine and mepacrine, are more effective than either alone.

HYDROXYCHLOROQUINE SULPHATE

Initial and maintenance dose: 200–400 mg daily; maximum dose: 400 mg daily or 6.5 mg/kg ideal body weight. In obese patients, it is important to calculate the ideal body weight in order to avoid excess dosage. Tablets are not scored, but due to a long half-life, the daily dosage can be varied (e.g. 200 mg day 1, then 400 mg day 2, etc.) to avoid exceeding recommended limits.

The onset of effects is slow because of tissue distribution in fat and the mode of action, and it may take up to 12 weeks. Beneficial effects take a similar period to wear off. Approximately 60% of patients with DLE respond within 6 months, but there may be some loss of efficacy with continued treatment, requiring the addition of mepacrine to regain disease control.

MEPACRINE HYDROCHLORIDE

The usual dose is 50–100 mg daily but doses up to 400 mg daily have been used. Yellow skin discolouration is inevitable and may be severe at higher doses. The onset of action is about 3–6 weeks. It may be used as monotherapy or combined with hydroxychloroquine.

CHLOROQUINE PHOSPHATE OR SULPHATE

Chloroquine base is usually given at a dose of 150 mg daily (= 200 chloroquine sulphate or 250 mg chloroquine phosphate). The maximum recommended dose is 2.5 mg/kg/d based on ideal body weight. Its onset of action is more rapid and may be as short as 1 month.

Chloroquine carries a higher risk of retinopathy (see Adverse Effects and Their Management) than hydroxychloroquine, possibly because it crosses the blood–retinal barrier more easily, so it should be used only after other antimalarials have failed. There are inadequate data on chloroquine to advise a safe maximum dose, and cumulative dosage may be important, so treatment is usually limited to courses of 6 months.

BASELINE INVESTIGATIONS AND CONSIDERATIONS

The clinical history and baseline investigations should screen the patient for the following:

- Contraindications and underlying conditions exacerbated by antimalarials (see Cautions).
- Underlying haematological, hepatic and renal disease (full blood count, liver function tests and renal profile).

The most recent guidelines from the Royal College of Ophthalmologists no longer recommend baseline screening for underlying ocular disease (see Monitoring).

MONITORING

The Royal College of Ophthalmologists' Hydroxychloroquine and Chloroquine Retinopathy: Recommendations on Monitoring 2020 guidelines recommend that patients with the following risk factors should have annual ophthalmic eye screenings (fundus photography and spectral domain optical coherence tomography):

- Impaired renal function (eGFR <60 mL/min/1.73 m^2).
- Concomitant use of tamoxifen.
- Chloroquine use.
- Hydroxychloroquine dose >5 mg/kg per day.

In patients who do not have any of these risk factors, eye screening should commence 5 years after initiation of hydroxychloroquine. Patients on mepacrine do not need eye screening.

CONTRAINDICATIONS

Hydroxychloroquine and chloroquine should be avoided in individuals with a history of hypersensitivity to either drug. (Mepacrine is not contraindicated.)

CAUTIONS

- Pre-existing maculopathy: Avoid if possible and if treatment is needed then close liaison with an ophthalmologist is advised.
- Hepatic impairment.
- Renal impairment: In mild to moderate renal impairment the doses should be reduced (hydroxychloroquine, for example, may be reduced to 200 mg three times a week). Avoid in severe renal impairment (glomerular filtration rate [GFR] <10 mL/min). Routine therapeutic blood monitoring is not currently available for antimalarials.
- Neurological disorders, especially epilepsy.
- Glucose-6-phosphate dehydrogenase (G6PD) deficiency: Hydroxychloroquine has been reported to induce haemolytic anaemia in G6PD deficient patients although the evidence supporting this is conflicting.
- Myasthenia gravis may be exacerbated.
- Intermittent and variegate porphyria.

IMPORTANT DRUG INTERACTIONS

- Antacids and calcium carbonate reduce the absorption of hydroxychloroquine and chloroquine.

- Chloroquine and hydroxychloroquine increase the risk of ventricular arrhythmias with amiodarone.
- Cimetidine may decrease the metabolism of chloroquine and hydroxychloroquine, resulting in reduced plasma levels.
- There may be an increased risk of methemoglobinemia when chloroquine is administered with dapsone.
- Penicillamine plasma concentration and toxicity may be increased by both chloroquine and hydroxychloroquine.
- The effects of remdesivir may be potentially reduced by chloroquine and hydroxychloroquine.
- Co-administration of azithromycin or other systemic macrolide antibiotics (including erythromycin or clarithromycin) with hydroxychloroquine or chloroquine may be associated with an increased risk of cardiovascular events (including angina or chest pain and heart failure) and cardiovascular mortality.

ADVERSE EFFECTS AND THEIR MANAGEMENT

- Ocular adverse effects, specifically an irreversible retinopathy with blindness, are the major risks associated with chloroquine and hydroxychloroquine treatment. The maculopathy may progress even after the cessation of the drug. Low-dose hydroxychloroquine carries a small risk of this complication, while mepacrine has negligible ocular toxicity.

  Early retinopathy with antimalarials takes the form of a non-specific fine pigmentary stippling in the macular area and loss of the foveal light reflex. This may develop into irreversible bull's-eye maculopathy and widespread retinal pigment epithelial atrophy, associated with a central scotoma, loss of visual acuity and peripheral visual field loss. Corneal deposits and impairment of accommodation are reversible, dose-related side effects.

  The overall prevalence of hydroxychloroquine retinopathy among users is approximately 7.5%, but it ranges from 2% in patients on <5 mg/kg/day for less than 10 years to 20% in those treated for more than 20 years. Strategies to reduce cumulative doses are therefore beneficial, and many patients with cutaneous lupus can be adequately managed by limiting antimalarial therapy to the spring and summer seasons. Risk factors are listed in Table 7.1.

  If visual abnormalities or symptoms occur, the drug should be discontinued and the patient monitored for possible progression after cessation of therapy.
- Common adverse effects include gastrointestinal (GI) disturbance, headache and pruritus. These are usually mild. More serious but rare adverse effects include hepatic damage, myopathy, neuropathy and psychosis.

TABLE 7.1

Risk Factors for Hydroxychloroquine Retinopathy

Duration	>5 years
Dose	>5 mg/kg/d
Age	Older people
Co-morbidities	Renal, hepatic impairment, obesity
Ocular disease	Retinal or macular complaints
Concurrent medication	Tamoxifen

- Cutaneous adverse effects include skin and mucous membrane pigmentation, depigmentation of hair, alopecia and exfoliative dermatitis. Serious cutaneous adverse reactions, including acute generalized exanthematous pustulosis (AGEP) and toxic epidermal necrolysis, have been reported with hydroxychloroquine. Mepacrine causes reversible yellow discolouration of the skin when used in maintenance doses of 100 mg daily and may occasionally cause severe lichenoid eruptions (preceded by itch). Psoriasis may be worsened by chloroquine and hydroxychloroquine.
- Haematological adverse effects of antimalarials include a small but significant risk of marrow suppression and haemolysis in G6PD deficiency has been reported.
- When taken as an overdose, antimalarials are very toxic especially in infants, so safe storage is essential.

USE IN SPECIAL SITUATIONS

PREGNANCY

The use of hydroxychloroquine (formerly FDA Category C) in pregnancy is controversial. The manufacturers recommend avoidance of hydroxychloroquine in pregnancy and breastfeeding because of a theoretical risk of cochlear damage. However, stopping hydroxychloroquine when pregnancy is discovered makes little sense because of the long half-life. Separate studies in the UK and North America have found that continuation of hydroxychloroquine in pregnant patients with SLE is probably safe. There is considerable experience of pregnancy in patients safely receiving antimalarials as prophylaxis in malaria-endemic regions, and UK obstetricians are happy to continue hydroxychloroquine in patients in in vitro fertilization (IVF) programmes.

Chloroquine (formerly FDA Category D) is contraindicated in pregnancy, except for treating and preventing malaria. Because mepacrine is unlicensed, the manufacturers have no data on its use in pregnancy and breastfeeding.

LACTATION

Small amounts of antimalarials are excreted in breast milk; therefore, mothers taking these drugs should not breastfeed. However, the same is true for lactation as pregnancy, in terms of experience obtained from malarial prophylaxis.

CHILDREN

Quinolones and mepacrine are not licensed for use in children. When essential, hydroxychloroquine should be used at the minimum effective dose and should not exceed 6.5 mg/kg/d or 400 mg. Tablets of 200 mg therefore cannot be used in children weighing <31 kg. Chloroquine is sometimes used in specialist units at a daily dose of 4 mg/kg/d for ease of administration.

ESSENTIAL PATIENT INFORMATION

- Patients should be warned to stop treatment and seek advice from the prescribing doctor if they develop visual symptoms, such as reduced acuity, abnormal colour vision or blurred vision.
- Patients prescribed chloroquine should be specifically counselled about the risk of permanent visual loss.

FURTHER READING

Andreoli L, Bertsias GK, Agmon-Levin N et al. EULAR recommendations the management of family planning, assisted reproduction, pregnancy and menopause in patients with systemic lupus erythematosus and/or antiphospholipid syndrome. Ann Rheum Dis. 2017 Mar;76(3):476–85.

Melles RB, Marmor MF. The risk of toxic retinopathy in patients on long-term hydroxychloroquine therapy. JAMA Ophthalmol. 2014;132(12):1453–60.

Royal College of Ophthalmology, Hydroxychloroquine and chloroquine retinopathy: Recommendations on monitoring. 2020.

Ruiz-Irastorza G, Martín-Iglesias D, Soto-Peleteiro A. Update on antimalarials and systemic lupus erythematosus. Curr Opin Rheumatol. 2020;32(6):572–82.

Schrezenmeier E, Dörner T. Mechanisms of action of hydroxychloroquine and chloroquine: Implications for rheumatology. Nat Rev Rheumatol. 2020;16(3):155–66.

Shipman WD, Vernice NA, Demetres M et al. An update on the use of hydroxychloroquine in cutaneous lupus erythematosus: A systematic review. J Am Acad Dermatol. 2020 Mar;82(3):709–22.

8 Antivirals for Herpesviruses

Hannah Cookson

CLASSIFICATION AND MODE OF ACTION

Herpesviruses are members of a large family of DNA viruses that cause disease in humans and animals. At least five species are extremely widespread in humans, namely herpes simplex virus (HSV-1 and HSV-2, both of which can cause orolabial and genital infections), varicella zoster virus (VZV, which causes chickenpox and shingles), Epstein–Barr virus (EBV, the cause of infectious mononucleosis), and cytomegalovirus (CMV, which can have cutaneous presentations, such as ulcers, in the immunocompromised). HSV and VZV are neurotropic and, following primary infection, establish long-term asymptomatic latency in the ganglia of sensory nerves. Reactivation of latent viruses leads to enhanced replication and cell lysis and disease symptoms. Other human herpesviruses establish latency in lymphoid cells and can play a role in oncogenesis.

Most viral illnesses, including HSV and VZV, are self-limiting and do not require specific antiviral therapy. However, occasionally serious complications such as encephalitis and disseminated infections can occur, especially in neonates or immunocompromised patients (such as transplant recipients, cancer patients and those with human immunodeficiency virus [HIV] infection), and exposure to VZV infection in early pregnancy results in congenital varicella syndrome in up to 5% of pregnancies.

Antiherpes drugs inhibit viral DNA synthesis and viral replication by inhibiting viral DNA polymerase, which results in premature chain termination. Aciclovir (acyclovir) is the prototype guanosine analogue antiherpes drug and requires activation by viral thymidine kinase. It has a low water solubility and poor gastrointestinal (GI) absorption, with low oral bioavailability (15–30%), so IV administration is required to achieve consistent high plasma levels. The poor oral bioavailability is improved by esterification to the pro-drug valaciclovir (valacyclovir), which is hydrolysed to aciclovir via hepatic first-pass metabolism and increases the bioavailability 3–5-fold to approximately 70%. The superior pharmacokinetics of valaciclovir allow a reduced dosage frequency that may improve clinical efficacy and compliance. The therapeutic activity of aciclovir against herpesviruses is as follows: HSV>VZV>EBV>CMV.

Penciclovir has a similar spectrum of activity and potency against HSV and VZV, but due to a very low oral bioavailability, it is only used topically. Famciclovir is a pro-drug of penciclovir that improves the oral bioavailability of penciclovir to over 70%. The active triphosphate form of penciclovir has been shown to have more persistent antiviral activity in HSV-infected cells than aciclovir, and this may lead to an increase in efficacy. Ganiciclovir and its ester valganciclovir are licensed for the treatment of CMV in immunocompromised patients requiring treatment.

Drug resistance is an emerging threat to the clinical utility of antiviral drugs, especially following their long-term use in immunocompromised patients. Aciclovir resistance in HSV is usually associated with mutations in the viral thymidine kinase gene rather than DNA polymerase, as this enzyme is not essential for viral replication. Strains resistant to aciclovir are almost always cross-resistant to penciclovir and famciclovir. Resistant infections can be managed by foscarnet or cidofovir, but both are more toxic than aciclovir. Foscarnet is inhibitory for all herpesviruses and HIV, and it inhibits viral nucleic acid synthesis by interacting directly with viral DNA polymerase or reverse transcriptase. Foscarnet-resistant strains of herpesvirus have been described, and in this situation IV cidofovir should be considered (an unlicensed use).

DOI: 10.1201/9781003016786-8

INDICATIONS AND DERMATOLOGICAL USES

- Aciclovir is licensed for use in HSV and VZV infection.
- Valaciclovir is licensed for HSV and VZV infection and CMV prophylaxis in organ transplant recipients.
- Famciclovir is licensed for use in shingles and genital herpes.
- Ganciclovir and valganciclovir are licensed for the treatment of CMV in immunocompromised patients, including CMV retinitis in HIV patients.
- Foscarnet is licensed for unresponsive HSV infection in immunocompromised patients and CMV retinitis in HIV patients.

HSV INFECTION

Primary HSV infection of the mouth and lips (gingivostomatitis) or eyes in immunocompetent individuals is usually managed with topical aciclovir or penciclovir. Oral aciclovir may provide modest clinical benefit in preventing subsequent recurrent orolabial herpes. Severe infection, neonatal HSV and immunocompromised individuals require systemic therapy.

Primary and recurrent genital HSV infection is usually treated with an oral antiviral drug. This reduces virus shedding, symptoms and healing time, but does not significantly reduce the risk of further recurrence. Long-term prophylactic therapy with aciclovir or valaciclovir may be considered in patients with frequently recurring, debilitating genital herpes that is impairing the quality of life. It reduces the rate of clinical recurrence by about 90%, and subclinical shedding is markedly reduced but not eliminated. Aciclovir has been used safely for up to 10 years. Shorter-term prophylaxis (e.g. special events or risk periods) reduces the overall risk of recurrence by about 70% in those with sun-induced recurrences of HSV.

Long-term HSV prophylactic regimes may also be useful in the treatment of disabling recurrences of herpetic whitlow and HSV-related erythema multiforme.

Prophylactic oral aciclovir is used in late pregnancy (from 36 weeks) to reduce viral shedding in females with recurrent genital herpes and before organ transplantation.

VZV INFECTION

In healthy children, primary infection with VZV (chickenpox) is usually benign and self-limiting. However, in adolescents and adults, chickenpox is more severe, and oral antiviral therapy should be started within 24 hours of onset of the rash. This shortens the healing time and duration of fever and symptoms. Starting aciclovir after this time point appears to be of no value in uncomplicated adult varicella.

Systemic therapy is recommended for immunocompromised patients to reduce the risk of pneumonitis. Pregnant females and immunocompromised patients who are not immune to VZV require specialist advice and may require urgent treatment with varicella zoster immunoglobulin following exposure to chickenpox.

Oral antiviral treatment is indicated in herpes zoster (shingles) to reduce the severity and duration of acute pain, complications (post-herpetic neuralgia) and viral shedding. Treatment is recommended in patients over 50 years of age, those with non-truncal involvement, immunocompromised patients and patients with moderate-to-severe rash or pain. Ideally, treatment should be started within 72 hours of the onset of the rash, but it can be started up 1 week after onset of the rash in those patients at a higher risk of complications. Immunocompetent children with herpes zoster infection do not usually require antiviral treatment.

Additional treatment with prednisolone may accelerate resolution of acute pain but does not reduce post-herpetic neuralgia. Valaciclovir and famciclovir have been shown to be superior to aciclovir in reducing herpes zoster-associated pain and are generally preferred due to their more convenient dosing regimens. Administration of aciclovir IV increases the rate of healing and resolution of acute neuritis in immunocompetent patients with shingles compared with oral therapy, but IT does not appear to confer any improved long-term benefits.

Immunocompromised patients require IV therapy for 7 days to reduce the risk of disseminated VZV infection. In those who are severely immunocompromised, oral therapy may be administered for 6 months.

FORMULATIONS/PRESENTATION

- Aciclovir: 200 mg and 800 mg tablets; 200 mg, 400 mg and 800 mg dispersible tablets; and suspensions of 200 mg/5 mL, 400 mg/5 mL (with sugar-free versions available). Powder to reconstitute for slow IV infusion. Topical aciclovir 5% cream and 3% eye ointment.
- Valaciclovir: 250 mg and 500 mg tablets.
- Famciclovir: 125 mg, 250 mg and 500 mg tablets.
- Penciclovir: 1% cream for herpes labialis. Not recommended under 12 years.
- Foscarnet sodium: Solution for IV infusion.
- Ganciclovir: Solution for IV infusion.
- Valganciclovir: 900 mg tablets.

DOSAGES AND SUGGESTED REGIMENS

NON-GENITAL HSV INFECTION (PRIMARY GINGIVOSTOMATITIS/HERPES LABIALIS)

Oral aciclovir:

- Adults and children over 2 years: 200 mg 5×/day for 5 days (double the dose if immunocompromised or absorption-impaired).
- Infants aged 1 month–2 years: Half adult dose.

Intravenous aciclovir is recommended to achieve higher blood levels than oral aciclovir in severe infections (disseminated infection, extensive eczema herpeticum, neonatal infection and HSV encephalitis):

- Adults and children over 12 years: 5 mg/kg Tds for 5 days. Obese individuals should receive a dosage based on their ideal body weight.
- Neonates, infants and children up to 12 years: See children's formulary for dosage according to body surface area or body weight.

Valaciclovir:

- Adults: 500 mg Bd for 5 days (up to 10 days if new lesions appear or healing is incomplete; double the dose in immunocompromised).
- Adults and children over 12 years: Two 2 g doses with a 12-hour interval for treatment of acute herpes labialis.

PRIMARY GENITAL HSV INFECTION

- Oral aciclovir: 200 mg 5×/day or 400 mg Tds for 5 days (longer if new lesions appearing). Increase dose to 400 mg 5×/day in immunocompromised.
- Valaciclovir: 500 mg Bd for 5 days (up to 10 days if new lesions appear or healing is incomplete; double the dose in the immunocompromised patient).
- Famciclovir: 250 mg Tds for 5 days.

RECURRENT GENITAL HSV INFECTION

- Oral aciclovir: 200 mg 5×/day, 400 mg Tds for 3–5 days or 800 mg Tds for 2 days. In the immunocompromised patient, give 400 mg Tds for 5–10 days.
- Valaciclovir: 500 mg Bd for 3–5 days (double the dose and treat up to 10 days in immunocompromised).
- Famciclovir: 125 mg Bd for 5 days or 1 g Bd for 1 day (500 mg Bd for 5–10 days in immunocompromised).

Alternatively, topical therapy with aciclovir or penciclovir may be used for recurrent HSV. Treatment should be commenced at the onset of symptoms. Penciclovir is not recommended in children under the age of 12 years.

PROPHYLACTIC REGIMENS FOR FREQUENTLY RECURRING GENITAL HERPES

- Short-term prophylaxis: Aciclovir 400 mg Bd for 1 week.
- Long-term prophylaxis: Aciclovir (400 mg Bd or 200 mg Tds); valaciclovir 500 mg once daily (increase to twice daily for very frequent recurrences); famciclovir 250 mg Bd. Long-term prophylactic therapy is usually interrupted after 6–12 months to assess recurrence frequency.

PRIMARY VZV INFECTION (CHICKENPOX)

- Oral aciclovir: 800 mg 5×/day for 7 days, in both normal and immunocompromised patients.

HERPES ZOSTER (SHINGLES)

- Oral aciclovir: 800 mg 5×/day for 7 days for adults and children over 12 years. In younger children, 20 mg/kg (up to 800 mg) qds (unlicensed).
- Intravenous aciclovir: 10 mg/kg Tds for acute herpes zoster affecting the trigeminal nerve (forehead and eyelids).
- Valaciclovir: 1g Tds for 7 days in adults and immunocompromised children over 12 years.
- Famciclovir: 500 mg Tds for 7 days (or 10 days in the immunocompromised patient) or 750 mg 1–2×/day for 7 days.

In immunocompromised patients, antiviral therapy should be continued for at least 7 days and for 2 days after the lesions have crusted.

ACICLOVIR-RESISTANT HSV AND VZV

- Intravenous Foscarnet Sodium: 40 mg/kg Tds by slow infusion for 2–3 weeks or until lesions have healed. It is licensed for use in acyclovir-resistant mucocutaneous HSV infections and may also be effective in acyclovir-resistant VZV infections.

SPECIAL POINT

Chickenpox vaccination with live attenuated VZV is not part of the current routine UK childhood immunization programme. It is recommended for non-immune healthcare workers, older children/adults and close family contacts of immunocompromised individuals.

Passive immunity is conferred by administration of varicella zoster immunoglobulin, which should be given to high-risk individuals within 4 days of contact (British National Formulary [BNF] advises 10 days) with chickenpox or herpes zoster. High-risk individuals include neonates, non-immune pregnant females and immunocompromised patients – including those who have received systemic corticosteroids in the previous 3 months (>40 mg prednisolone daily for more than 1 week).

Despite recent attempts, no effective vaccine has yet been developed for HSV infection.

BASELINE INVESTIGATIONS AND CONSIDERATIONS

- Routine monitoring is not required for aciclovir, valaciclovir and famciclovir.
- For IV foscarnet the renal profile, calcium and magnesium levels should be monitored during treatment.

MONITORING

Renal indices, electrolytes, calcium and magnesium should be monitored frequently during foscarnet therapy.

CONTRAINDICATIONS

A known hypersensitivity to the antiviral agent.

CAUTIONS

- Aciclovir IV: Maintain adequate hydration and reduce dose in renal failure. Dose-limiting toxicities of IV aciclovir are renal insufficiency and CNS side effects.
- Valaciclovir: Caution with high doses in hepatic impairment and reduce dose of IV infusion in renal failure.
- Famciclovir: Reduce dose in renal impairment.
- Aciclovir and penciclovir: Aciclovir and penciclovir creams can cause transient stinging, burning or numbness. They should not be used in the mouth.

IMPORTANT DRUG INTERACTIONS

The concomitant use of aciclovir or valaciclovir, with ciclosporin and possibly tacrolimus, may increase nephrotoxicity.

- The plasma concentrations of aciclovir are increased with mycophenolate mofetil.
- Excretion of aciclovir is reduced by probenecid.
- Plasma concentrations of theophylline may be increased with aciclovir and valciclovir.
- Excretion of famciclovir is possibly reduced by probenecid.
- Foscarnet with pentamidine isethionate increases the risk of hypocalcaemia.
- Ganciclovir and valganciclovir increase risk of seizures when given with imipenem.

ADVERSE EFFECTS AND THEIR MANAGEMENT

Oral anti-herpesvirus drugs are generally well-tolerated.

- Aciclovir has been infrequently associated with nausea, diarrhoea, rash, headache, pruritus, photosensitivity and, very rarely, renal insufficiency, hepatitis, jaundice, neuropsychiatric effects (dizziness, confusion, drowsiness, hallucinations psychosis and convulsions), tremor and fever. Anaemia, thrombocytopenia or leukopenia have been described.

- Valaciclovir has similar adverse effects but in higher doses may be associated with confusion, hallucinations, nephrotoxicity and, uncommonly, severe thrombocytopenic syndromes, especially in immunocompromised patients.
- Famciclovir may be associated with headache, diarrhoea and nausea. Urticaria, rash and hallucinations or confusion (predominantly in older people) have been reported.
- Intravenous foscarnet may cause a range of adverse effects, including GI effects, neuropsychiatric disturbance, renal impairment and bone marrow toxicity. It requires careful monitoring for electrolyte disturbance, especially hypocalcaemia.
- Aciclovir and penciclovir creams can cause transient stinging, burning or numbness. Ophthalmic use of aciclovir can give rise to local irritation and, rarely, blepharitis or, very rarely, hypersensitivity.
- Ganciclovir and valganciclovir can cause a range of side effects, including gastrointestinal side effects, bone marrow toxicity, neuropsychiatric disturbance, hepatic function derrangement, renal impairment and skin reactions.

USE IN SPECIAL SITUATIONS

Pregnancy

- Aciclovir and valaciclovir: Not known to be harmful in pregnancy, but the manufacturers advise to use only when potential benefits outweigh risk. No increase in the frequency of congenital abnormalities has been recognized in infants born to females who took aciclovir during pregnancy, and the drug has been used safely in neonates.
- Famciclovir: Avoid but use only when potential benefits outweigh risk.
- Foscarnet: Avoid use.
- Ganciclovir and valganciclovir: Avoid use.

Lactation

- Aciclovir and valaciclovir: Significant amounts are found in milk; it is not known to be harmful but should be used with caution.
- Famciclovir: Insufficient data exist.
- Foscarnet: Avoid use.
- Ganciclovir and valganciclovir: Avoid use.

Children

- Aciclovir is licensed for use in children and is the treatment of choice.
- Valaciclovir is licensed for use in children over 12 years for CMV infection.
- Famciclovir is not licensed for children and not generally recommended due to limited safety data.
- Foscarnet is not licensed for use in children. Doses of 40 mg/kg Tds can be given for severe mucocutaneous HSV infection.

ESSENTIAL PATIENT INFORMATION

Patients should be advised about additional symptomatic treatment of their infection with oral analgesics and to maintain adequate fluid intake. It should be explained that a person who has not had chickenpox or the varicella vaccine can catch chickenpox from a person with shingles and that the person is infectious until their lesions have dried (usually 5–7 days). While chickenpox is spread by respiratory droplets and skin contact, only direct skin contact with shingles carries the risk of infection.

Seek urgent specialist advice for ocular infection with cold sores or shingles.

FURTHER READING

Andrei Snoek G. Advances in the treatment of varicella-zoster virus infections. Adv Pharmacol. 2013;67:107–68.

Foley E, Clarke E, Beckett VA, Harrison S, Pillai A, FitzGerald M, Owen P, Low-Beer N, Patel R. Management of genital herpes in pregnancy. Royal College of Obstetricians and Gynaecologists. 2014. https://www. rcog.org.uk/globalassets/documents/guidelines/management-genital-herpes.pdf.

McDonald EM, deKock J, Ram FS. Antivirals for management of herpes zoster including ophthalmicus: A systematic review of high-quality randomized controlled trials. Antivir Ther. 2012;17:255–64.

NICE. Clinical knowledge summary of shingles. National Institute for Health and Care Excellence. 2022. CKS.nice.org.uk/topics/shingles/management.

Sacks S, Aoki FY. Famciclovir for the management of genital herpes simplex in patients with inadequate response to aciclovir or valaciclovir. Clin Drug Invest. 2005;25:803–9.

9 Apremilast

Gayathri K. Perera

CLASSIFICATION AND MODE OF ACTION

Apremilast (Otezla) is a sulfonyl isoindole type compound with a similar structure to crisaborole. Its chemical formula is $C_{22}H_{24}N_2O_7S$.

Apremilast is an oral, small-molecule inhibitor of phosphodiesterase 4 (PDE4), an enzyme that breaks down cyclic adenosine monophosphate (cAMP). The resulting increase in cAMP within cells reduces, but does not completely inhibit, a variety of inflammatory cytokines, such as interleukin (IL)-1α, IL-6, IL-8, IL-10 MCP-1, MIP-1β, MMP-3, IL-17 and TNF-α. An increase in cAMP is reported to increase the levels of IL-10, an anti-inflammatory cytokine.

Apremilast is well absorbed orally and extensively metabolised by cytochrome oxidative metabolism, primarily CYP3A4. The half-life is 6–9 hours, and it is eliminated by the kidneys and in faeces.

INDICATIONS AND DERMATOLOGICAL USE

Apremilast was first licensed by the FDA for use in psoriatic arthritis in early 2014. Later that year, a license was extended to adults with moderate-to-severe chronic plaque psoriasis who qualified for phototherapy or systemic therapy. It was the first oral medication for the treatment of psoriasis and psoriatic arthritis in 20 years. It was granted a European license for use in the treatment of psoriasis and psoriatic arthritis in January 2015, and the UK approved its use in 2016. In 2019, it was also approved for oral ulceration associated with Behçet's disease in adults. It was initially produced by Celgene, and the company was taken over by Amgen Europe B.V. in 2019.

FORMULATIONS/PRESENTATION

Apremilast is still within patent, and so there is no generic formulation. It is available as 10 mg (pink-coloured and diamond-shaped), 20 mg (brown, diamond-shaped) and 30 mg (beige, diamond-shaped) film-coated tablets.

DOSAGES AND SUGGESTED REGIMENS

The initial titration schedule is 10 mg once a day on day 1, then 10 mg twice daily on day 2, then 10 mg in the morning and 20 mg in the evening on day 3, then 20 mg twice daily on day 4, then 20 mg in the morning and 30 mg in the evening on day 5, then maintenance dosing of 30 mg twice daily (at least 12 hours apart) from day 6 onward.

DOI: 10.1201/9781003016786-9

If the eGFR is <30 mL/minute/1.73 m^2, then the dose should be reduced 30 mg once a day (dose titration is available in the product literature).

BASELINE INVESTIGATIONS AND CONSIDERATIONS

Although the pharmaceutical company does not require baseline or monitoring blood tests, UK dermatologists recommend:

- Full blood count (FBC) (complete blood count [CBC]).
- Urea, electrolytes and creatinine/renal indices.
- Liver function tests (LFTs).
- TB evaluation.
- HIV and hepatitis screening if at risk.

MONITORING

During therapy repeat FBC, renal indices and LFTs after 8 weeks then every 6 months thereafter.

CONTRAINDICATIONS AND CAUTIONS

In January 2017, the MHRA/CHM released an alert, following post-marketing reporting, cautioning a causal relationship between Apremilast and depression and insomnia. Instances of suicidal ideation and behaviour, including suicide, have been observed in patients with or without a history of depression.

The value of Apremilast in treating patients who may be already psychologically affected by chronic plaque psoriasis and debilitating psoriatic arthritis needs to be evaluated, and patients need to be counselled and followed closely for signs of increased mental health issues such as depression or suicidal ideation. Baseline and during treatment depression scores should be taken for signs of increased anxiety or depression if the benefit of Apremilast is thought to outweigh the risk in these patients. Patients and carers should be advised to notify the prescriber of any changes in behaviour or mood and any suicidal ideation.

Patients who have galactose intolerance, total lactase deficiency or glucose/galactose malabsorption should not take Apremilast.

IMPORTANT DRUG INTERACTIONS

Any medications or over-the-counter products that increase the activity of cytochrome P450/CYP3A4 will lead to a decrease in the effect of Apremilast. Such medications include rifampicin, phenobarbital, carbamazepine, phenytoin and St John's wort.

Although it does not suppress the immune system directly and there are limited data on the question of vaccinations, experts recommend against giving live attenuated vaccines to patients on Apremilast. Live attenuated vaccines include: BCG; intranasal influenza; measles, mumps and rubella; oral polio; oral typhoid; varicella zoster (VZIg) (chickenpox); and yellow fever.

ADVERSE EFFECTS AND THEIR MANAGEMENT

- Gastrointestinal: Diarrhoea, nausea and vomiting are the commonest side effects, affecting at least 34% of all patients compared to placebo. These side effects are most often within the first 2–6 weeks. A few patients have been hospitalized due to severe diarrhoea.

   Weight loss of 5–10% of body weight has been reported in 1 in 10 patients in clinical trials. If this is not due to nausea and subsequent reduction of food intake, and not due to diarrhoea, Apremilast may need to be discontinued and further investigations undertaken.
- Respiratory: Upper respiratory tract infections, runny nose, sneezing and nasal stuffiness have all be reported.
- Neurology: Headaches are one of the commonest adverse events in real-world data. Ensure adequate hydration, sleep, and use simple analgesia as needed. Depression has already been discussed.
- Skin: Urticaria and angioedema can occur with the medication.
- General: Back pain and fatigue can occur with the medication.

USE IN SPECIAL SITUATIONS

PREGNANCY AND PRE-CONCEPTION

As there is limited information on fertility and pregnancy, it is not recommended that patients conceive while on Apremilast, and females of childbearing potential should use effective contraception.

LACTATION

Avoid as animal studies have shown presence of Apremilast in breast milk.

CHILDREN

Apremilast is not approved for use in children (i.e. those aged under 18 years).

ESSENTIAL PATIENT INFORMATION

Advise patients that this is a relatively new drug and that real-world data about side effects is still being collected. Any unexpected adverse effect should be reported to the prescriber and the regulatory authority informed (for example MHRA Yellow Card system in the UK).

   Advise patients to stop treatment and seek help if affected by mood swings, severe depression or suicidal ideation.

FURTHER READING

Afra TP, Razmi TM, Dogra S. Apremilast in psoriasis and beyond: Big hopes on a small molecule. Indian Dermatol Online J. 2019 Jan–Feb;10(1):1–12. doi: 10.4103/idoj.IDOJ_437_18.
Hsu S, Papp KA, Lebwohl MG, et al. Consensus guidelines for the management of plaque psoriasis. Arch Dermatol. 2012;148:95–102.

Menter A, Korman NJ, Elmets CA, et al. Guidelines of care for the management of psoriasis and psoriatic arthritis. Section 6: Case-based presentations and evidence-based conclusions. J Am Acad Dermatol. 2011;65:137–74.

Papp K, Cather JC, Rosoph L, et al. Efficacy of Apremilast in the treatment of moderate to severe psoriasis: A randomised controlled trial. Lancet. 2012;380:738–46.

Papp K, Reich K, Leonardi CL, et al. Apremilast, an oral phosphodiesterase 4 (PDE4) inhibitor, in patients with moderate to severe plaque psoriasis: Results of a phase III, randomized, controlled trial (efficacy and safety trial evaluating the effects of Apremilast in psoriasis [ESTEEM] 1). J Am Acad Dermatol. 2015 Jul;73(1):37–49. doi: 10.1016/j.jaad.2015.03.049. PMID: 26089047.

10 Azathioprine

Sarah H. Wakelin and Simon Meggitt

CLASSIFICATION AND MODE OF ACTION

The synthetic purine analog azathioprine (AZA) was initially developed as an immunosuppressant in the 1960s, but is now most widely prescribed for its immunomodulatory, steroid-sparing actions, especially in the treatment of inflammatory skin and bowel disease and lupus.

AZA is a pro-drug, and after oral ingestion and absorption, it is rapidly hydrolysed non-enzymatically to an imidazole derivative (methlynitroimidazole) and 6-mercaptopurine (6-MP). Although 6-MP is also available for oral administration, AZA is usually preferred, as its bioavailability is more reliable. 6-MP undergoes metabolism by competing enzymatic pathways to form various active metabolites (thioguanine nucleotides) and inactive metabolites (Figure 10.1). Thioguanine nucleotides function as rogue nucleic acids and disrupt DNA replication with antiproliferative effects, especially on lympho-cytes and other haemopoietic cells. The principal deactivating pathways are regulated by the enzymes thiopurine S-methyltransferase (TPMT) and xanthine oxidase (XO). Impairment of these pathways, due to inherent low enzyme activity or drug interactions, can lead to accumulation of potentially toxic levels of thioguanine nucleotides and the risk of life-threatening bone marrow suppression. Tests to measure TPMT activity are now widely available and play a key role in the safe and effective prescribing of AZA. The nucleotide diphosphatase 15 (NUDT15) converts thioguanine nucleotides to inactive metab-olites, and reduced activity of this enzyme is also associated with a risk of severe myelosuppression.

INDICATIONS AND DERMATOLOGICAL USES

The UK licensed indications for AZA are listed below. There are no FDA approved dermatological indications in the United States.

- Pemphigus vulgaris.
- Systemic lupus erythematosus.
- Dermatomyositis/polymyositis.

AZA has also been widely used as a steroid-sparing treatment for bullous pemphigoid, and in this context it appears to have similar efficacy to mycophenolate mofetil. Good clinical evidence sup-ports its use as an oral monotherapy in the treatment of atopic dermatitis, and it has been shown to be of benefit in chronic actinic dermatitis and parthenium allergic contact dermatitis.

AZA is also used to treat a range of vasculitides, including granulomatosis with polyangiitis (Wegener's granulomatosis), Behçet's disease, Henoch–Schönlein purpura and severe cutaneous leukocytoclastic vasculitis. Small studies have reported benefit in severe alopecia areata, lichen planus, pyoderma gangrenosum and sarcoid.

FORMULATIONS/PRESENTATION

- Generic and branded formulation tablet sizes of 25 mg and 50 mg.

DOSAGES AND SUGGESTED REGIMENS

The onset of action is slow, and therapeutic effects may take 6–8 weeks. An empirical dose of 1–3 mg/kg/d is recommended in the package insert, adjusting within these limits according to response and side effects. However, UK dermatology and gastroenterology guidelines advise dosing

DOI: 10.1201/9781003016786-10

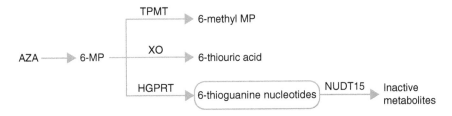

FIGURE 10.1 Simplified metabolism of azathioprine via different enzyme pathways. Active metabolites are boxed. AZA, azathioprine; HGPRT, hypoxanthine-guanine phosphoribosyl transferase; MP, mercaptopurine; NUDT15, nucleotide diphosphate 15; TPMT, thiopurine methyltransferase; XO, xanthine oxidase.

according to pre-treatment TPMT levels as in Table 10.1. Red blood cell TPMT phenotype testing is generally preferred to genotyping in these populations, as it detects all patients with absent activity whether they have a known variant of TPMT genotype or not. (Genotyping is used in haemato-oncology, as it is not affected by previous blood transfusions). Patients with absent TPMT activity should not receive AZA (see Baseline Investigations and Considerations). In exceptional situations, a greatly reduced dose (5%) has been used with very close haematological and metabolite monitoring.

The Clinical Pharmacogenetics Implementation Consortium guidelines recommend additional NUDT15 genotype testing, particularly for individuals of Asian and Hispanic ethnicity, due to the higher frequency of loss-of-function gene variants in these groups. Those affected should receive a lower starting dose of AZA with close monitoring.

Tablets should be swallowed whole, and the daily dose may be divided and taken with food to reduce gastric upset.

Dose adjustment may be needed depending on tolerability, efficacy and routine blood monitoring, particularly the full blood count (FBC) and white cell count (WCC). Measurement of thiopurine metabolites may also be considered after a steady state is reached at 4 weeks (see Monitoring). When a therapeutic response is achieved, the dose should be reduced to the lowest possible maintenance dose.

The effects of treatment may be slow to wear off after treatment ceases, due to persistence of active drug metabolites. Therapy should be discontinued if there is no improvement after 3 months.

CONTRAINDICATIONS AND CAUTIONS

- Hypersensitivity to AZA or 6-MP is an absolute contraindication, as AZA hypersensitivity syndrome is potentially life-threatening.

TABLE 10.1

Recommended Dosages of Azathioprine (AZA) Based on Thiopurine Methyl-Transferase (TPMT) Activity

TPMT Range (pmol/h/mg HB)	Maintenance AZA Dose mg/kg
Absent <10	Contraindicated
Intermediate/carrier 10–25	1.0–1.5
Normal/high >26	2.0–3.0

Units of measurement and category boundaries may vary, and prescribers are advised to contact their laboratory for further advice.

- Very low/absent or unknown TPMT levels (see Baseline Investigations and Considerations).
- Severe infection.
- Pancreatitis.
- Severely impaired hepatic function or bone marrow depression.
- Use with caution in pregnancy – see below.
- Malignancy is a contraindication to any form of immunosuppression, including AZA, due to the possible increased risk of disease progression.

Human immunodeficiency virus (HIV) infection is not a contraindication, and there is growing experience of safe use of AZA and other immunosuppressive drugs in HIV-positive patients. In this situation, it is used in those who are stabilized on highly active antiretroviral therapy (HAART). HIV status should be checked before starting AZA and close liaison carried out with infectious disease specialists before initiating therapy in HIV-positive individuals.

Hepatitis B virus (HBV) is an important consideration as up to one-third of the world's population has evidence of past or active infection with this virus. HBV carriers are at risk of a disease flare on treatment with immunosuppressants and acute liver failure on drug withdrawal. Pretreatment screening should include measurement of HBV surface antigens (HBsAg) and anti-HBV core antibodies (anti-HBc), and non-immune individuals at risk of infection should receive immunization against HBV. Liver function tests (LFTs) alone are inadequate as these may be normal in infected individuals. The risk for hepatitis C virus (HCV)-infected individuals is unclear, but management of all patients seropositive for HBV and HCV should be discussed with a hepatologist or infectious disease specialist as prophylactic antiviral therapy may be required.

COVID-19, influenza and pneumococcal vaccination are recommended for all people who are on immunosuppressant medication. Ideally, vaccination should take place at least 2 weeks before therapy is started. Prescribers are advised to consult the latest recommendation on COVID-19 vaccine and booster scheduling (see e.g. https://www.nhs.uk/conditions/coronavirus-covid-19/coronavirus-vaccination/health-conditions/).

Current COVID-19 guidelines should be consulted for dermatology patients with immune-mediated inflammatory disorders (IMID) who are eligible for treatment with neutralising monoclonal antibodies or antivirals.

IMPORTANT DRUG INTERACTIONS

- Xanthine oxidase inhibitors (allopurinol, oxypurinol and febuxostat) lead to accumulation of active metabolites with potentially life-threatening myelotoxicity. If co-administration is essential, the dose of AZA should be reduced to 1/4–1/3 of the routine dose, with very careful haematological monitoring.
- Drugs that can cause bone marrow depression should be avoided, including other immunosuppressants, clozapine and antifolate drugs (trimethoprim, cotrimoxazole, dapsone and sulphasalazine).
- Ribavirin (used for hepatitis C) inhibits an enzyme in the purine salvage pathway and has been reported to cause severe pancytopenia.
- Warfarin resistance has been reported, so anticoagulation needs monitoring, and an increased warfarin dose may be required.

SPECIAL POINT – VACCINATION

- Live-attenuated vaccines may be given to patients who are stable on doses of AZA up to 3 mg/kg/day (with or without prednisolone up to 20 mg/day), as this is not considered sufficiently immunosuppressive to risk severe infection. Killed vaccines are safe but are likely

to be less effective. The package insert does not concur on the use of live vaccines stating that these are contraindicated in patients receiving AZA.
- See the Department of Health Green Book for latest UK recommendations on vaccines and vaccination.

BASELINE INVESTIGATIONS AND CONSIDERATIONS

- Full blood count (FBC) (complete blood count [CBC]).
- Urea, electrolytes and creatinine.
- LFTs.
- TPMT activity (see Dosages and Suggested Regimens).
- NUDT15 genotype (consider for at-risk groups if available).
- Hepatitis B and C serology.
- HIV testing.
- Varicella zoster virus (VZV) serology in patients without a reliable history of chickenpox, shingles or varicella vaccination. VZV vaccine should ideally be given to the non-immune several weeks before starting AZA.
- See above under Contraindications and Cautions for COVID-19.
- Cervical screening should be up-to-date. A pretreatment gynaecological review is recommended in females with a history of cervical intraepithelial neoplasia (CIN), as immunosuppressants increase the risk of progression to invasive disease and reduce the success of treatment.
- Dermatological examination and treatment of skin cancer and actinic keratoses is recommended for transplant recipients and seems appropriate for all patients in whom long-term treatment is likely.
- TPMT activity testing may be unreliable for up to 60 days after red cell transfusions due to interference by donor TPMT activity. Diuretics, some non-steroidal anti-inflammatory drugs (NSAIDs) and aminosalicylates such as sulfasalazine may have inhibitory effects on TPMT, but the clinical relevance of these is unclear.

MONITORING

- Fortnightly FBC, renal indices and LFTs for the first 8 weeks then at 12 weeks. Thereafter, when on a stable dose, no less than every 3 months, as toxicity can occur at any stage in therapy. Any downward trend in the neutrophil count should be noted, as an early decrease that is still within the normal total WBC range may herald more severe neutropenia.
- Measurement of (active) TGN and (hepatotoxic) meMP thiopurine metabolites may be useful to assess adherence, optimize dosing and guide-dose adjustment, for example, in those with unusually high TPMT activity ('hyper-methylators') who are at risk of a poor response and hepatotoxicity. Administration of low-dose AZA with allopurinol 100 mg daily is advocated in UK gastroenterology guidelines for patients who develop abnormal LFTs, particularly in those with high levels of meMP. TGN levels have been found to correlate with clinical remission rates in patients with inflammatory bowel disease (IBD), but their role in dermatology is unclear.

ADVERSE EFFECTS AND THEIR MANAGEMENT

- Gastrointestinal: Nausea is the commonest adverse effect of AZA and often limits tolerability. It may be helped by dividing the daily dose and taking medication with food or co-prescription of an antiemetic. Severe nausea is a feature of AZA hypersensitivity, so if affected, especially if accompanied by other symptoms as below, treatment should be stopped.
- Hypersensitivity: Idiosyncratic hypersensitivity to AZA is common in clinical practice. It usually presents within the first few weeks of treatment. Symptoms are often non-specific and flu-like, with nausea, malaise, arthralgia and may be misinterpreted as infection. Urticarial, maculopapular, vasculitic rashes, erythema nodosum, AGEP and Sweet

syndrome have been described. In severe cases, life-threatening shock may occur with possible fatality. Treatment should be stopped immediately if hypersensitivity is suspected. Rechallenge is not recommended.

- Hepatitis: Mild abnormalities of transaminases (<2 times upper limit of normal) are not uncommon and may settle with continued treatment. Measure thiopurine metabolites if available. Deteriorating or sustained elevations of LFTs require dose reduction or discontinuation of therapy. Acute drug-induced liver injury may be hepatocellular (high transaminases) or cholestatic (high bilirubin and alkaline phosphatase). The latter usually takes longer to resolve. A chronic pattern of liver injury termed nodular regenerative hyperplasia has been reported in transplant recipients and patients with IBD.

- Haematological: Bone marrow suppression is one of the most serious adverse effects and can be fatal. Measurement of baseline TPMT does not identify all patients at risk of severe bone marrow suppression, so it is essential that all patients are carefully monitored by regular measurement of FBC. Leukopenia is commonest, but anaemia or thrombocytopenia may also occur. These may develop suddenly or slowly over several months. Mild lymphopenia ($0.5–1.0 \times 109/L$) is often observed and does not usually lead to complications. Macrocytosis is also common; B12 and folate deficiency should be excluded.

    There are no specific guidelines for dose reduction according to haematological parameters. Mild reductions in haemoglobin, leukocyte count $3–4 \times 109/L$ or platelet count of $70–100 \times 109/L$, may be managed by reducing the dose of AZA by 50% and further close monitoring. The original dose can be resumed if values normalize, but treatment should be discontinued if indices continue to fall.

- Malignancy: Evidence varies according to the type of malignancy and patient population (e.g. an increased risk of post-transplant lymphoma and hepatosplenic T-cell lymphoma in patients with IBD) which may not be relevant to dermatology patients.

    There is clear evidence that AZA is associated with an increased risk of non-melanoma skin cancer (NMSC). In transplant recipients, long-term use of AZA combined with other immunosuppressants raises the risk of NMSC development more than 200-fold. AZA may carry a proportionally higher risk than other immunosuppressants, as the absorption spectrum of 6-TG peaks at 340 nm (within the ultraviolet A [UVA] spectrum). Irradiation of 6-TG–substituted DNA induces free radical formation and irreparable DNA damage. In the short term, this manifests as increased UVA sensitivity; in the longer term, carcinogenesis. It is therefore important that those treated with AZA are advised about sun protection, self-examination and the need to report any suspicious skin lesions.

- Infection: AZA may increase the risk of infection even in the absence of neutropenia. In practice, this does not appear to be a common clinical problem among dermatology patients. However, patients taking AZA may be susceptible to more severe infection with VZV. Non-immune individuals may require VZ immunoglobulin or prophylactic acyclovir if they have significant exposure to chickenpox or herpes zoster.

- Pancreatitis: This has been reported in up to 4% of patients with IBD. It is usually mild, resolving after cessation of therapy.

USE IN SPECIAL SITUATIONS

Pregnancy

There is no conclusive evidence that thiopurines are teratogenic; they are usually continued in patients established on therapy during pregnancy to prevent disease relapse/transplant rejection. However, thiopurines cross the placenta, so the decision to start AZA in females who are planning pregnancy should be careful considered. Human studies have shown that AZA does not affect sperm quality or male fertility.

LACTATION

Negligible amounts of AZA and its metabolites are present in breast milk, and although the World Health Organization (WHO) has advised that the risks to the infant outweigh any benefit, recent evidence does not support this.

CHILDREN

AZA is licensed for use in childhood and has been reported to be safe and effective for severe atopic eczema. High doses may be needed (2.5–3.5 mg/kg) to achieve remission. Long-term use needs careful consideration, as the risk of skin cancer increases with treatment duration, so photo-protection is essential in this age group. Nausea and loss of appetite can be a problem in children and may be helped by taking medication with food in the evening.

OLDER PEOPLE

Older people often take more medication and are therefore at increased risk of drug interactions. They are also more susceptible to the adverse effects of AZA, so lower dosages should be considered.

ESSENTIAL PATIENT INFORMATION

Patients should be informed whether the drug is being used for a licensed indication or not. It should be explained that the onset of action is slow and that benefits may not appear until after 2–3 months of treatment.

The dermatologist should ensure that patients clearly understand the need for regular blood monitoring in order to minimize the risk of adverse effects and are able to comply with this. Patients should be warned that they are at increased risk of infection and should seek urgent medical attention if they develop the following symptoms and signs:

- High fever/severe flu-like illness.
- Severe sore throat.
- Unexplained bruising or bleeding.
- Jaundice.

The increased risk of skin cancer should be discussed, and patients should be given practical information about sun protection and skin surveillance.

FURTHER READING

Fuggle NR, Bragoli W, Glover M, et al. The adverse effect profile of oral azathioprine in pediatric atopic dermatitis and recommendations for monitoring. J Am Acad Dermatol. 2015;72:108–14.

Meggitt S, Anstey AV, Mohd Mustapha MF, et al. British Association of Dermatologists guidelines for the safe and effective prescribing of azathioprine. Br J Dermatol. 2011;165:711–34.

Milsop JW, Heller MM, Eliason MJ, et al. Dermatological medication effects on male fertility. Dermatol Ther. 2013;26:337–46.

Public Health England. Immunisation against infectious disease: The Green Book. Accessed at: https://www.gov.uk/government/collections/immunisation-against-infectious-disease-the-green-book.

Schram ME, Borgonjen RJ, Bik CM, et al. Off label use of azathioprine in dermatology: A systematic review. Arch Dermatol. 2011;147:474–88.

Warner B, Johnston E, Arenas-Hernandez M, et al. A practical guide to thiopurine prescribing and monitoring in IBD. Frontline Gastroenterol. 2018;9:10–5.

11 Azole Antihelminths

Mahreen Ameen

CLASSIFICATION AND MODE OF ACTION

The antihelminth drugs that are most commonly used in dermatology are the two benzimidazole carbamates, albendazole, which was first approved in 1983, and mebendazole, which was introduced in 1972. These long-established agents are used in both human and veterinary medicine. Tiabendazole (thiabendazole) is no longer used systemically due to its adverse effects. Its topical use is only advocated for treatment of cutaneous larva migrans if systemic therapy is contraindicated.

Both albendazole and mebendazole have broad-spectrum antihelminth activity. They are most commonly prescribed for the treatment of nematode infestations, including roundworm, whipworm, threadworm and hookworm. Albendazole and mebendazole have a number of mechanisms of action: They act as vermicidals by causing selective degenerative alterations in the tegument and intestinal cells of the worm and by impairing cellular metabolism, thereby leading to immobilization and death of the parasite.

Albendazole and mebendazole are poorly absorbed following ingestion, and absorption is greatly enhanced if taken with food, especially a fatty meal. Administration on an empty stomach is only appropriate when intraluminal parasites are targeted. Both drugs undergo extensive first-pass metabolism in the liver, and metabolic activation and detoxification depend on cytochrome P450 (CYP450) 2C and flavin mono-oxygenases. The oral bioavailability of mebendazole is reported to be less than 20%, which is significantly less than that of albendazole and is a consequence of both poor absorption and rapid first-pass metabolism.

INDICATIONS AND DERMATOLOGIC USES

Soil-transmitted helminthiasis, which can parasitize the human gastrointestinal (GI) tract, is responsible for GI infection in millions of people worldwide. In comparison, helminths are uncommon causes of skin diseases. Azole antihelminth drugs are indicated as treatment for the following infestations:

- Mebendazole: Pinworm (threadworm), roundworm, whipworm and hookworm. Licensed in the UK and approved by the FDA.
- Albendazole: Approved by the FDA for pork tapeworm (trichinosis) hydatid disease caused by dog tapeworm (Echinococcus granulosus). Unlicensed in the UK.

The following are off-label uses:

- Cutaneous larva migrans: This is the most common helminth infestation of the skin. It is characterized by an intensely pruritic, serpiginous rash and is acquired from direct contact of the skin with soil or sand contaminated by dog or cat hookworms, followed by percutaneous penetration and migration of larvae within the epidermis.
- Gnathostomiasis: This is caused by the nematode Gnathostoma spp. and is endemic in southeastern Asian and Latin American countries. It is acquired by consuming raw or insufficiently cooked meat or fish. Ingested larvae cause cutaneous or, less frequently, visceral disorders.

DOI: 10.1201/9781003016786-11

- Trichinosis: Similarly, this is caused by eating undercooked pork or wild game and is caused by the nematode Trichinella spiralis. It is endemic worldwide and presents with facial oedema, particularly peri-orbitally, splinter haemorrhages, fever and myalgia.

FORMULATIONS/PRESENTATION

Availability differs according to country. Generally, albendazole is the treatment of choice, and mebendazole is usually only considered as a second-line drug if albendazole is unavailable.

Albendazole (200 mg and 400 mg) and mebendazole (100 mg and 500 mg) are formulated as chewable tablets and as an oral suspension (100 mg/5 mL).

DOSAGES AND SUGGESTED REGIMENS

- Cutaneous larva migrans: Albendazole 400–800 mg daily for 3–5 days. Treatment up to 7 days is sometimes given, and a second course may be required in cases of relapse. Single-dose ivermectin is an alternative treatment and is associated with higher cure rates (see Chapter 23). When systemic therapy is contraindicated, solitary or a limited number of lesions can be treated with 10–15% tiabendazole solution/ointment Tds for 15 days to affected areas.
- Gnathostomiasis: Albendazole 400–800 mg daily for 21 days or single-dose ivermectin 0.2 mg/kg, which may be repeated after 7 days. Cure rates are high and comparable for both drugs, but the relapse rate may be higher with albendazole.
- Trichinosis: Albendazole 400 mg Bd for 8–14 days or mebendazole 200–400 mg Tds for 3 days.

BASELINE INVESTIGATIONS AND CONSIDERATIONS/MONITORING

- None routinely required.
- Full blood count (FBC) (complete blood count [CBC]) and liver function tests (LFTs) if underlying haematological or hepatic abnormalities are suspected or when high-dose/long-term therapy is considered. Repeat during treatment if abnormal.

CONTRAINDICATIONS AND CAUTIONS

- Albendazole and mebendazole are not recommended for use during pregnancy or for children under the age of 2 years.
- Hepatic impairment: Both drugs must be used with caution in those with hepatic impairment as they are metabolized in the liver, and therefore severe liver disease may result in higher plasma levels of the parent drug and metabolites. In cutaneous larva migrans, alternative topical treatments should be considered to avoid the risks associated with systemic therapy.

IMPORTANT DRUG INTERACTIONS

- Cimetidine, an inhibitor of CYP450, may suppress the metabolism of benzimidazoles and increase the bioavailability of the active metabolites of albendazole. Cimetidine does not appreciably raise serum mebendazole levels, as these are low due to its poor systemic absorption.
- Anticonvulsants: Carbamazepine, phenobarbitone (phenobarbital) and phenytoin can decrease the half-life of albendazole and mebendazole, leading to a decrease in their serum concentration.

- Dexamethasone can increase plasma levels of albendazole by up to 50%.
- Metronidazole: There have been reports of Stevens–Johnson syndrome and toxic epidermal necrolysis occurring when high doses of either metronidazole or mebendazole are given concomitantly.

ADVERSE EFFECTS AND THEIR MANAGEMENT

Albendazole and mebendazole have a similar adverse effect profile, with fewer effects reported for mebendazole, probably because of very low absorption. In spite of these, albendazole is considered a safe drug, given the extensive clinical experience using it over decades.

- Gastrointestinal adverse effects (>1%) include nausea, vomiting, diarrhoea and abdominal pain. This is usually self-limiting and does not require special treatment. However, children especially must be monitored for dehydration, which may require active treatment if the individual is not able to tolerate oral fluids.
- Headaches and dizziness are the next most commonly reported side effects and can be managed with simple analgesics.
- Hypersensitivity reactions, including rash, pruritus and urticaria, have been reported less frequently. These are usually not severe and can be managed with antihistamines and/or topical steroids. Telogen effluvium may also occur.
- Hepatitis elevation of liver enzymes may occur (with a frequency of only 0.035%) but is usually self-limiting without serious sequelae. The risk is increased with long-term therapy. Mild abnormalities seldom necessitate discontinuation of drug therapy. Closer monitoring is recommended in patients with underlying liver disease. There have been very rare reports of acute liver failure.
- Haematological toxicity/marrow suppression with agranulocytosis and aplastic anaemia have been reported rarely.

USE IN SPECIAL SITUATIONS

PREGNANCY

Albendazole and mebendazole (both formerly FDA Category C) are not recommended in pregnancy because animal studies showed teratogenic and embryotoxic effects. It is advised that females of childbearing potential should avoid conception during and for one month after completing treatment. However, clinical trials have demonstrated a lack of adverse birth outcomes after deworming pregnant females with mebendazole. Therefore, pregnancy is not an absolute contraindication to benzimidazoles, but it is advised that treatment should be avoided in the first trimester of pregnancy.

LACTATION

Low concentrations of albendazole and its active metabolite are detectable in breast milk after a single dose of albendazole 400 mg. However, these are not considered to be harmful to the infant. Therefore, there is no absolute contraindication to the use of albendazole in breastfeeding mothers. There are very limited data on the presence of mebendazole in breast milk, but given its low bioavailability, it is unlikely to be significant.

CHILDREN

The benzimidazoles are generally not recommended in children under the age of 2 years. However, clinical data suggest that the incidence of adverse effects is likely to be the same in young children as in older children. Therefore, both albendazole and mebendazole can be used from the age of 12 months if the risks of not treating outweigh the risks of drug-related adverse effects.

FURTHER READING

Albanese G, Venturi C. Albendazole: A new drug for human parasitoses. Dermatol Clin. 2003;21(2):283–90.

Caumes E. Treatment of cutaneous larva migrans. Clin Infectious Dis. 2000;30:811–14.

Montresor A, Awasthi S, Crompton DW. Use of benzimidazoles in children younger than 24 months for the treatment of soil-transmitted helminthiasis. Acta Trop. 2003;86(2–3):223–32.

Van den Bossche H, Rochette F, Hörig C. Mebendazole and related antihelmintics. Adv Pharmacol Chemother. 1982;19:67–128.

Van den Enden E. Pharmacotherapy of helminth infection. Expert Opin Pharmacother. 2009;10(3):435–51.

12 Bexarotene

Julia J. Scarisbrick

CLASSIFICATION AND MODE OF ACTION

Synthetic retinoic acid receptor agonists, including isotretinoin and acitretin, have been used in the treatment of primary cutaneous T-cell lymphoma (CTCL) since the 1990s. The synthetic retinoid Bexarotene is a member of a subclass of retinoids called rexinoids. It is an agonist of the retinoid X receptors and has a distinct biological activity from retinoic acid receptor agonists. Bexarotene binds to and activates RXR-α, -β and -γ, which act as transcription factors to regulate a range of cellular processes, including differentiation and proliferation, apoptosis and insulin sensitization. It produces dose-dependent apoptosis of CTCL cell lines and also down-regulates CCR4 and E-selectin expression, affecting malignant T-cell trafficking to the skin. The original multinational clinical trial assessing efficacy in advanced-stage CTCL (mycosis fungoides and Sezary syndrome) showed an overall response rate of 45–55% according to dose and a median duration of response of 299 days. Similar response rates have been confirmed in patients with early-stage disease.

Bexarotene has a peak plasma concentration 2 hours after ingestion and a half-life of 7 hours. It is 99% protein-bound and metabolized by cytochrome P450 3A4 (CYP3A4) to hydroxybexarotene and oxybexarotene, which are excreted in bile.

INDICATIONS AND DERMATOLOGICAL USES

- Bexarotene was approved by the Food and Drug Administration (FDA) in 1999 and licensed in Europe in 2002 for the treatment of patients with advanced CTCL refractory to at least one systemic treatment.

Bexarotene has also been shown to be an effective and safe treatment for refractory early-stage CTCL both as monotherapy and combination therapy. It requires careful monitoring and should only be prescribed by those with special expertise in the management of CTCL.

FORMULATIONS/PRESENTATION

- Bexarotene is available as 75 mg soft capsules (containing sorbitol).
- Bexarotene 1% gel is also available and used for early-stage CTCL in patients with refractory disease but is not European Medical Agency (EMA) approved.

DOSAGES AND SUGGESTED REGIMENS

The 2013 UK consensus statement outlines a bexarotene dosing schedule and recommended blood monitoring protocols, as well as management of adverse effects.

Dosage is based on body surface area. The manufacturer recommends an initial dose of 300 mg/m^2/day, but UK guidelines recommend a lower dose of 150 mg/m^2/day, increasing after 4 weeks to 300 mg/m^2/day according to toxicity and results of blood monitoring. Dose increments of bexarotene by 75 mg/day (1 capsule every 2–4 weeks) are advised in patients with unstable lipids or other dose-related adverse effects.

A maximal dose of bexarotene 450 mg/m^2/day may be used if tolerated, as a higher dosage may improve clinical response. Medication should be swallowed whole and taken with food. See Figure 12.1 for bexarotene dose increments and monitoring.

DOI: 10.1201/9781003016786-12

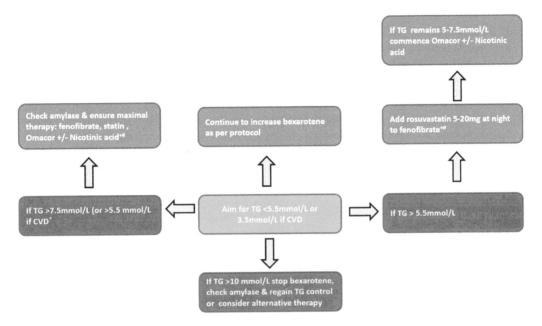

FIGURE 12.1 Management of hypertriglyceridaemia during bexarotene therapy. [+] If CK rises stop fenofibrate. [#] If statin intolerant switch to Omacoromacor (omega-3). [*] Hypertriglyceridaemia is dose dependent and reduction of bexarotene dose by 1 capsule od may regain TG control. Patients may be safely started on triple therapy (fibrate, statin and omega-3) but addition of nicotinic acid should be monitored by a lipid specialist. (Modified from: Scarisbrick JJ, et al. U.K. consensus statement on safe clinical prescribing of bexarotene for patients with cutaneous T-cell lymphoma. Br J Dermatol. 2013;168:192–200.)

Clinical response may take up to 6 months, so treatment should be continued in all patients for this duration, provided there is no disease progression or severe adverse effects. Responses must be measured in all 'compartments' that may be affected by CTCL; this includes skin tumour burden (using a modified severity weighted assessment tool [mSWAT]). The lymph nodes and viscera are assessed by imaging of the neck, chest, abdomen and pelvis. Circulating lymphocytes are assessed for an aberrant CTCL phenotype with typical loss of one, or both, of CD7 and CD26 on the malignant lymphocytes (e.g. a circulating $CD4^+$ $CD7^-$ $CD26^-$ population) by flow cytometry. A 50% reduction in a compartmental score is considered a partial response and is detailed in the Global Response Criteria. A 25% increase in the skin or 50% in any other compartment is considered to be a progressive disease with intermediate values considered as a stable disease. Clinical responses are rarely complete, and anti-CTCL therapies may be continued in patients with stable disease (improvement <50%) who show an improved quality of life.

Patients deriving benefit should remain on bexarotene indefinitely, which may be for several years. Loss of response may necessitate dose increase or adjuvant therapy such as PUVA, alpha interferon, methotrexate, denileukin difitox or extra corporeal photopheresis or switching from bexarotene to an alternative CTCL therapy.

Safe prescribing requires use of lipid-lowering agents and thyroxine. If bexarotene therapy is permanently withdrawn, these should be stopped immediately or reverted to pre-bexarotene therapy. If bexarotene is withheld temporarily, lipid-lowering therapy may be continued, but thyroxine should be stopped and reintroduced when bexarotene is restarted. Topical therapy does not require blood monitoring.

BASELINE INVESTIGATIONS AND CONSIDERATIONS

- Full blood count (FBC) (complete blood count [CBC]).
- Serum urea and electrolytes (U&Es).

- Liver function tests (LFTs).
- Fasting lipids (triglycerides [TG] and cholesterol) and glucose.
- Thyroid function (thyroid-stimulating hormone [TSH]), free thyroxine (fT4) and optimally free tri-iodothyronine (fT3).
- Creatine kinase.

Lipid-lowering medication should be started one week before bexarotene therapy and continued throughout treatment with regular monitoring of lipids. Fenofibrate 160–200 mg should be commenced, and if patient is already on a statin or has pre-existing hypercholesterolaemia, 5 mg/day of Rosuvastatin should be added and increased up to a maximum of 20 mg with careful monitoring for muscle pain (worse on exercise), or raised creatinine kinase. Simvastatin has a known interaction with CYP3A4 and is contraindicated. A low-fat diet and moderation of alcohol intake should also be encouraged.

Thyroxine supplements (levothyroxine 25–50 micrograms/day) should be initiated on day 1 of bexarotene treatment and the dose adjusted according to thyroid hormone levels.

CONTRAINDICATIONS AND CAUTIONS

Contraindications to bexarotene include:

- History of pancreatitis.
- Hypervitaminosis A.
- Uncontrolled hyperlipidaemia.
- Uncontrolled thyroid disease.
- Pregnancy and lactation.
- Depression.

Like all synthetic retinoids, bexarotene is highly teratogenic and absolutely contraindicated in pregnancy. Females of childbearing potential must be counselled about this risk and given guidance on the use of highly effective contraception. Due to a theoretical reduction in efficacy of hormonal contraception, this should include reliable non-hormonal contraception. Pregnancy should be avoided for a minimum of one month after treatment is discontinued. There is no known risk to the offspring of males taking bexarotene.

Hyperlipidaemia should be treated before initiation of bexarotene, and the manufacturer advises that the triglyceride level should be below 4.52 mmol/L. It should be used with caution in people with diabetes mellitus receiving insulin or agents that enhance insulin secretion or sensitivity, as their actions may be enhanced, leading to hypoglycaemia.

The risks associated with bexarotene-induced hyperlipidaemia require careful consideration in patients with ischaemic heart disease.

IMPORTANT DRUG INTERACTIONS

Bexarotene is metabolised by CYP3A4, and a full medication history should be taken, as drugs that induce CYP3A4 may reduce bexarotene levels with loss of efficacy. Similarly, bexarotene toxicity may be increased by other CYP3A4 substrates. Bexarotene may also induce CY34A and auto-induce its own metabolism at high doses as well as enhancing metabolism of tamoxifen and hormonal contraceptives.

- Gemfibrozil increases bexarotene levels, so co-administration should be avoided.
- Vitamin A supplements should be limited to <15,000 IU/day.

MONITORING

Hyperlipidaemia and TSH suppression are dose-dependent effects of bexarotene, and continual monitoring is required notably during dose escalations.

- Fasting lipids and glucose should be checked weekly and until stable, then monthly throughout treatment.

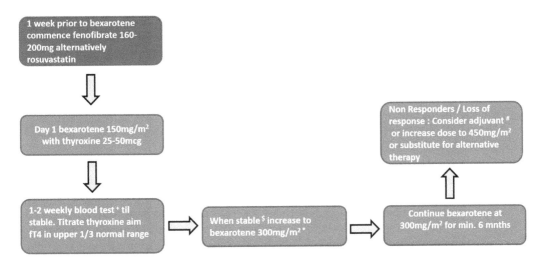

FIGURE 12.2   Bexarotene dose increments and monitoring in patients with CTCL. + Bloods to be monitored – FBC, U&Es, LFTs, fasting lipid, free T4 level, fasting glucose and CK. * Dose dependent side effects may require a dose reduction typically 1 capsule. $ Stable blood results are defined as 2 consecutive blood tests with results within acceptable parameters. # Adjuvant therapy may include PUVA, interferon, radiotherapy, denileukin difitox or ECP. (Modified from: Scarisbrick JJ, et al. U.K. consensus statement on safe clinical prescribing of bexarotene for patients with cutaneous T-cell lymphoma. Br J Dermatol. 2013;168:192–200.)

- LFTs should be checked weekly during the first month and until stable, then monthly.
- Free thyroxine 3 (fT3) and free thyroxine 4 (fT4) levels should be checked weekly until stable, then every month and if symptoms of hypothyroidism occur.
- Serum creatine kinase should be checked weekly at initiation, then monthly when stable.
- Blood should be checked every 1–2 weeks after dose escalations until stable dose is achieved when bloods may be checked monthly.

'Stable' is defined as 2 consecutive blood tests, with results within acceptable parameters at an optimised dose.

Management of hypertriglyceridemia is outlined in Figure 12.2. Patients with persistently elevated TG may also be given omega-3-acid ethyl esters and/or ezetimibe. If TG levels are not controlled, a reduction in bexarotene dose should be considered. A persistently high TG level (>6.0 mmol/L) despite lipid-lowering therapy is a relative contraindication to continuing treatment. Serum amylase should be measured in all patients with TG >7.5 mmol/L. Severe hypertriglyceridemia with TG >10 mmol/L is an absolute contraindication to bexarotene therapy due to the high risk of pancreatitis.

- The pregnancy prevention plan must be followed by all females of childbearing potential 1 month before starting, throughout treatment and 1 month after cessation of treatment. All men should also use effective contraception and prevent conception for the same time period.

ADVERSE EFFECTS AND THEIR MANAGEMENT

- Hyperlipidaemia occurs in the majority of patients and is dose-related. As with other dose-related adverse effects, it may be managed by dose reduction, typically by 75 mg (1 capsule) per day, but larger reductions or withdrawal may be necessary in uncontrolled hypertriglyceridemia. The total cholesterol (TC) levels should be kept below 7 mmol/L, and ideally below 4 mmol/L with LDL-cholesterol <2 mmol/L. In patients with known coronary heart disease, aim to normalise TG with levels <3.5 mmol/L. Rosuvastatin lowers both triglycerides and cholesterol.
- Hypothyroidism: Bexarotene suppresses TSH, leading to primary hypothyroidism, and supplements are required, aiming to maintain and free T3/T4 in the upper third of the

normal range to facilitate lipid control. TSH suppression is dose-dependent, and continued monitoring is required, particularly during dose escalations. The dose of levothyroxine should be increased by 25–50 mcg increments up to a maximum dose of 225 mcg/day.

- Hepatitis: Abnormal liver blood tests have been reported, and frequent monitoring is required. Increases in aspartate transaminase (AST) and alanine transaminase (ALT) can usually be managed with a dose reduction of 1 capsule and repeated testing. If AST or ALT levels are ≥3× the upper limit of normal, bexarotene should be withdrawn. Increases in bilirubin of ≥2 the upper limit of normal require immediate attention and consideration of underlying cholestasis.
- Hyperglycaemia may occur, so fasting glucose levels should be checked regularly. If raised (>6.5 mmol/L), consider adding metformin. A lower threshold for introducing insulin should be considered with appropriate advice from a diabetologist/endocrinologist.
- Eye disorders include dry eyes, conjunctivitis, cataracts and abnormal vision.
- Phototoxicity is usually mild and causes easy sunburn. Patients should be advised to minimize exposure to sunlight and artificial ultraviolet light and to wear protective clothing and high sun protection factor sunscreens.
- Leukopenia (mainly neutropenia) can occur at any time, but mostly occurs as a late side effect after 10–15 months. It is more common at higher doses or when bexarotene is given in combination with interferon or systemic chemotherapy. Dose reduction by 1 capsule of bexarotene is recommended if the neutrophil count drops below 1.0×10^9/L. Reduce the dose by 50% if $<0.5 \times 10^9$/L. Rarely, granulocyte/macrophage colony-stimulating factor may be required.
- Mental health adverse effects of bexarotene, like other oral retinoids, may include depression and anxiety.

USE IN SPECIAL SITUATIONS

PREGNANCY

Bexarotene is absolutely contraindicated during pregnancy, and females should not become pregnant for at least 1 month before, during and 1 month after stopping therapy. As advanced CTCL is rare in females of childbearing potential, this is seldom an issue in clinical practice. Males should also use contraception 1 month before, during and 1 month after stopping bexarotene therapy.

OLDER PEOPLE

The majority of patients in CTCL clinical studies are 60 years and older, so it has been widely tested in older people.

FURTHER READING

Gilson D, Whittaker S, Child F, et al. British Association of Dermatologists and UK Cutaneous Lymphoma Group guidelines for the management of primary cutaneous lymphomas. Br J Dermatol. 2019;180(3):496–526.

Olsen EA, Whittaker S, Kim YH, et al. Clinical end points and response criteria in mycosis fungoides and Sézary syndrome: A consensus statement of the International Society for Cutaneous Lymphomas, the United States Cutaneous Lymphoma Consortium, and the Cutaneous Lymphoma Task Force of the European Organisation for Research and Treatment of Cancer. J Clin Oncol. 2011 June 20;29(18):2598–2607.

Olsen EA, Whittaker S, Willemze R, et al. Primary cutaneous lymphoma: Recommendations for clinical trial design and staging update from the ISCL, USCLC, and EORTC. Blood. 2022 Aug 4;140(5):419–43.

Scarisbrick JJ, Morris S, Azurdia R, et al. U.K. Consensus statement on safe clinical prescribing of bexarotene for patients with cutaneous T-cell lymphoma. Br J Dermatol. 2013;168:192–200.

13 Ciclosporin

Murtaza Khan and John Berth-Jones

CLASSIFICATION AND MODE OF ACTION

Ciclosporin (cyclosporin, cyclosporine) is a lipophilic cyclic polypeptide comprised of 11 amino acid residues with a molecular weight of 1202 daltons. It is the original calcineurin inhibitor and was first isolated in 1970 from the soil fungus Tolypocladium inflatum during a search for antifungal agents. The drug was found to have immunosuppressive actions, and its use revolutionized solid organ transplant medicine. It was inadvertently found to be effective in the treatment of psoriasis in 1979.

Ciclosporin exerts immunosuppressant effects mainly by preventing the activation of T lymphocytes, which are implicated in the pathogenesis of inflammatory skin disorders such as psoriasis and atopic dermatitis. It binds to a cytoplasmic protein, cyclophilin, forming a complex that inhibits the activity of calcineurin. In T-cells, calcineurin activates the nuclear factor of activated T-cells (NFAT), which promotes the production of interleukin-2 (IL-2) and numerous other cytokines that initiate the activation and proliferation of T-cells. In addition, the drug inhibits the release of histamine from mast cells, which may in part explain its usefulness in urticaria.

Gastrointestinal (GI) absorption varies according to food intake and gut motility, and plasma levels vary between individuals. This variation is reduced by the use of microemulsion formulations. Ciclosporin is metabolized by the cytochrome P450 (CYP450) enzyme system (predominantly CYP3A4 and CYP3A5) in the liver and therefore has many potential drug interactions. Its metabolites are predominantly eliminated in the bile, so alteration in renal function does not increase blood levels significantly.

INDICATIONS AND DERMATOLOGICAL USES

Ciclosporin is licensed as an immunosuppressant following solid organ transplantation and in the prevention and treatment of graft-versus-host disease following bone marrow transplantation. It is also licensed as a treatment of nephrotic syndrome and severe rheumatoid arthritis. The licensed dermatological indications in the UK for the use of ciclosporin are severe psoriasis and severe atopic eczema.

Ciclosporin has been shown to greatly improve the quality of life in patients with psoriasis in randomized controlled trials. It is effective in the management of severe chronic plaque psoriasis, erythrodermic psoriasis and pustular psoriasis. In addition, it improves joint disease in psoriatic arthritis. In the United States, ciclosporin is approved for the treatment of adult patients with severe or recalcitrant psoriasis. It leads to an approximate PASI 75 of 70% at 12 weeks. Ciclosporin is widely used for the treatment of severe atopic dermatitis (atopic eczema), although it is not FDA approved for this indication. The rapid onset of action of ciclosporin is particularly useful for short-term control of atopic dermatitis, and it has been shown to be effective and well-tolerated in children aged 2–16 years.

There are numerous reports of off-label uses of ciclosporin in dermatology. Dermatoses in which it can be useful include:

- Pyoderma gangrenosum.
- Lichen planus and lichen planopilaris.

DOI: 10.1201/9781003016786-13

- Palmo–plantar pustulosis.
- Nodular prurigo (prurigo nodularis).
- Chronic spontaneous (idiopathic) urticaria.
- Photodermatoses, such as chronic actinic dermatitis and solar urticaria.
- Behçet's disease.
- Toxic epidermal necrolysis.

FORMULATIONS/PRESENTATION

There are differences in the bioavailability of the various formulations and brands of ciclosporin. For dermatological use, the modified microemulsion forms of ciclosporin, e.g. Neoral or Gengraf (in the United States), are usually prescribed, as they offer more consistent bioavailability than the original formulation (Sandimmun), which was a solution of ciclosporin in olive oil. Ciclosporin has a narrow therapeutic index (small differences in dosage and absorption can make large differences to efficacy and toxicity), so physicians should specify the brand when prescribing it and should not switch randomly between brands. Several brands are available as:

- Capsules of 10, 25, 50 and 100 mg.
- Oral solution: Sugar-free solution containing ciclosporin 100 mg/mL. This may be mixed with orange or apple juice to improve the taste but not with grapefruit juice. Avoid milk due to the unpleasant taste.
- Concentrate for IV infusion, containing 50 mg/mL.

DOSAGES AND SUGGESTED REGIMENS

- Dosage is usually calculated using body weight as mg per kg body weight per day (mg/kg/d). In obese patients, it is safer to use ideal (lean) body weight for dose calculation.
- It is usually taken as two divided doses per day (licensed regimen). Once daily dosing has also been used in dermatology.

For psoriasis: In non-urgent cases, the recommended starting dose is 2.5–3.0 mg/kg/d, which can be titrated up to 5 mg/kg/d over 6–8 weeks. For severe or urgent cases in which a rapid effect is required, treatment should be initiated at 5 mg/kg/d. Improvement is usually apparent within 6 weeks, and the drug should be discontinued if there is an inadequate response after 3 months of therapy. Once sufficient improvement is observed, the dose should be slowly reduced by 0.5–1 mg/kg/d to the lowest effective dose.

Treatment should be limited to intermittent short courses lasting 3–6 months, which are usually sufficient for the control of most cases of psoriasis. However, some patients with severe disease may require therapy for several years, exceeding the limit of 1 year of continuous therapy recommended in the FDA guidelines. In this situation, the lowest effective dose should be used with meticulous monitoring for side effects. Due to the risk of renal toxicity, continuous use of ciclosporin for more than 2 years is not generally recommended.

For atopic dermatitis: Ciclosporin is licensed in the UK for short-term treatment (usually up to 8 weeks). Although it is not FDA approved for this indication, there are similar guidelines for its use in the United States. Ciclosporin is effective and well-tolerated in adults and is highly effective and probably better-tolerated in children. Ciclosporin can be used at a starting dose of 5 mg/kg/d for the first 2–4 weeks, by which time a clinical response is expected. Thereafter, the dose is gradually tapered. An alternative approach is to start with a lower dose (e.g. 2.5 mg/kg/d). The use of ciclosporin for a longer term, i.e. up to 12 months, for adults and children with severe atopic dermatitis has been studied and shown to be generally safe and effective with appropriate monitoring.

BASELINE INVESTIGATIONS AND CONSIDERATIONS

- Blood pressure should be monitored on at least two occasions, preferably 2 weeks apart.
- Physical examination to exclude infection and skin malignancy.
- Mean baseline value of creatinine should be recorded on at least 2 occasions 2 weeks apart.
- Full blood count (FBC) (complete blood count [CBC]), electrolytes, uric acid, liver function tests (LFTs), fasting lipids and urinalysis.
- Consider screening for viral hepatitis, human immunodeficiency virus (HIV), and latent tuberculosis and for immunity to varicella, depending on the patient's history and risk factors.
- Flu and pneumococcal vaccination are recommended for people who are on immuno-suppressant medication; ideally these inactive vaccines should be administered at least 2 weeks before therapy is started. Prescribers are advised to consult the latest recommendation on COVID-19 vaccine and booster scheduling (see e.g. https://www.nhs.uk/conditions/coronavirus-covid-19/coronavirus-vaccination/health-conditions/). During treatment with ciclosporin, vaccination may be less effective. The use of live attenuated vaccines should be avoided. Consider arranging vaccinations before starting ciclosporin when indicated.
- Current COVID-19 guidelines should be consulted for dermatology patients with immune-mediated inflammatory disorders (IMID) who are eligible for treatment with neutralizing monoclonal antibodies or antivirals.
- Patients should be advised to follow recommended guidelines for cancer screening, e.g. cervical smear and breast imaging.

MONITORING

- Blood pressure (BP) should be monitored every 2 weeks for the first 2 months of treatment and monthly thereafter. This should be maintained below 140/90 mmHg.
- Serum creatinine should be measured every 2 weeks for the first 2 months, then every 2 months if there is no cause for concern. A rise in creatinine of 25% above baseline, even if within the normal range, should prompt dose reduction by 1 mg/kg/day and retesting after 2 weeks. If values do not improve, treatment should be discontinued.
- Additional investigations such as fasting lipids, liver function, potassium and urate levels can be monitored at less frequent intervals, depending on patient comorbidities and the results.
- Drug levels are not routinely monitored in dermatology. However, this can sometimes be useful, e.g. to assess suspected non-adherence or drug interaction.

SPECIAL POINTS

There is considerable spontaneous fluctuation in serum creatinine. It is strongly recommended that at least two measurements are obtained before treatment so that the mean can then be used as a baseline. Individual measurements during treatment often give rise to anxiety, which may resolve when repeated.

The serum creatinine is related to muscle mass. Patients with a low muscle mass may have significant nephrotoxicity, even though their serum creatinine remains within the normal range, so change relative to baseline is the key parameter to monitor.

CONTRAINDICATIONS AND CAUTIONS

Ciclosporin should generally be avoided in the following circumstances:

- Impaired renal function.
- Uncontrolled hypertension.
- Malignancy.
- Active infection.

- Concomitant ultraviolet (UV) B or psoralen and ultraviolet A (PUVA) therapy.
- Severe hepatic dysfunction.
- Immunodeficiency.

HIV-associated psoriasis is often severe and refractory to first-line therapies. Ciclosporin may be used in special cases after careful evaluation and with the expert advice of an infectious disease specialist.

IMPORTANT DRUG INTERACTIONS

Ciclosporin interacts with a large number of drugs, and a database for drug interactions such as the current British National Formulary (BNF) should be consulted for a full list. Some of the important interactions are listed below:

- Nephrotoxic drugs: Other nephrotoxic drugs should be avoided as far as possible, although the concomitant use of non-steroidal anti-inflammatory drugs (NSAIDs) often occurs.
- Statins: These should generally not be co-administered with ciclosporin, as there are metabolic interactions including inhibition of the metabolism of statins by CYP450, increasing the risk of myopathy. However, some statins (e.g. pravastatin) are not metabolized by CYP450 and the use of these medications reduces the risk.
- CYP450 inducers and inhibitors: Ciclosporin is metabolized by the hepatic CYP450 system, primarily CYP3A4 and CYP3A5. This leads to a number of potential drug interactions that may increase or decrease levels of ciclosporin (Table 13.1). The interaction with erythromycin is especially noteworthy.
- Grapefruit juice: This is also a CYP450 inhibitor and should be avoided while taking ciclosporin. It also increases the absorption of ciclosporin from the gut.
- Methotrexate and ciclosporin require caution when co-prescribed, as each drug can reduce the elimination of the other.
- Aciclovir and other antiviral drugs may increase the risk of nephrotoxicity (see Chapter 8).
- Antimalarials (chloroquine and hydroxychloroquine) increase the plasma concentration of ciclosporin (see Chapter 7).

ADVERSE EFFECTS AND THEIR MANAGEMENT

- Hypertension: Ciclosporin raises BP largely through a peripheral vascular effect. If the systolic BP rises above 140 mmHg or diastolic BP rises above 90 mmHg, the BP should be checked again in 2 weeks. If it remains elevated, the dose of ciclosporin should be reduced

---

TABLE 13.1

Cytochrome P450 (CYP450) Inducers and Inhibitors

CYP450 Inducers (Reduce Ciclosporin Levels)	CYP450 Inhibitors (Increase Ciclosporin Levels)
Rifampicin	Macrolide antibiotics (erythromycin, clarithromycin)
Phenobarbital	Ciprofloxacin
Carbamazepine	Fluoxetine
Phenytoin	Ketoconazole, itraconazole, fluconazole
St John's wort	Omeprazole
	Cimetidine

---

or treatment should be commenced with an antihypertensive agent. Nifedipine is a useful drug as it has a nephroprotective effect when used in combination with ciclosporin. However, both drugs may cause gingival hyperplasia, so monitor for this at each visit.

- Nephrotoxicity: Ciclosporin causes nephrotoxicity by mechanisms thought to include renal vasoconstriction and hypoxia, leading to the formation of free radicals. The effects are related to dose and duration of treatment, so intermittent short courses are preferable. It also upregulates transforming growth factor-beta (TGF-β) expression in juxtaglomerular cells, which promotes renal fibrosis. A rise in creatinine of >25% requires dose reduction (see Monitoring). The creatinine level usually normalizes within 4–8 weeks of cessation of the drug. Continued use can result in irreversible chronic renal impairment.
- Metabolic: Hyperkalaemia, hypercalciuria and hypomagnesaemia (which may cause muscle cramps). Hyperkalaemia is thought to be due to renal tubular resistance to aldosterone. The risk is increased when ciclosporin is administered with potassium-sparing diuretics and aldosterone antagonists.
- Hyperuricaemia: This may occur due to reduced urate clearance.
- Malignancy: Patients treated with ciclosporin are at increased risk of non-melanoma skin cancers, especially squamous cell carcinoma. This risk is significantly increased in patients previously exposed to PUVA therapy. Some studies have also reported an increased incidence of lymphoma. Patients taking ciclosporin on a long-term basis should have examinations of their skin, lymph nodes and abdomen every 6 months.
- Gingival hyperplasia: Gum hypertrophy is a known side effect of ciclosporin. It is worsened by poor oral hygiene. If gingival hyperplasia develops, patients should be advised to see a dentist, and in severe cases it may be necessary to withdraw ciclosporin.
- Neurological: Patients taking ciclosporin often report paraesthesia or tremor, and the seizure threshold may be lowered.
- Hypertrichosis is common and is most problematic in dark-haired female patients.
- Miscellaneous: Sebaceous hyperplasia has mainly been reported in transplant recipients. Fatigue, headache, flu-like symptoms and GI disturbances occur occasionally. Nausea and reflux may be helped by changing to a liquid formulation.

USE IN SPECIAL SITUATIONS

Pregnancy

Ciclosporin is not considered teratogenic. There is considerable experience of its use in pregnancy following organ transplantation without any established serious hazard to the unborn child. There are also reports of successful use of ciclosporin in generalized pustular psoriasis of pregnancy.

Lactation

Ciclosporin is excreted in breast milk. Mothers taking the drug should be informed about this, and they are generally advised against breastfeeding, although there are reports of this being done without adverse outcome.

Children

Ciclosporin is not licensed in the UK for use in children less than 16 years, or FDA approved for psoriasis patients less than 18 years. However, in addition to its use in childhood atopic dermatitis, it has been used in patients as young as 1 year of age in nephrotic syndrome, juvenile dermatomyositis and organ transplantation without serious side effects. As in adults, the main risks are renal toxicity and hypertension.

OLDER PEOPLE

Older patients often do not tolerate ciclosporin and should be monitored with particular care for nephrotoxicity.

ESSENTIAL PATIENT INFORMATION

The important side effects should be explained and supplemented with written information. Patients should be advised to attend appointments for clinical assessments and blood tests on a regular basis. Advice should be given regarding the avoidance of sunlight, interacting drugs and grapefruit juice. Patients should also be warned that any change in formulation should only be done under physician supervision.

FURTHER READING

Berth-Jones J, Exton LS, Ladoyanni E, et al. British Association of Dermatologists guidelines for the safe and effective prescribing of oral ciclosporin in dermatology 2018. Br J Dermatol. 2019;180:1312–38.
Berth-Jones J, Finlay AY, Zaki I, et al. Cyclosporin in severe childhood atopic dermatitis: A multicentre study. J Am Acad Dermatol. 1996;34:1016–21.
Lebwohl M, Heymann W, Berth-Jones J, et al. Treatment of Skin Disease. 5th Edn. Elsevier; London; 2018.

14 Colchicine

Esther A. Hullah and Michael P. Escudier

CLASSIFICATION AND MODE OF ACTION

Colchicine is a naturally occuring alkaloid, obtained from plants of the lily family, including Colchicum autumnale, which has been used for medicinal purposes since the time of ancient Greece. It occurs as pale to greenish yellow crystals, is irritating to skin lipid soluble and oxidizes rapidly on light exposure, so it must be stored in the dark.

Following oral administration, colchicine is rapidly absorbed in the jejunum and ileum, and it undergoes significant hepatic first-pass metabolism. While there is wide individual variability in bioavailability, primarily due to differing expression of protein targets, including CYP34A and P-glycoprotein, peak plasma levels are generally achieved after 30–120 minutes and within leucocytes at around 48 hours.

Colchicine is primarily metabolized in the liver, by the cytochrome P450 enzyme CYP3A4, via demethylation before hepatobiliary excretion in the stool. The remaining 10–20% is excreted unchanged in the urine, such that renal impairment may prolong the half-life and increase the risk of toxicity.

The cellular effects of colchicine, including its anti-inflammatory action, are primarily accounted for by its inhibition of microtubule polymerisation and the resultant effects on cell division and migration, signal transduction, gene expressions and cellular transport. Other mechanisms which may play a role include inhibition of cyclooxygenases COX-1 and COX-2.

Colchicine is seen at particularly high concentrations in leucocytes and impairs neutrophil function, macrophage activation and mast cell degranulation.

INDICATIONS AND DERMATOLOGICAL USES

Colchicine is licensed only for use in gout and familial Mediterranean fever (FMF), with all other uses being off-licence.

- Gout and pseudogout

  The inflammation in gout is mediated by neutrophil and macrophage activation, leucocyte adhesion molecules, inflammasome activation and IL-1β production, all of which are inhibited by colchicine.

  Colchicine is used in the management of acute gout and also as a prophylactic agent against acute flares when initiating allopurinol in patients with chronic gout. It is also recommended for pseudogout or calcium pyrophosphate crystal arthritis prophylaxis and for acute episodes.

- FMF

  This condition is associated with a mutation in the gene that encodes the protein pyrin, which regulates inflammasome activation, resulting in increased IL-1β production and inflammation resulting in fever, arthritis and serositis.

  Colchicine is the primary treatment for FMF and has good long-term efficacy and safety and proven safety in children, during pregnancy and with nursing patients.

DOI: 10.1201/9781003016786-14

At daily doses of 1.0–2.0 mg, it reduces the frequency of FMF attacks and prevents the development of amyloidosis and subsequent chronic renal failure. It can also induce remission of proteinuria and nephrotic syndrome in patients with established amyloid nephropathy.

- Additional indications
  The range of potential uses of colchicine has broadened significantly, particularly within dermatology and oral medicine. However, in many cases the current evidence base is limited to case series or case reports.

The following are the exceptions, having been the subject of controlled trials.

- Behçet's Disease: Colchicine significantly reduces the frequency of oral and genital ulceration, pseudofolliculitis and erythema nodosum.
- Chronic Urticaria: Over half of patients treated for a mean period of 7 months achieved a partial or complete response.
- Epidermolysis Bullosa Acquisita: Colchicine is an effective monotherapy and acts through its inhibition of secretion of anti-type VII collagen antibody, with improvement in dysphagial symptoms, mucosal erosions, oesophageal stenosis and cutaneous erosions.
- Leucocytoclastic Vasculitis: While several case reports support the efficacy of colchicine in this group of conditions, a prospective randomized controlled trial using 0.5 mg per day did not confirm this.
- Recurrent Aphthous Stomatitis: Colchicine at a dose of 0.5–1.5 mg per day is often effective in reducing the severity (symptoms, size and durations of lesions) as well as the frequency of attacks over a period of 3 months.
- Sweet's Syndrome (Acute Febrile Neutrophilic Dermatosis): Over half of patients show regression of lesions at a dose of 1.0–2.0 mg per day with the remainder responding with the addition of prednisolone.

FORMULATION/PRESENTATION

Oral administration is the most common route of administration. Intravenous delivery, while quicker-acting, is associated with a significantly increased risk of toxicity. In contrast topical use is less well evidenced in the literature.

The starting dose is 0.5 mg daily, increasing to 1–1.5 mg in divided (0.5 mg) doses, as tolerated. The dose tolerated by the patient is usually dependent on gastrointestinal (GI) side effects.

The usual maintenance dose is 0.5–2.0 mg, daily although dosage adjustment is required in patients with moderate-to-severe renal impairment or hepatobiliary dysfunction. Tolerance is improved by delivering the drug in divided doses, while long-term studies have confirmed its safety in chronic use.

Special Point

Colchicine has a narrow therapeutic window and a significant variation in the dose required to cause morbidity or mortality, and as little as 6–7 mg has caused death. Toxicity typically manifests as GI symptoms, with the later development of widespread organ dysfunction including renal failure, arrhythmias and heart failure.

As mentioned above, its hepatobiliary and renal excretion means that impairment of either pathway can result in its accumulation and toxicity. Similarly, colchicine overdose can arise from drug interactions, e.g. antibiotics, antifungals, calcium channel blockers, immunosuppressants and statins. Acute toxicity manifests as cholera-like symptoms and signs of dehydration, electrolyte disturbance, metabolic acidosis, renal failure and shock. Convulsions, muscle paralysis, neuropathy and respiratory distress are common.

BASELINE INVESTIGATIONS AND CONSIDERATIONS

- Full blood count (FBC) (complete blood count [CBC]).
- Urea, electrolytes and creatinine.
- Liver function tests (LFTs).

MONITORING

- FBC (CBC) and differential white cell count every month.
- LFTs and renal indices every 3 months.

CONTRAINDICATIONS

- Haematological disease.
- Severe renal impairment or haemodialysis (colchicine cannot be removed by dialysis or exchange transfusion).

CAUTIONS

Care should be exercised in patients who:

- Are older or debilitated as they may be especially susceptible to cumulative toxicity, which leads to GI, renal, hepatic, cardiac or haematological complications.
- Have gastrointestinal hepatic or cardiac disease who are at increased risk of developing toxicity.
- Have renal impairment or are concurrently using nephrotoxic drugs as they are at a greater risk of toxicity.
- Have chronic kidney disease i.e. stage 5 with a glomerular filtration rate (GFR) <15 mL/min.

IMPORTANT DRUG INTERACTIONS

- Macrolide antibiotics (erythromycin, clarithromycin and others) increase the risk of colchicine toxicity, due to interactions with the cytochrome P450 (CYP450) 3A4 microsomal enzyme system.
- Ciclosporin (cyclosporine) concentrations are increased by colchicine, with an increased risk of nephrotoxicity and neuromuscular adverse effects.
- Vitamin B12 absorption may be impaired by colchicine, resulting in megaloblastic anaemia.
- Statins and fibrates may cause acute myopathy when given with colchicine. Patients should be advised to report any muscular pain or weakness.
- Other potential interactions include drugs metabolized by CYP3A4, including azole antifungals, antiviral drugs and cardiac medication.

ADVERSE EFFECTS AND THEIR MANAGEMENT

Colchicine is generally well-tolerated. The most common unwanted effects are:

- Gastrointestinal: Nausea, vomiting and diarrhoea, which may worsen with increasing dosage, and occur in 5–10% of patients. Less commonly elevation of liver transaminases can also occur as malabsorption syndrome, affecting B12, fat, protein, actively transported sugars and electrolytes. Other gastrointestinal effects include paralytic ileus.
- Bone marrow suppression: Agranulocytosis, thrombocytopenia and aplastic anaemia can occur after prolonged treatment. Administration of granulocyte colony stimulating factor (G-CSF) should be considered in such cases.
- Myopathy and neuropathy: This occurs especially in patients with renal impairment. The myopathy is proximal, with elevated serum creatinine phosphokinase, and the neuropathy is axonal. Myopathy recovers on withdrawal of colchicine, but neurological recovery may be slow.
- Dermatological: These include urticaria; rarely, Stevens–Johnson syndrome, toxic epidermal necrolysis and alopecia universalis; and very rarely, porphyria cutanea tarda.

There have been isolated reports of bladder spasms, renal damage and haematuria, and hypothyroidism.

USE IN SPECIAL SITUATIONS

PREGNANCY

The use of colchicine in pregnancy is controversial as a result of the potential risks and should only be considered if the potential benefits to the mother outweigh the possible risk to the fetus, e.g. FMF.

A systematic review and meta-analysis of four papers addressing the use of colchicine throughout pregnancy, for FMF, did not reveal an increased incidence of miscarriage or major fetal malformations. In fact, the incidence of miscarriage was significantly lower in patients who took colchicine compared with those who did not. There was also no significant difference in birth weight or gestational age between those who did and did not take colchicine. However, when not limited to FMF, colchicine use was associated with a significantly lower birth weight and gestational age compared with a control group including, healthy patients who did not take colchicine.

LACTATION

While colchicine is excreted into breast milk, there are no reported adverse effects in breastfed infants and it is therefore considered compatible with breastfeeding.

CHILDREN

Safe use of colchicine in children has been reported in a number of case reports, e.g. as an adjuvant treatment with systemic corticosteroids in children with linear IgA disease.

ESSENTIAL PATIENT INFORMATION

Patients should be advised:

- To reduce dosage of colchicine if weakness, anorexia, nausea, vomiting or diarrhoea occurs.
- Of the dangers of overdosage.
- That as colchicine can adversely affect the fetus, pregnancy should be avoided during treatment.

FURTHER READING

Bhattacharyya B, Panda D, Gupta S, et al. Anti-mitotic activity of colchicine and the structural basis for its interaction with tubulin. Med Res Rev. 2008;28:155–83.

Cocco G, Chu DC, Pandolfi S. Colchicine in clinical medicine. A guide for internists. Eur J Intern Med. 2010;21:503–8.

Indraratna PL, Virk S, Gurram D, et al. Use of colchicine in pregnancy: A systematic review and meta-analysis. Rheumatology. 2018;57:382–7.

Robinson KP, Chan JJ. Colchicine in dermatology: A review. Australas J Dermatol. 2018;59:278–85.

Slobodnick A, Shah B, Pillinger MH, et al. Colchicine: Old and new. Am J Med. 2015;128:461–70.

15 Corticosteroids

Clive B. Archer

CLASSIFICATION AND MODE OF ACTION

Synthetic corticosteroids (glucocorticoids, glucocorticosteroids and steroids) are analogues of endogenous adrenal steroid hormones and are widely used in dermatology. They have anti-inflammatory, immunosuppressive, antiproliferative and vasoconstrictor actions. The effects of steroids are mediated predominantly by binding to intracellular glucocorticoid receptors, which then bind to specific DNA sequences that regulate gene transcription. Corticosteroids also have non-genomic actions, such as interactions with cellular membranes and receptors. Corticosteroids thereby reduce inflammation via several molecular mechanisms, suppressing the many inflammatory genes that are activated in chronic inflammatory diseases and repressing the expression of pro-inflammatory proteins.

After absorption corticosteroids bind to the carrier protein, transcortin (cortisol-binding globulin) and albumin. Transcortin levels are decreased in liver disease, kidney disease, hypothyroidism and obesity. This may therefore increase the level of free corticosteroids in these conditions. Liver disease also results in decreased albumin levels and potentially increased steroid side effects. Steroids are metabolized by the liver to water-soluble metabolites that are excreted by the kidneys.

The relative potencies and approximate equivalent doses of steroids compared with hydrocortisone are shown in Table 15.1.

Prednisolone and methylprednisolone are the steroids most commonly used in medicine. The relatively high mineralocorticoid activity of cortisone and hydrocortisone with consequent fluid retention makes them unsuitable for long-term therapy.

Prednisone is generally used instead of prednisolone in the United States. It is a pro-drug that is converted to prednisolone in the liver. However, there is 20% less on conversion, and liver failure may impair conversion further. The onset of action is also slower.

TABLE 15.1

Relative Potencies and Approximate Equivalent Doses of Corticosteroids Compared with Hydrocortisone

Drug	Relative Glucocorticoid (Anti-Inflammatory) Potency	Relative Mineralocorticoid Potency	Equivalent Anti-Inflammatory Dose[a] (mg)
Hydrocortisone (Cortisol)	1	1	100
Prednisolone	4	0.8	25
Methylprednisolone	5	0.5	20
Triamcinolone	5	0	20
Betamethasone	25	0	4
Dexamethasone	25	0	4

[a] Applies only to oral or IV administration.

Source: Reproduced with the permission of Guy's and St Thomas' Hospitals NHS Foundation Trust.

DOI: 10.1201/9781003016786-15

INDICATIONS AND DERMATOLOGICAL USES

The following corticosteroids are licensed for systemic use in the suppression of inflammatory and allergic disorders:

- Betamethasone.
- Deflazacort.
- Dexamethasone.
- Methylprednisolone.
- Prednisolone.
- Triamcinolone.

Parenteral hydrocortisone is indicated for the treatment of anaphylactic shock and severe angioedema.

Corticosteroids have been widely used in dermatology since the 1950s. Some of the diseases for which they are commonly prescribed are as follows:

- Dermatitis: Acute contact dermatitis (allergic or irritant), atopic dermatitis, chronic actinic dermatitis and exfoliative dermatitis due to drugs.
- Connective tissue diseases: Lupus erythematosus (all types), dermatomyositis, mixed connective tissue disease, relapsing polychondritis and eosinophilic fasciitis.
- Immunobullous diseases: Pemphigus (all types), bullous pemphigoid, cicatricial pemphigoid, pemphigoid gestationis, linear IgA disease and epidermolysis bullosa aquisita.
- Vasculitis: Hypersensitivity vasculitis, polyarteritis nodosa and granulomatosis with polyangiitis (GPA, Wegener's granulomatosis).
- Neutrophilic dermatoses: Acute febrile neutrophilic dermatosis (Sweet syndrome), pyoderma gangrenosum and Behçet's disease.
- Other dermatoses: Lichen planus, sarcoidosis, acute severe urticaria, angioedema, Stevens–Johnson syndrome (but not toxic epidermal necrolysis [TEN]), large haemangiomas (required less often now that beta-adrenoceptor blockers are used in this context).

FORMULATIONS/PRESENTATION

Includes the following:

- Prednisolone: 1 mg, 2.5 mg, 5 mg and 25 mg tablets; 2.5 mg, 5 mg enteric-coated tablets (note decreased gastric absorption); 5 mg scored soluble tablets.
- Betamethasone: 0.5 mg scored tablets; 0.5 mg scored soluble tablets.
- Triamcinolone: Aqueous suspension for injection. As acetonide, 10 mg/mL, 40 mg/mL; as hexacetonide, 5 mg/mL, 20 mg/mL.
- Deflazacort: 1 mg, 6 mg and 30 mg tablets.
- Dexamethasone: 0.5 mg (500 microgram) tablets.
- Methylprednisolone: 2 mg, 4 mg, 16 mg, 100 mg tablets; 40 mg, 125 mg, 500 mg, 1 g and 2 g powder for reconstitution with water (as sodium succinate).
- Hydrocortisone: 100 mg/mL solution for injection (as sodium phosphate); 100 mg powder for reconstitution with water (as sodium succinate).

DOSAGES AND SUGGESTED REGIMENS

Steroids given for immunosuppression are usually given as a single daily dose in the morning to minimize adrenal suppression. Prednisolone has predominant glucocorticoid activity and is used for most purposes. It has the advantage over more potent steroids of allowing fine dose adjustment.

The starting dose of prednisolone varies according to the skin disease, its severity and concurrent disorders such as hepatic impairment. The BNF recommends a daily starting dose of 10–20 mg, up to 60 mg in severe disease. In dermatological practice, it may be necessary to use higher doses to gain initial disease control, e.g. 60–100 mg prednisolone daily in pemphigus.

In children, a typical short-course, high-dose regimen is 1–2 mg/kg/d for 3–5 days. If treatment is required for >7 days, the dose is usually reduced gradually.

A high-dose pulsed IV regimen with 500 mg^{-1} g methylprednisolone daily for 3 days may be faster-acting and more effective than oral therapy, but these advantages have yet to be fully validated, and controlled prospective studies are lacking.

For androgen excess syndromes, a unique regimen is indicated, involving nighttime suppressive therapy with low-dose treatment (below physiological levels) to suppress the early-morning peak of adrenocorticotrophic hormone (ACTH) that stimulates adrenal androgen production (see Chapter 4).

The rate of drug withdrawal depends mostly on disease activity. Rapid withdrawal may precipitate disease flares in some disorders. The maintenance dose should be kept at the minimum required for the shortest length of time in order to minimize side effects. Alternate-day dosing may reduce adverse effects by allowing time for the hypothalamic–pituitary–adrenal (HPA) axis to recover.

Soluble formulations of prednisolone or betamethasone may be of advantage in treating severe oral inflammatory disease (lichen planus, pemphigus), as they can be held in the mouth before swallowing to obtain a local anti-inflammatory effect.

SPECIAL POINT: ADRENAL SUPPRESSION

The approximate physiological daily secretion of cortisol by the adrenal cortex is 20 mg (equivalent to about 5 mg prednisolone daily). Short courses of high-dose prednisolone (2 weeks or less) do not require tapering as, although suppressed, the HPA axis recovers promptly.

In patients on long-term prednisolone therapy, once a daily dose of 7.5 mg has been reached, dose reduction should be slower to allow the HPA axis to recover, e.g. 1–2.5 mg weekly.

Patients taking oral corticosteroids must continue systemic therapy during periods of stress, such as infection, trauma or surgery, either orally or by injection. Extra steroids are needed for up to 3 days during periods of acute illness to prevent an acute adrenal crisis. Patients who have been taking 5 mg or more of prednisolone for more than 4 weeks are at risk of an adrenal crisis during periods of high stress. Patients who have completed a short course of treatment (3 weeks or less) within the previous week also require corticosteroid replacement during acute stress.

BASELINE INVESTIGATIONS AND CONSIDERATIONS

- Full blood count (FBC) (complete blood count [CBC]).
- Urea, electrolytes and creatinine.
- Liver function tests (LFTs).
- Urinalysis for glucose and/or blood glucose, if at risk of diabetes.
- Fasting lipid profile, if at risk of hyperlipidaemia.
- Dual energy x-ray absorptiometry (DEXA) scan of the lumbar spine and hips, if long-term treatment is required.
- Blood pressure (BP) and weight.
- Growth chart for height and weight for children.

MONITORING

After 1 month, then every 2–3 months:

- BP.
- Urinalysis for glucose.

- Urea and electrolytes.
- DEXA scan after 6 months, then 12 months, then yearly.
- Consider ophthalmological review for cataracts and raised intraocular pressure.

CONTRAINDICATIONS

Systemic infection, including latent tuberculosis (unless specific antimicrobial therapy is given).

CAUTIONS

Corticosteroids should be used with caution in patients with the following pre-existing diseases, which might be exacerbated:

- Diabetes mellitus.
- Hypertension or congestive heart failure.
- Glaucoma.
- Osteoporosis.
- Active peptic ulcer disease.
- Liver failure.
- Severe affective disorders/history of corticosteroid-induced psychosis.
- Previous steroid myopathy.
- Kidney failure.
- Recent myocardial infarction (risk of cardiac rupture).

During the COVID-19 pandemic, people in the UK were advised to shield if on high-dose corticosteroids (equivalent to prednisolone 20 mg per day or more) for 4 weeks or longer, or on lower-dose corticosteroids (equivalent to prednisolone 5 mg per day) for 4 weeks or longer, in combination with other disease modifying medication.

Flu and pneumococcal vaccination are recommended for people who are on immunosuppressant medication; ideally these inactive vaccines should be administered at least 2 weeks before therapy is started. Prescribers are advised to consult the latest recommendation on COVID-19 vaccine and booster scheduling (see e.g. https://www.nhs.uk/conditions/coronavirus-covid-19/coronavirus-vaccination/health-conditions/).

Current COVID-19 guidelines should be consulted for dermatology patients with immune-mediated inflammatory disorders (IMID) who are eligible for treatment with neutralising monoclonal antibodies or antivirals.

IMPORTANT DRUG INTERACTIONS

- Antacids: These can reduce the absorbtion of prednisolone if given in high doses.
- Anticonvulsants: Increased clearance of corticosteroids occurs with carbamazepine, phenytoin and phenobarbitone.
- Antibiotics: Increased clearance of corticosteroids occurs with rifampicin and isoniazid.
- Ciclosporin (cyclosporine): This increases the plasma concentration of prednisolone.
- Coumarin anticoagulant efficacy may be enhanced by high-dose corticosteroids, so closer monitoring is required to avoid bleeding.
- The therapeutic effects of hypoglycaemic agents (including insulin), antihypertensive therapy and diuretics are antagonized by corticosteroids.
- Corticosteroids may increase the risk of benign intracranial hypertension if given with retinoids and tetracyclines.

ADVERSE EFFECTS AND THEIR MANAGEMENT

- Fluid and electrolyte imbalance (mineralocorticoid) effects are slight with prednisolone, methylprednisolone and triamcinolone, and negligible with betamethasone and dexamethasone. They include hypertension, sodium and water retention and potassium loss. The risk of hypokalaemia is increased when given with acetazolamide, loop diuretics and thiazide diuretics.
- Sudden death and life-threatening ventricular arrhythmias have been associated with pulsed methylprednisolone therapy, possibly as a consequence of rapid electrolyte shifts. All patients receiving such therapy should preferably have cardiac monitoring and daily monitoring of electrolytes.
- Glucocorticoid effects are the main problem associated with long-term corticosteroid therapy. They include osteoporosis, diabetes mellitus and Cushing syndrome.
- Corticosteroid myopathy typically affects the proximal muscles of the pelvic girdle then shoulder girdle. The patient should be asked if they have difficulty rising from chairs and climbing stairs. Exercising and slow tapering of the corticosteroid dose may help.
- Peptic ulcer disease: It is uncertain if corticosteroids increase the risk of peptic ulcer disease, and if so, the effect is modest. There is clearer evidence that they increase the risk of peptic ulceration when given with non-steroidal anti-inflammatory drugs (NSAIDs). Treatment with a proton pump inhibitor or an H2-antagonist seems appropriate in patients with a history of peptic ulcer disease or those who develop symptoms of gastritis. The potential advantage of soluble or enteric-coated preparations (with consequent reduced gastric absorption) versus plain tablets to reduce the risk of peptic ulceration remains uncertain. As corticosteroid therapy may mask the signs of a perforated peptic ulcer or other visceral perforation, patients taking these drugs who develop significant abdominal pain warrant urgent specialist attention.
- Neuropsychiatric adverse effects include euphoria, irritability, anxiety, sleep disturbance, cognitive impairment, depression, labile mood and suicidal thoughts. Psychotic symptoms include mania, delusions and aggravation of schizophrenia. Particular care is required when systemic corticosteroids are given to patients with existing or a previous history of severe affective disorders.
- Cardiovascular disease risk is increased in those on long-term corticosteroids. Thrombophlebitis may also occur.
- Cutaneous adverse effects include atrophy, telangiectasia and striae. Truncal acne may occur but usually clears on corticosteroid withdrawal. Corticosteroids impair fibroblast production of type 1 collagen and delay wound healing.
- Ocular adverse effects include corneal thinning, glaucoma and posterior subcapsular cataracts. Children are at increased risk of cataracts, and regular slit lamp examinations should be considered in those on long-term treatment.
- Leucocytosis is a common finding due to reduced neutrophil margination.
- Infection: Susceptibility is increased and infections may be more severe. Clinical signs and symptoms of opportunistic infections and tuberculosis may be suppressed. Chickenpox is of particular concern, since this usually minor illness may be fatal in immunosuppressed patients. Patients taking corticosteroids without a definite history of chickenpox should avoid close personal contact with chickenpox or herpes zoster, and if exposed, they should seek urgent medical attention. Passive immunization with varicella/zoster immunoglobulin (VZIG) is required in non-immune patients who are receiving systemic corticosteroids or who have used them within the previous 3 months; this should ideally be given within 3 days of exposure. If a diagnosis of chickenpox is confirmed, the illness warrants special care and urgent treatment. Corticosteroids should not be stopped, and the dose may need to be increased. Similarly, patients should be advised to avoid contact with measles, and if exposed without prior immunity, to seek prompt medical attention for prophylaxis with normal immunoglobulin. (See Cautions.)
- Hypersensitivity reactions, including anaphylaxis, may occur rarely.

Special Point: Osteoporosis

Bone loss is one of the most important adverse effects of corticosteroid therapy, even in low doses. Mechanisms include glucocorticoid inhibition of osteoblast function and induction of osteoclast and osteocyte apoptosis. Bones with a high trabecular content like vertebrae are most vulnerable. Asymptomatic fractures may occur in up to 50% of patients receiving long-term glucocorticoid therapy, and minimal trauma fractures occur at higher bone mineral density (BMD) than with other primary or secondary causes of osteoporosis. The greatest rate of bone loss occurs during the first 6–12 months of therapy, so early preventative measures are important. A DEXA scan is the investigation of choice to assess BMD.

A computerised tool, FRAX®, developed in 2008 at the University of Sheffield, is available online (www.shef.ac.uk/FRAX). It provides an assessment of fracture risk in those aged 40 and over, taking into account different osteoporosis risk fractures, including long-term (>3 months) corticosteroid therapy and BMD, if available. Clinical risk factors for the assessment of fracture probability are shown in Table 15.2. The World Health Organization (WHO) classification of bone densitometry results is based on comparison with the mean value for adults of the same age and sex:

- A normal value for BMD is within 1 standard deviation of the score (T score 0 to −1).
- Osteopenia is defined as BMD value 1–2.5 standard deviations below the mean (T score −1 to −2.5).
- Osteoporosis is diagnosed when the T score is −2.5 or lower.

Intervention to prevent osteoporosis should start as soon as corticosteroids are prescribed. Lifestyle measures, such as exercise, stopping smoking and restricting alcohol consumption, should be recommended for all patients.

Bisphosphonates are the agents of choice for treatment and prevention of osteoporosis. They slow the rate of bone turnover. Alendronic acid or risedronate sodium (given daily or once a week) are first-choice drugs, and disodium etidronate is an alternative (given in 2-week cycles every 13 weeks).

TABLE 15.2

Clinical Risk Factors Used for the Assessment of Fracture Probability

- Age
- Sex
- Low body mass index ($\leq 19\ kg/m^2$)
- Previous fragility fracture, particularly of the hip, wrist and spine, including morphometric vertebral fracture
- Parental history of hip fracture
- Current smoking
- Alcohol intake of three or more units daily

Secondary Causes of Osteoporosis Include
- Rheumatoid arthritis
- Untreated hypogonadism in men and women
- Prolonged immobility
- Organ transplantation
- Type 1 diabetes
- Hyperthyroidism
- Gastrointestinal disease
- Chronic liver disease
- Chronic obstructive pulmonary disease

Calcium and vitamin D supplementation should be considered, especially in patients whose dietary intake is unreliable. The recommended doses are 1,000–1,500 mg calcium and 800 IU vitamin D daily. Milk, hard cheese and yogurt are good sources of calcium. Vitamin D-rich foods include salmon, mackerel and tuna. Ultraviolet exposure is another consideration, as individuals who avoid the sun or expose little skin are at increased risk of vitamin D deficiency.

Calcitonin also inhibits osteoclastic bone reabsorption and may be a more suitable option in children and young adults.

Gonadal hormone replacement therapy with oestrogen supplements for post-menopausal females reduces the risk of fractures. The oestrogen receptor modulator raloxifene, which has potent agonist effects on bone and antioestrogen effects on the uterus and breast, may be a good alternative. Testosterone replacement should be considered in males with low testosterone levels.

- Avascular necrosis (osteonecrosis) of the bone may occur with high-dose or prolonged corticosteroid therapy. The femoral head is most commonly affected, and disease may occur bilaterally. Other sites include the femoral condyles and head of humerus. Symptoms of pain or reduced movement at one or more joints should prompt further investigation. Magnetic resonance imaging (MRI) is more sensitive for diagnosing early avascular necrosis than radiography. Specialist referral is warranted in suspected cases.

USE IN SPECIAL SITUATIONS

PREGNANCY AND PRE-CONCEPTION

All corticosteroids cross the placenta to a variable degree. Betamethasone and dexamethasone cross the placenta readily, while 88% of prednisolone is inactivated. In humans, there is no convincing evidence that systemic corticosteroids cause an increase in fetal abnormalities such as cleft lip. The main risk when they are administered for prolonged periods or repeatedly during pregnancy is intrauterine growth retardation. There is also a theoretical risk of neonatal adrenal suppression, but this usually resolves spontaneously after birth.

Menstrual irregularities may follow depot IM corticosteroid therapy but are uncommon with oral therapy. Sperm counts may be decreased, but this does not usually impair fertility.

LACTATION

Corticosteroids are excreted in small amounts in breast milk. However, doses of up to 40 mg daily of prednisolone are unlikely to cause systemic effects in the infant. Infants of mothers taking higher doses than this should be monitored for signs of adrenal suppression.

CHILDREN

Long-term corticosteroids cause growth suppression in children. Full catch-up growth may not be attained after medication is discontinued. Normal growth is achieved on 5 mg prednisolone per day for a child with 1 m^2 surface area. Alternate day dosing may reduce growth suppression but can have reduced therapeutic effectiveness against the disease being treated.

ESSENTIAL PATIENT INFORMATION

The Medicines Control Agency has documented the recommended advice that should be given to patients who are prescribed long-term systemic corticosteroids (see below). It is important to tell patients prescribed systemic corticosteroids (especially for >7 days) about the possible adverse effects and of the actions they may need to take. It is also important to inform patients about the benefits of treatment. Specifically, they should be advised:

- Not to stop taking corticosteroids suddenly.
- To see a doctor if they become unwell.
- Of the increased susceptibility to infections, especially chickenpox.
- Of the serious side effects that may occur.
- To read and keep the patient information leaflet.
- Always to carry the steroid treatment card and to show it to any health professional involved in their treatment. Patients may also be advised to wear a medical alert bracelet.

(Reproduced with kind permission of the Medicines Control Agency.)

FURTHER READING

Barnes PJ. Glucocorticosteroids: Current and future directions. Br J Pharmacol. 2011;163:29–43.

Buckley L, Guyatt G, Fink HA, et al. 2017 American College of Rheumatology guideline for the prevention and treatment of glucocorticoid-induced osteoporosis. Arthritis Rheumatol. 2017;69:1521–37.

Compston J, Cooper A, Cooper C, et al. UK clinical guideline for the prevention and treatment of osteoporosis. Arch Osteoporos. 2017;12:43.

Mitra R. Adverse effects of corticosteroids on bone metabolism: A review. Phys Med Rehab. 2011;3:466–71.

16 Cyclophosphamide

Matthew Scorer, Olga Golberg and Karen Harman

CLASSIFICATION AND MODE OF ACTION

Cyclophosphamide is an antineoplastic drug from the nitrogen mustard group of alkylating agents, which also include melphalan and chlorambucil. The primary mechanism of action is DNA cross-linking, by irreversibly binding an alkyl group to the guanine base of DNA. This leads to the inhibition of DNA replication and cell division. Cyclophosphamide causes immunosuppression by affecting T-cell–mediated and humoral immunity, mainly proliferating B-lymphocytes. It is well-absorbed after oral administration, with a bioavailability of greater than 75%. The drug undergoes hepatic conversion by specific cytochrome P450 (CYP450) isoenzymes to active metabolites, such as phosphoramide mustard and toxic compounds. Its half-life is 4 to 8 hours. Metabolites of cyclophosphamide, including acrolein, are excreted in the urine and have an irritant effect on the bladder mucosa.

INDICATIONS AND DERMATOLOGICAL USES

The main use of cyclophosphamide is in combination with other agents in the treatment of lymphomas, leukaemias and solid tumours. It is also used as an immunosuppressant in severe, refractory autoimmune disorders.

The only approved primary dermatologic indication is advanced mycosis fungoides; all the other dermatological uses of cyclophosphamide are unlicensed, other than where skin manifestations are part of a systemic, life-threatening, progressive autoimmune disease. The main uses in dermatology include:

- Immunobullous diseases: Pemphigus (vulgaris and foliaceus), pemphigoid (bullous and mucous membrane).
- Vasculitides: Refractory cutaneous vasculitis, polyarteritis nodosa, ANCA-associated vasculitides (e.g. granulomatosis with polyangiitis), cryoglobulinaemic vasculitis and autoimmune connective tissue disease-associated vasculitis.
- Connective tissue diseases: Systemic and cutaneous lupus erythematosus, dermatomyositis, Behçet's disease.
- Pyoderma gangrenosum.

FORMULATIONS

- Tablets contain 50 mg cyclophosphamide.
- Vials contain 500 mg, 1000 mg and 2000 mg of cyclophosphamide powder to reconstitute for intravenous injection and infusion. These may be used to prepare an elixir for oral use.

No special action is required if skin extravasation occurs following intravenous injection.

DOSAGES AND SUGGESTED REGIMENS

High doses and complex regimens are used in the treatment of malignant diseases before bone marrow transplantation and for severe autoimmune disease. Dermatological diseases are usually managed with lower doses of 50–200 mg/day and seldom require more than 2.5 mg/kg/day.

DOI: 10.1201/9781003016786-16

Cyclophosphamide is commonly used in conjunction with systemic corticosteroids. Regimens vary from daily oral administration to fortnightly or monthly pulses, or a combination of these. Studies comparing pulsed intravenous and daily oral cyclophosphamide therapies in vasculitis suggest equal efficacy but a lower cumulative dosage and rate of complications with pulsed regimens. However, the risk of relapse may be higher. Large comparative trials of differing doses and regimens are lacking for dermatological conditions.

The co-prescription of mesna to reduce the risk of haemorrhagic cystitis and antimicrobial prophylaxis should be considered with intravenous cyclophosphamide (see Adverse Effects and Their Management).

In the treatment of pemphigus, a well-established pulse and oral regimen with corticosteroids, reported by Parischa and coworkers, is as follows:

- Days 1–3: 100 mg dexamethasone in 500 mL of 5% glucose as an intravenous infusion over 2 hours.
- Day 2: 500 mg cyclophosphamide added to the dexamethasone intravenous infusion.

This constitutes 1 dexamethasone-cyclophosphamide pulse (DCP).

- Days 4–28: Oral cyclophosphamide 50 mg daily with conventional daily doses of oral corticosteroids.

The cycle is repeated every 28 days until clinical remission is achieved and oral steroids are withdrawn (phase I: typically 3–4 months). DCPs continue in 28-day cycles with 50 mg oral cyclophosphamide in between the pulses for a further 9 months (phase II), then oral cyclophosphamide 50 mg daily continued for another 9 months (phase III). Treatment is then withdrawn (phase IV) and patients followed up for 10 years.

This protocol has been reported to induce long-term remission and possible cure of pemphigus, indicating a disease-modifying effect. It has also been used for other dermatological diseases. Modifications to this regimen include using intravenous methylprednisolone (250–1000 mg for 3–5 days) instead of dexamethasone. Another approach is to combine conventional daily oral corticosteroids with monthly intravenous cyclophosphamide pulses (15 mg/kg).

To induce remission in ANCA–associated systemic vasculitis, cyclophosphamide is often used as a first-line drug as follows:

- Oral cyclophosphamide 2 mg/kg/day (up to 200 mg/day) for 3 months, then continued or reduced to 1.5 mg/kg/day if remission achieved.

or

- Intravenous cyclophosphamide 15 mg/kg (max 1500 mg) given in 250–500 mL of 0.9% saline or 5% dextrose over 1–2 hours. Requires pre-hydration with 1 L normal saline and oral intake of 3 L/day for 3 days. The first 3 pulses are given at 2-week intervals, thereafter at 3-week intervals.

In this context, cyclophosphamide is discontinued after 3–6 months, and alternative maintenance therapy established with azathioprine, rituximab, methotrexate or mycophenolate mofetil due to the risks of bladder and gonadal toxicity with prolonged therapy. A reduced dose should be used in older patients and renal impairment.

In lupus nephritis, 'low-dose' intravenous treatment is a recommended induction therapy (the Euro-Lupus regimen is cyclophosphamide IV 500 mg on weeks 0, 2, 4, 6, 8 and 10). In organ- or life-threatening systemic lupus erythematosus (SLE), or as rescue therapy in patients who do not respond to other immunosuppressants, the recommended regimen is cyclophosphamide IV 0.75–1 g/m^2 BSA monthly for 6 months (National Institutes of Health regimen). Continuation after this period should be avoided.

In cutaneous lupus erythematosus (CLE), cyclophosphamide has not been commonly used or studied due to the adverse effect profile. Case series describe successful use of the National Institutes of Health regimen (as described above for SLE) in severe, refractory CLE.

In Behçet's syndrome with arterial involvement, monthly intravenous pulses of cyclophosphamide are recommended in combination with corticosteroids. Cyclophosphamide may also be used in the management of extensive venous thrombosis due to Behçet's syndrome.

Cyclophosphamide should be given early in the day and a high fluid intake should be maintained throughout the day to encourage frequent bladder voiding.

SPECIAL POINT

Several rheumatological guidelines advise dose reduction in older people or those with impaired renal function to reduce the risk of toxicity.

Dose reductions for continuous low-dose oral cyclophosphamide:

- Age >60 years: Reduce the dose by 25%.
- Age >75 years: Reduce the dose by 50%.

Dose reductions for pulsed cyclophosphamide are shown in Table 16.1.

CONTRAINDICATIONS

- Previous urinary malignancy (urinary tract transitional cell carcinoma).
- Haemorrhagic cystitis.
- Bone marrow depression/severe leucopenia (see Figure 16.1).
- Pregnancy and lactation.
- Hypersensitivity to cyclophosphamide.
- Serious underlying infection.

CAUTIONS

- Previous or concurrent mediastinal irradiation; risk of cardiotoxicity.
- Hepatic impairment; reduce dose.
- Hepatitis B and C virus.
- Previous tuberculosis (TB) or risk of TB.
- Renal impairment; reduce dose if creatinine >300 μmol/L.
- Older people; reduce dose.

TABLE 16.1

Dose Reductions for Pulsed Cyclophosphamide

Age (Years)	Creatinine <300 μmol/L	Creatinine 300–500 μmol/L
<60	15 mg/kg/pulse	12.5 mg/kg/pulse
60–70	12.5 mg/kg/pulse	10 mg/kg/pulse
>70	10 mg/kg/pulse	7.5 mg/kg/pulse

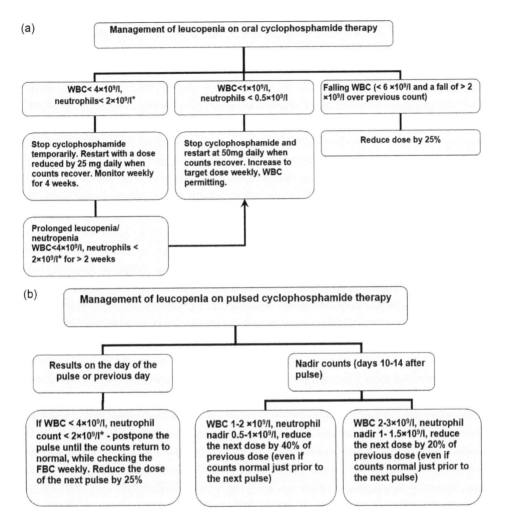

FIGURE 16.1   Management of leucopenia on (a) oral and (b) pulsed cyclophosphamide therapy. (Data from Lapraik C, Watts R, Bacon P, et al., 2007). NB: The lower value of the normal neutrophil range may vary from centre to centre. Check your local laboratory reference range.

- Influenza vaccine (annual) and pneumococcal vaccine (once) recommended, ideally 2 weeks before therapy started.
- Consult latest recommendations on COVID-19 vaccine and booster scheduling (see e.g. https://www.nhs.uk/conditions/coronavirus-covid-19/coronavirus-vaccination/health-conditions/).

IMPORTANT DRUG INTERACTIONS

The risk of toxicity may be potentiated if cyclophosphamide is used concomitantly with any drug with similar toxicities, such as myelosuppression. A large number of potential interactions are detailed in the summaries of product characteristics. Careful individual assessment of the risk and benefits of concomitant or sequential administration of cyclophosphamide with potential interactants is required.

Particular caution is required for drugs that increase or decrease the activity of CYP450 due to the potential effect on cyclophosphamide metabolism.

Interactions with a good evidence base and theoretical interactions with specific recommendations are listed below.

- General anaesthesia may need to be modified if cyclophosphamide has been used within 10 days (as it enhances effects of suxamethonium).
- Live vaccinations are contraindicated during and for 3 months after cyclophosphamide therapy.
- Netupitant (an antiemetic) increases the exposure to cyclophosphamide.

BASELINE INVESTIGATIONS AND CONSIDERATIONS

The following investigations and assessments should be considered before starting treatment:

- Full blood count (FBC) (complete blood count [CBC]) and differential white blood cell count to ensure normal neutrophil count.
- Liver function tests (LFTs) and renal indices.
- Urinalysis.
- Pregnancy test in females of childbearing potential.
- Hepatitis B and C serology (HBV and HCV carriers are at risk of a disease flare on immuno-suppressant treatment). All patients seropositive for HBV and HCV should be discussed with hepatology or infectious disease specialists, as prophylactic antiviral treatment may be required.
- Varicella zoster (VZV) serology.
- Human immunodeficiency virus (HIV) serology.
- Tuberculosis (TB) risk assessment in all patients by clinical examination, history of previous infection, chest radiograph (CXR) and, if appropriate, a tuberculin test or IGRA as with patients being screened for anti-TNF therapy (see Chapter 36).
- Cervical screening up-to-date and a gynaecological review undertaken in patients with a history of cervical intraepithelial neoplasia (CIN).

Contraception should be established in men and women before therapy and continued for at least 3 months after treatment.

MONITORING

Oral cyclophosphamide:

- FBC (CBC) weekly for the first month, every 2 weeks for the next 2 months, then monthly; consider decreasing to every 3 months if stable after 3–6 months.
- Renal indices, LFTs monthly for 3–6 months, then every 3 months if stable.
- Urinalysis monthly, after 3–6 months, every 3 months if stable.
- Urine cytology if haematuria or after a cumulative dose of 50 g.

Pulsed cyclophosphamide:

- Check FBC and renal indices before each pulse (on same or preceding day). Adjust dose if leucopenia/neutropenia (see Adverse Effects and Their Management and Figure 16.1).
- Nadir FBC should be checked on day 10 after the first pulse (the nadir in the white cell count occurs 8–14 days after pulsing, with recovery after 18–25 days). Adjust dose if leucopenia/neutropenia (see Adverse Effects and Their Management and Figure 16.1).
- Nadir FBC should be checked again (day 10) if the dose of cyclophosphamide or interval between pulses changes.
- Urinalysis should be performed monthly.

Lifelong urinalysis every 6 months has been recommended following prolonged treatment, due to the risk of bladder cancer.

ADVERSE EFFECTS AND THEIR MANAGEMENT

Alkylating agents are potent immunosuppressants, but their use is reserved for severe disease because of concerns about serious side effects.

- Bladder toxicity and haemorrhagic cystitis have been attributed to a toxic metabolite, acrolein, and appear to be related to the cumulative dose of cyclophosphamide. Reactivation of a human BK polyoma virus may also play a role. Haemorrhagic cystitis is associated with an increased risk of bladder cancer. Urine microscopy should be performed regularly to detect early problems. Microscopic non-glomerular haematuria is a significant risk factor for the development of bladder cancer. If five or more red blood cells/high power fields appear in the urine, cyclophosphamide should be discontinued. Haematuria often resolves after a few days, but if it persists or is macroscopic, urology referral is indicated. Vigorous hydration before and throughout therapy reduces the risk of haemorrhagic cystitis; the aim is for a minimal urine output of 100 mL/hour (2–3 L/day). Long-term sequelae of this cystitis are bladder fibrosis and contracture.

  Mesna protects the urinary epithelium by reacting with the toxic metabolite acrolein. It should be considered in patients treated with IV cyclophosphamide and is used routinely in those who receive high-dose treatment or have had previous urothelial toxicity. Mesna can be given orally or intravenously. When used with pulsed IV cyclophosphamide, the oral dose of mesna should be 40% of the cyclophosphamide dosage in mg, given 2 hours before the pulse and repeated 2 and 6 hours after the pulse of cyclophosphamide. The dose of intravenous mesna should be 20% of the cyclophosphamide dosage in mg and given with the pulse and then at 2 and 6 hours.

- Infection risk is related to the severity and duration of drug-induced leucopenia. A white blood cell nadir $\leq 3 \times 10^9$/L has been associated with severe and fatal infections in patients on cyclophosphamide therapy. Opportunistic infections such as Pneumocystis jirovecii (carinii) infection may occur and prophylactic antibiotic therapy with oral co-trimoxazole may be indicated. The risk of infection is greater in older people and those receiving simultaneous treatment with high-dose steroids. Current COVID-19 guidelines should be consulted for dermatology patients with immune-mediated inflammatory disorders (IMID) who are eligible for treatment with neutralizing monoclonal antibodies or antivirals.

- Haematological effects include leucopenia, which is dose-related and can be used as a dosage guide during treatment (Figure 16.1). Following a single dose, spontaneous recovery usually occurs within 21 days. Anaemia and thrombocytopenia may occur.

- Malignancy risk is increased, specifically bladder cancer. Studies suggest the risk is dose-related, and it is recommended that lifelong exposure should not exceed 25 g. The risk of acute leukaemia, non-melanoma skin cancer and other solid tumours may also be increased. These can develop several years after treatment is discontinued.

- Chickenpox or shingles contact in non-immune patients may lead to severe infection, and VZV immune globulin or post-exposure prophylaxis with an antiviral therapy should be considered.

- Gastrointestinal effects such as nausea, vomiting and anorexia are common and dose-related complications of cyclophosphamide therapy. They can be managed with dose reduction and effective antiemetic medications, e.g. ondansetron before pulse therapy. Abdominal pain, diarrhoea and oral mucositis may occur. Haemorrhagic colitis and hepatotoxicity are rare.

- Dermatological effects include alopecia (anagen effluvium), which occurs in 5–30% of patients and is dose-dependent. Hair regrowth occurs in most patients even with continued treatment. Diffuse hyperpigmentation, especially of palmoplantar skin and nail pigmentation, may occur. Severe cutaneous adverse drug reactions (including SJS/TEN) have been reported.
- Cardiac and pulmonary toxicity in the form of pulmonary fibrosis, interstitial pneumonitis and cardiomyopathy are rare and associated with high doses of cyclophosphamide used in the treatment of malignancy. The drug should be discontinued if cardiac or pulmonary toxicity is suspected.
- Hypersensitivity to cyclophosphamide may rarely occur, including anaphylaxis. Possible cross-reactivity with other alkylating agents has been reported.
- Infertility is a risk as cyclophosphamide interferes with spermatogenesis and oogenesis. Amenorrhea, azoospermia and irreversible sterility may occur with prolonged therapy. Risk factors for cyclophosphamide-induced infertility include: Age >30 years, long-term therapy and cumulative dose >10 g. Expert advice should be sought for patients of reproductive potential to discuss the option of sperm or oocyte banking.
- Minor adverse effects have been observed with pulsed intravenous cyclophosphamide, and some are thought to be specific to this method of administration. These include facial flashing, palpitations and hiccups, which occurred during intravenous infusions, whereas malaise, headache and taste alteration developed soon after DCP.

USE IN SPECIAL SITUATIONS

CHILDREN

- Cyclophosphamide is not recommended for treatment of skin disease in children, as it may cause irreversible loss of fertility.

PREGNANCY AND LACTATION

- Cyclophosphamide is a known teratogen (formerly FDA Category D) and should not be used in pregnancy except in life-threatening situations. Prenatal exposure in the first trimester has been associated with absent digits, abnormal facies, cleft palate and hernias. Pregnancy should be avoided for at least 3 months after cyclophosphamide treatment in females and males, and some authorities advise 12 months.
- Cyclophosphamide is contraindicated in lactation, as large quantities of active metabolites are excreted in milk. Breastfeeding should not commence for 36 hours after stopping the treatment.

ESSENTIAL PATIENT INFORMATION

Patients should be informed of possible side effects and the need for regular blood monitoring. They should be specifically advised:

- To take cyclophosphamide in the morning and ensure good hydration (2–3 litres of fluid a day) and frequent bladder voiding.
- To seek immediate medical help if they develop symptoms such as a sore throat, fever, easy bruising/bleeding, pallor, shortness of breath and cough.
- To use effective contraception during and for at least 3 months after the treatment.
- About the risk of infertility.
- To report any contact with VZV if non-immune.
- To ensure sun protection.

FURTHER READING

Fanouriakis A, Kostopoulou M, Alunno A, et al. 2019 update of the EULAR recommendations for the management of systemic lupus erythematosus. Ann Rheum Dis. 2019;78:736–45.

Harman K, Brown D, Exton L, et al. British Association of Dermatologists' guidelines for the management of pemphigus vulgaris 2017. Br J Dermatol. 2017;177:1170–201.

Hatemi G, Christensen R, Bang D, et al. 2018 update of the EULAR recommendations for the management of Behçet's syndrome. Ann Rheum Dis. 2018;77:808–18.

Lapraik C, Watts R, Bacon P, et al. BSR and BHPR guidelines for the management of adults with ANCA associated vasculitis. Rheumatology. 2007;46:1–11.

Pasricha JS, Poonam. Current regimen of pulse therapy for pemphigus: Minor modifications, improved results. Indian J Dermatol Venereol Leprol. 2008;74:217–21.

17 Dapsone

Charles Archer and Antonia Lloyd-Lavery

CLASSIFICATION AND MODE OF ACTION

Dapsone (4',4'-diaminodiphenyl sulphone) was first introduced in the 1940s for treatment of leprosy and remains an important therapy against Mycobacterium leprae. It is structurally related to the sulfonamides (Figure 17.1) and shares their antimicrobial action, i.e. impairing microbial synthesis of folate from para-aminobenzoic acid (PABA) by competitive inhibition of the enzyme dihydropteroate synthesase.

Dapsone also has anti-inflammatory actions that account for much of its use in dermatological diseases. The mechanism of this action is unclear, but it is thought to be due to inhibition of neutrophil function (chemotaxis and myeloperoxidase activity) and release of inflammatory mediators. It may also have a local anti-inflammatory effect. Dapsone inhibits the signal transduction cascade common to chemotactic stimuli, suppressing neutrophil recruitment and local production of toxic products.

Dapsone is readily absorbed with good bioavailability (>85%), and a relatively long half-life (14–18 hours) allows once-daily dosing. It is distributed across all body organs and crosses the blood–brain barrier and placenta. Dapsone is metabolized in the liver through a combination of hydroxylation (cytochrome P450 [CYP450]-dependent) into hydroxylamines, which are toxic and implicated in the haematological side effects of the drug, and acetylation (N-acetyl transferase dependent) into mono-acetyl dapsone, which is non-toxic. These products are then conjugated and excreted through the urine (Figure 17.2).

INDICATIONS AND DERMATOLOGICAL USES

Dapsone is licensed for the treatment of leprosy and dermatitis herpetiformis and Pneumocystis jiroveci (carinii) pneumonia prophylaxis in immunodeficient subjects (especially acquired immunodeficiency syndrome [AIDS]). It is also of benefit in a number of dermatoses characterized by neutrophilic infiltrates:

- Immunobullous dermatoses: Dermatitis herpetiformis (DH), linear IgA disease, chronic bullous dermatosis of childhood, bullous pemphigoid, mucous membrane pemphigoid and epidermolysis bullosa acquisita.
- Neutrophilic dermatoses: Erythema elevatum diutinum, Sweet syndrome, subcorneal pustular dermatosis (Sneddon–Wilkinson syndrome), leukocytoclastic vasculitis, pyoderma gangrenosum and delayed pressure urticaria.
- Other inflammatory dermatoses including acne and rosacea, Behçet's disease, relapsing polychondritis and granuloma faciale.
- Severe, necrotic brown recluse spider bites.

FORMULATIONS/PRESENTATION

Dapsone is available as white scored 50 mg and 100 mg tablets.

DOI: 10.1201/9781003016786-17

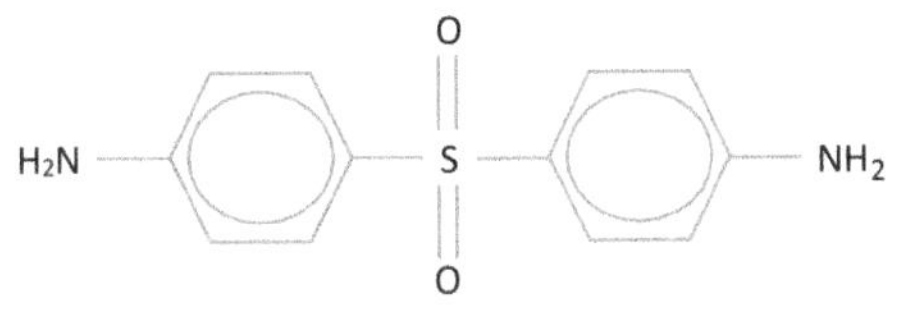

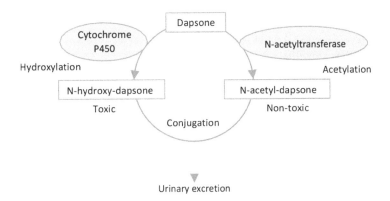

FIGURE 17.1   Chemical structure of dapsone.

FIGURE 17.2   Metabolism of dapsone.

DOSAGES AND SUGGESTED REGIMENS

The World Health Organization (WHO) recommended dose for leprosy is 100 mg daily for adults as follows:

- Multibacillary leprosy: Regimens combining 3 drugs are recommended to avoid develop-ment of resistant strains, using dapsone with rifampicin and clofazimine for 12 months.
- Paucibacillary leprosy: Dapsone combined with rifampicin for 6 months.

For most dermatological conditions, an initial dose of 50 mg daily should be given for the first 2 weeks, to ensure there is no immediate adverse effect, and then adjusted according to the clinical response. In older patients, a smaller starting dose of 25 mg daily may be used. The minimum drug requirement for the majority of conditions lies between 1–2 mg/kg/day. In practice the dose is usually increased by weekly 50 mg increments to achieve control of the symptoms. The clinical response in dermatitis herpetiformis is prompt, and skin lesions start to resolve within 48 hours. However, some patients with DH are resistant to dapsone and require higher doses. The maximum dose should not exceed 300 mg/day. Once the condition is controlled, the dose should be reduced to the lowest dose required for maintenance, which may be continued in the long term. If side effects are not tolerated or if adverse effects develop, then use of sulfapyridine or sulfamethoxypyridazine should be considered.

The rash of DH is gluten-dependent, and the mainstay of therapy in the long term is a strict gluten-free diet (GFD). Patients who adhere to a strict GFD are slowly able to reduce their minimum dapsone requirement and eventually wean off dapsone altogether, though it takes 2 years on average for the rash to be controlled by GFD alone. Dapsone has no effect on the associated gluten-sensitive enteropathy.

BASELINE INVESTIGATIONS AND CONSIDERATIONS

- Full blood count (FBC) (complete blood count [CBC]) and reticulocyte count.
- Urea, electrolytes and creatinine.
- Liver function tests (LFTs).

- Assess all patients for glucose-6-phosphate dehydrogenase level (G6PD) deficiency (see below).
- Assess patients for any pre-existing medical condition (e.g. cardiorespiratory) that might be exacerbated by a minor reduction in haemoglobin level.
- Urinalysis.

MONITORING

- FBC, reticulocytes, urea and electrolytes and LFTs weekly for first month, then monthly for 3 months, then every 3 months if there is no increase in dosage.
- Urinalysis every 3 months.
- Measure methaemoglobin levels if patients are symptomatic.
- Urgent FBC if patients develop symptoms suggesting agranulocytosis.

SPECIAL POINT

G6PD deficiency is the most common disease producing enzyme deficiency worldwide. It is an X-linked inherited disorder and most commonly affects persons of African, Asian, Mediterranean and Middle Eastern descent. Prevalence of the deficiency is correlated with the geographic distribution of malaria, and it is thought that the defect may confer some protection against this infection. Sporadic gene mutations may affect all populations, and different mutations result in different levels of enzyme deficiency and disease manifestations. Some people with G6PD deficiency are asymptomatic. G6PD catalyses the reduction of NADP to NADPH via the pentose phosphate pathway, which is the only method of NADPH generation in erythrocytes (Figure 17.3). They are therefore more susceptible to oxidative stress in the context of infection and certain drugs and dietary triggers. Deficiency of G6PD greatly increases this vulnerability and can lead to neonatal hyperbilirubinemia and acute or chronic haemolysis.

CONTRAINDICATIONS

- Dapsone hypersensitivity.
- Previous hypersensitivity reaction to sulfonamides.
- Acute porphyria.
- Severe ischaemic heart disease or pulmonary disease.
- Severe anaemia: Treat before starting dapsone.
- Severe G6PD deficiency.

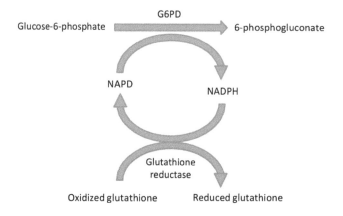

FIGURE 17.3   Glutathione maintenance in erythrocytes.

CAUTIONS

- Cardiac, peripheral vascular and pulmonary disease, particularly in older people who may not tolerate minor reductions in haemoglobin concentration.
- Other conditions predisposing to haemolysis.
- Dapsone can artifactually lower glycosylated haemoglobin levels in patients with Type II diabetes and impair disease monitoring.
- Dapsone can be used with great caution at low doses and with close monitoring in those with mild degrees of G6PD deficiency.
- Pregnancy: Dapsone has been used safely in pregnancy, but neonatal haemolysis and methemoglobinemia have been reported in the third trimester. If dapsone is necessary, folic acid supplementation (5 mg/day) should be prescribed to the mother before conception and throughout pregnancy.
- Breastfeeding: Dapsone is present in breast milk, and a case of haemolytic anaemia in a breastfed infant has been reported. Risks to the infant are thought to be very small unless the infant is G6PD-deficient.

IMPORTANT DRUG INTERACTIONS

- Anti-epileptics (fosphenytoin, phenytoin, phenobarbital and primidone): Use with caution due to increased risk of side effects.
- Antimalarials (chloroquine and primaquine): Use with caution due to increased risk of side effects.
- Clozapine: Contraindicated due to the risk of blood dyscrasias.
- Folic acid antagonists (e.g. methotrexate) increase dapsone levels with increased risk of side effects.
- Nitrofurantoin: Use with caution due to increased risk of side effects.
- Probenecid reduces urinary excretion of dapsone, increasing plasma concentration with increased risk of toxicity.
- Rifampicin induces dapsone metabolism and enhances urinary excretion.
- Saquinavir: Contraindicated due to the risk of cardiac arrhythmias.
- Sulphonamides: Use with caution due to increased risk of haemolysis.
- Trimethoprim and co-trimoxazole decrease renal clearance of dapsone and increases the risk of toxicity.

ADVERSE EFFECTS AND THEIR MANAGEMENT

- Haemolysis and haemolytic anaemia are dose-related and due to reduced erythrocyte survival. Mild haemolysis with a drop in haemoglobin of 1–2 g/dL (10–20 g/L) occurs in most patients at a standard therapeutic dose. Hydroxylated metabolites of dapsone cause oxidation of glutathione, which, in its reduced state, plays an important role in maintaining erythrocyte cell membrane integrity. Underlying G6PD deficiency impairs the ability to maintain adequate reserves of reduced glutathione, and therefore predisposes individuals to severe haemolysis (see above).
- Methemoglobinemia is caused by the reaction of hydroxylated metabolites of dapsone with oxyhaemoglobin (containing Fe^{2+}) in the presence of oxygen, leading to formation of a ferric compound (Fe^{3+}) that has reduced capacity for oxygen transport. Raised levels of methaemoglobin can lead to symptoms of headache, shortness of breath and lethargy and a bluish discolouration of the lips and fingertips. Methaemoglobin normally undergoes reduction by a NADPH-dependent enzyme methaemoglobin reductase, and there is an adaptive increase with time. Patients with a deficiency of the enzyme are more susceptible.

- Methemoglobinemia does not need treatment unless patients are symptomatic. If the level is >20%, then dapsone should be discontinued; at a level >30%, additional measures can be taken. Cimetidine can reduce methaemoglobin levels by inhibition of CYP450, which reduces synthesis of the toxic hydroxylated metabolites (Figure 17.2). It can be prescribed at a dose of 400 mg Tds for mild methemoglobinemia. More severe cases may require treatment with oxygen and IV methylene blue 1% solution to restore the iron in haemoglobin to its reduced oxygen-carrying state.
- Agranulocytosis is a rare side effect occurring in about 1 in 10,000 prescriptions due to a direct toxic effect of hydroxylated metabolites. It is usually gradual in onset, occurring within 2–16 weeks of starting therapy, but may be sudden. It may also arise late in the course of treatment. A significant drop in neutrophil count can present with fever, mouth ulcers and a sore throat. It may be accompanied by thrombocytopenia. Regular monitoring of the blood count is therefore mandatory.
- Sulfhaemoglobinaemia arises from a direct combination of dapsone with haemoglobin. It is rarely of clinical relevance.
- Dapsone hypersensitivity syndrome is a serious side effect and usually takes the form of a drug reaction (or rash) with eosinophilia and systemic symptoms (DRESS)-type reaction. It is estimated to occur in approximately 1% of patients. The onset is usually within 4–6 weeks of starting therapy, but it may be delayed up to 6 months. Patients present with fever, a morbilliform rash that can progress to erythroderma, lymphadenopathy, hepatitis with elevated liver enzymes, peripheral eosinophilia and atypical lymphocytes. If not recognized, the condition deteriorates, and there is a significant risk of death. The drug should be withdrawn immediately.
- Severe cutaneous reactions, including toxic epidermal necrolysis and Stevens–Johnson syndrome, have also been reported.
- Gastrointestinal adverse effects such as anorexia, nausea and vomiting are common and can limit patients' ability to tolerate and continue treatment. Hepatitis, jaundice, cholestasis and abnormal LFTs may occur.
- Peripheral motor and sensory neuropathies have been reported rarely. They are dose-related and caused by axonal damage. Headache, insomnia, malaise and, rarely, psychoses have been reported.
- Renal adverse effects include proteinuria and, very rarely, nephrotic syndrome.

USE IN SPECIAL SITUATIONS

PRE-CONCEPTION

Animal studies have shown that dapsone can reduce the number of sperm and their motility, potentially reducing male fertility, though there is no clear evidence for this in humans.

PREGNANCY

Dapsone can cross the placenta and should be avoided in pregnancy if possible. It has, however, been used safely with no evidence of teratogenicity since its introduction in 1947. Folic acid 5 mg daily should be given to females who are pregnant. The greatest risk is in the last trimester, when it may lead to neonatal haemolysis and methemoglobinemia.

LACTATION

Dapsone is secreted in breast milk and absorbed by the infant, giving rise to mild haemolytic anaemia. The risk to the infant is considered small unless it has G6PD deficiency.

<small>CHILDREN</small>

Dapsone has been used safely in infants and children at doses of 1–2 mg/kg/day.

ESSENTIAL PATIENT INFORMATION

Patients should be advised of the need to attend for regular monitoring and to seek urgent medical attention if affected by the following:

- Sore throat, mouth ulcers, purpura and bleeding: May indicate agranulocytosis/bone marrow suppression.
- Shortness of breath, headache, light-headedness, chest pain, blue discolouration of skin and yellow discolouration of skin/jaundice: May indicate significant haemolysis or methemoglobinemia.
- Widespread rash, itching, fever, and enlarged lymph nodes: May indicate dapsone hypersensitivity syndrome.

FURTHER READING

Agarwalla A, Agrawal S. Dapsone hypersensitivity syndrome: A clinical-epidemiological review. J Dermatol. 2005;32:883–9.

Frank JE. Diagnosis and management of G6PD deficiency. Am Fam Phys. 2005;72(7):1277–82.

Piette EW, Werth VP. Dapsone in the management of autoimmune bullous diseases. Immunol Allergy Clin North Am. 2012;32(2):317–22.

Wolverton SE, Remlinger K. Suggested guidelines for patient monitoring: Hepatic and haematological toxicity attributable to systemic dermatologic drugs. Dermatol Clin. 2007;25(2):195–205.

Zhu YI, Stiller MJ. Dapsone and sulfones in dermatology: Overview and update. J Am Acad Dermatol. 2001;45:420–34.

18 Dimethyl Fumarate

Oonagh Molloy and Brian Kirby

CLASSIFICATION AND MODE OF ACTION

Fumaric acid esters (FAE) have been used in the treatment of psoriasis for many years. Their use was proposed by Schweckendiek, a German chemist, in 1959. An oral formulation containing mono-ethylfumarate and dimethylfumarate (DMF) was later licensed as Fumaderm® in Germany in 1994 and used several European countries as an unlicensed drug with good results. A novel formulation of the active salt, DMF, called Skilarence® is now widely licensed for use in psoriasis and has largely replaced Fumaderm. Following oral administration, DMF is rapidly metabolized by esterases in the small intestine to monomethyl fumarate (MMF), the active metabolite.

Fumaric acid is a component of the tricarboxylic (Krebs) cycle, but the therapeutic mechanism of action of DMF remains unclear. DMF has many effects on immune function with a relative reduction in IL-17 producing T-cells and an increase in regulatory (anti-inflammatory) T-cells being relevant for psoriasis.

The efficacy and long-term safety of DMF as used in Fumaderm is well-established. Long-term survival rates in real use of around 60% are similar to psoriasis biological drugs. Moreover, a subset of patients (approximately 10%) have been found to show excellent long-term efficacy at low doses (<240 mg/day).

INDICATIONS AND DERMATOLOGICAL USES

- Moderate-to-severe psoriasis: DMF (as Skilarence) has been licensed in Europe for the treatment of moderate-to-severe psoriasis since 2017 and since 2014 (as Tecfidera) for the treatment of multiple sclerosis.
- The UK's National Institute for Health and Care Excellence (NICE) 2017 appraisal recommends DMF as a treatment option for psoriasis in adults only if the following criteria are met:
  - Psoriasis area and severity index (PASI) ≥10.
  - Dermatology life quality index (DLQI) >10.
  - Failed response to systemic therapy, including ciclosporin, methotrexate and psoralen UVA (PUVA) or where these are contraindicated or not tolerated.

This positions DMF as an alternative therapy to biological drugs and apremilast.

DMF has been reported as effective in granuloma annulare, cutaneous sarcoidosis, alopecia areata and pityriasis rubra pilaris, although it is used in these conditions in an off-licence manner, based on case reports and case series only.

FORMULATIONS/PRESENTATION

Dimethyl fumarate (Skilarence) is available as 30 mg and 120 mg gastro-resistant tablets.

DOSAGES AND SUGGESTED REGIMENS

The usual starting dose of Skilarence is 30 mg once daily, increased at weekly intervals up to a maximum dose of 720 mg a day. The average dose used is 3–4 tablets per day. A minority of patients (10%) will respond to very low doses of DMF. Tablets should be swallowed whole and taken with food to minimize gastric upset.

DOI: 10.1201/9781003016786-18

TABLE 18.1

Dosage Regiment for Dimethyl Fumarate (Skilarence) in Psoriasis

Week	Number of Tablets Morning	Midday	Evening	Total Daily Dose (mg) of Dimethyl Fumarate
Skilarence 30 mg				
1	0	0	1	30
2	1	0	1	60
3	1	1	1	90
Skilarence 120 mg				
4	0	0	1	120
5	1	0	1	240
6	1	1	1	360
7	1	1	2	480
8	2	1	2	600
9+	2	2	2	720

Note: A higher starting dose of 120 mg DMF twice daily, increased after a week to 240 mg twice daily, is used in the treatment of multiple sclerosis.

Source: Adapted from Skilarence® SPC.

The slowly escalating regime is aimed to improve tolerability (see Table 18.1). A clinical response is usually evident within 16 weeks, although the onset of action may be variable because of deviation from the usual escalation schedule.

NICE guidelines specify that treatment should be discontinued if there is insufficient response by 16 weeks as defined by:

• A 50% reduction in the PASI score (PASI50) and a 5-point reduction in DLQI from baseline.

Thereafter, the maintenance dose should be the lowest dose. Patient response does not appear to vary according to body weight or disease activity and is not predictable in advance.

BASELINE INVESTIGATIONS AND CONSIDERATIONS

• Full blood count (FBC) (complete blood count [CBC]).
• Urea, electrolytes, creatinine and urate.
• Liver function tests (LFTs) and bone profile.
• Urinalysis.
• Contraception for females of childbearing potential.

CONTRAINDICATIONS

SPECIAL POINT

In January 2021, MHRA/CHM in the UK issued updated advice on haematological contraindications to the initiation of DMF, following a European review of safety data as below:

• Leucocyte count $<3 \times 10^9$/L; Lymphopenia $<1.0 \times 10^9$/L.

Other contraindications are:

- Severe gastrointestinal disease.
- Severe renal dysfunction.
- Serious infection.
- Pregnancy and lactation.
- Allergic contact dermatitis to DMF.

DMF has been identified as an extremely potent contact allergen following its use as a mould-retarding agent in leather furniture and clothing. There is a risk of eliciting a severe cutaneous adverse reaction in patients sensitized by topical exposure who are given DMF.

CAUTIONS

- Renal impairment/proteinuria.

IMPORTANT DRUG INTERACTIONS

There are no data on drug interactions related to Skilarence. Caution is advised, however, in the setting of concomitant use of immunosuppressives and potentially nephrotoxic medication, such as NSAIDs. DMF does not appear to interact with the cytochrome P450 system.

ADVERSE EFFECTS AND THEIR MANAGEMENT

The most common reported side effects are gastrointestinal disturbance and flushing. The most common laboratory finding is lymphopenia. The incidence of serious bacterial infections while taking DMF is low.

- Gastrointestinal: In the phase III trial data on Skilarence, gastrointestinal symptoms (62.7%) including diarrhoea, abdominal bloating/distension and nausea were most prevalent in the first 3 months of treatment, with a reported attenuation in symptoms thereafter. A slower-dose escalation is advised in patients who experience gastrointestinal symptoms. Tablets should not be crushed or chewed, as this damages their protective enteric coating.
- Flushing: Flushing is a common side effect, with reported rates ranging from about 20–50%. It is thought to be due to MMF-induced prostaglandin release. A short course of low-dose non-enteric coated acetylsalicylic acid may help those who are more severely affected. Profound flushing associated with dyspnoea, angioedema or urticaria may indicate rare hypersensitivity or anaphylactoid reactions. If affected, patients should be advised to discontinue treatment and seek immediate medical care.
- Hepatotoxicity: Significant hepatotoxicity is rare; however, mildly raised transaminases are not uncommon. Drug-induced liver injury may occur shortly after initiation, several weeks later or beyond this time. A twofold rise in transaminases warrants dose reduction, investigation and monitoring.
- Nephrotoxicity: Nephrotoxicity is rare. Reversible proximal tubular dysfunction (Fanconi syndrome) has been reported and manifests as proteinuria, glycosuria, aminoaciduria and hyperphosphaturia. The serum creatinine and glomerular filtration rate may be normal. Early diagnosis is important, as untreated disease may lead to renal damage and osteomalacia. Monitoring of proteinuria, bone profile and urate levels is recommended at 3 monthly intervals.

- Haematological: Leukopenia and lymphopenia (10%) are very common, and eosinophilia is also a common laboratory abnormality during treatment. These are most apparent in the first three months of treatment and reversible with dose reduction or discontinuation. Lymphopenia is a potential risk factor for opportunistic infections. It is advised to manage as follows:
  - Lymphocyte counts <1.0 × 10^9/L but ≥0.7 × 10^9/L (grade 1 lymphopenia): Repeat monthly until the count >1.0 × 10^9/L on two consecutive tests, then resume every 3 months monitoring.
  - Lymphocyte count <0.7 × 10^9/L (grade 2 lymphopenia): Repeat and if the count remains <0.7 × 10^9/L, treatment must be stopped immediately.
- Lymphopenia may take 6–12 months to resolve after stopping treatment. Monitoring should continue until the lymphocyte count has returned to normal.
- Neurological: FAE and DMF therapy have been associated with very rare instances of progressive multifocal leukoencephalopathy (PML), a potentially fatal opportunistic infection caused by reactivation of latent John Cunningham virus. The risk of PML with FAEs has been estimated at <1/300,000 patient years. Symptoms include weakness or clumsiness on one side of the body or a limb, visual disturbance, memory loss, personality change and confusion. Persistent moderate or severe lymphopenia (<0.7 × 10^9/L) is the significant risk factor for the development of PML while taking DMF.
- Malignancy: There is no data to suggest a link between the use of DMF and the development of malignancy.

USE IN SPECIAL SITUATIONS

PREGNANCY

DMF was formerly classified as FDA Category C, as animal studies have shown evidence of embryo-fetal toxicity. There are no established studies of FAE in pregnancy, and the manufacturer advises that the drug is contraindicated.

LACTATION

The manufacturer advises to avoid.

CHILDREN

DMF is not licensed for use in patients under the age of 18. Small studies have reported benefit in the treatment of multiple sclerosis in this age group.

OLDER PEOPLE

The use of DMF in older populations is not precluded in the absence of contraindications.

ESSENTIAL PATIENT INFORMATION

Patients should be counselled about common side effects of DMF, particularly flushing and gastrointestinal effects, to mitigate against early, avoidable dropout. The importance of regular blood monitoring and the risk of rare but serious adverse effects should also be explained.

FURTHER READING

Ismail N, Collins P, Rogers S, et al. Drug survival of fumaric acid esters for psoriasis: A retrospective study. Br J Dermatol. 2014;171(2):397–402.

Kornberg MD, Bhargava P, Kim PM, et al. Dimethyl fumarate targets GAPDH and aerobic glycolysis to modulate immunity. Science. 2018;360(6387):449–53. doi:10.1126/science.aan4665.

Meissner M, Valesky EM, Kippenberger S, et al. Dimethyl fumarate – only an anti-psoriatic medication? J Dtsch Dermatol Ges. 2012 Nov;10(11):793–801.

Mrowietz U, Christophers E, Altmeyer P. Treatment of psoriasis with fumaric acid esters: Results of a prospective multicentre study. Br J Dermatol. 1998;138:456–60.

Mrowietz U, Sorbe C, Reich K, et al. Fumaric acid esters for the treatment of psoriasis in Germany: Characterising patients in routine care. Eur J Dermatol. 2020;30:41–8.

Reich K, Mrowietz U, Radtke MA, et al. Drug safety of systemic treatments for psoriasis: Results from the German psoriasis registry PsoBest. Arch Dermatol Res. 2015 Dec;307(10):875–83.

Sulaimani J, Cluxton D, Clowry J, et al. Dimethyl fumarate modulates the treg-Th17 cell axis in patients with psoriasis. Br J Dermatol. 2021;184:495–503.

19 Interleukin-4/13 Inhibitors

Alison Sears and Andrew Pink

CLASSIFICATION AND MODE OF ACTION

Dupilumab is an interleukin-4 (IL-4) receptor alpha inhibitor and is the first licensed biological therapy for use in the treatment of moderate-to-severe atopic dermatitis (AD). It is a fully human IgG4 monoclonal antibody that specifically binds to the IL-4 receptor alpha chain (IL-4Rα), which is shared by the IL-4 and IL-13 receptor complexes. Dupilumab thereby inhibits both IL-4 and IL-13 signalling. It was licensed in 2017. Tralokinumab is a fully human IgG4 monoclonal antibody which specifically binds to IL-13, preventing its interaction with the IL-13 receptor complex and downstream signalling (Figure 19.1). It was licensed in 2021.

IL-4 and IL-13 are T-helper type 2 (Th2) cytokines, produced primarily by Th2 lymphocytes, mast cells, eosinophils and basophils. IL-4 induces the differentiation of naive helped T-cells into Th2 cells. IL-4 and IL-13 play a key role in the pathogenesis of AD and allergic disorders, including the release of pro-inflammatory (Th2) cytokines, chemokines and immunoglobulin E.

INDICATIONS AND DERMATOLOGICAL USES

Dupilumab and tralokinumab are licensed for the treatment of adults with moderate-to-severe AD. Dupilumab is also licensed for use in children aged 6 years and above.

In the UK, patient eligibility for treatment is determined by the National Institute for Health and Care Excellence (NICE) criteria. Both drugs are NICE approved in the setting of documented failure

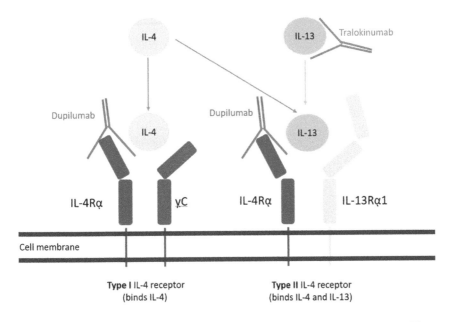

FIGURE 19.1 Dupilumab inhibits IL-4 and IL-13 signalling by binding to the shared IL-4Rα arm of the type 1 and type II IL-4 receptors. Tralokinumab inhibits IL-13 signalling by binding directly to IL-13, thereby blocking interaction with the type II receptor. (Adapted from Hamilton JD, Ungar B, Guttman-Yassky E. Drug evaluation review: Dupilumab in atopic dermatitis. Immunotherapy. 2015;7(10):1043–58.)

DOI: 10.1201/9781003016786-19

131

to and/or unsuitability for at least one other systemic therapy, such a ciclosporin, methotrexate, aza-thioprine and mycophenolate mofetil.

Adequate response to treatment, assessed at 16 weeks, is defined by at least a 50% reduction in the Eczema Area and Severity Index score (EASI50), an objective measure of disease severity, and at least a 4-point reduction in the Dermatology Life Quality Index (DLQI) from pre-treatment scores. Dupilumab is also licensed for the treatment of severe asthma with type 2 inflammation and severe chronic rhinosinusitis with nasal polyps. Tralokinumab was NICE approved for the treatment of adults with atopic dermatitis in 2022 with the same initiation and continuation criteria as for dupilumab.

FORMULATIONS/PRESENTATION

DUPILUMAB AND TRALOKINUMAB

- Dupilumab: 300 mg in a 2 mL solution (150 mg/mL) in a single-use pre-filled pen or syringe for SC injection.
- For children/adolescents: A 200 mg pre-filled syringe or pen. The pre-filled pen is not intended for use in children below 12 years of age; for children 6–11 years of age, the pre-filled syringe is recommended.
- Tralokinumab: 150 mg in 1 mL solution in pre-filled syringes.

Both solutions are clear to slightly opalescent, colourless to pale yellow.

The injection device should be kept in the outer carton in order to protect from light. They should be stored in a refrigerator (2–8°C). If removed from the refrigerator, it may be stored at room temperature (≤25°C) for up to 14 days.

Before use, the injection device should be removed from the refrigerator and left to stand at room temperature for about 30–45 minutes to allow the solution to come to a comfortable temperature. The product should not be shaken.

DOSAGES AND SUGGESTED REGIMENS

- Adult: 600 mg (2 × 300 mg injections) dupilumab or 600 mg (4 × 150 mg injections) tralokinumab loading dose administered SC at week zero (0), then 300 mg every other week.
- Children and adolescents (dupilumab): See Table 19.1.

It is recommended that treatment effectiveness should be reviewed at 16 weeks. In practice, the onset of action is often evident within 6 weeks. A 75% reduction in EASI (EASI75) occurs in around 50% of patients on dupilumab at 16 weeks, with sustained efficacy at 12 months. It can, however, take up to 6 months to reach maximum effect. After withdrawal, there is commonly a gradual relapse, and, from available data, the effectiveness on retreatment does not appear to be reduced.

TABLE 19.1

Dupilumab Dosing for Children and Adolescents

Age (Years)	Body Weight (kg)	Loading Dose	Subsequent Dose
12–17	15–59	400 mg	200 mg every 2 weeks
	≥60	600 mg	300 mg every 2 weeks
6–11	15–59	300 mg	300 mg at 2 weeks, then every 4 weeks[a]
	≥60	600 mg	300 mg every 2 weeks

[a] The dose may be increased to 200 mg every 2 weeks based on clinical judgement.

Pharmacokinetic studies showed a trend of reduced dupilumab exposure (the area under the concentration-time curve to the time of last measurable concentration), with increasing body weight at a dose of 300 mg SC. However, clinical trials (SOLO 1 and 2) demonstrated dupilumab treatment efficacy in subgroups (weight, age, gender, race, and background treatment, including immunosuppressants) to be consistent with the results in the overall study population, and no dose adjustment for weight is recommended for adults with atopic dermatitis.

Patients taking tralokinumab who achieve clear or almost clear skin after 16 weeks of treatment may be considered for maintenance dosing every 4 weeks; this may not be appropriate in patients weighing over 100 kg.

BASELINE INVESTIGATIONS AND CONSIDERATIONS

See Table 19.2 for suggested baseline investigations before initiating dupilumab or tralokinumab.

MONITORING

Not formally required in summary of product characteristics (SmPC), but consider full blood count (FBC) (complete blood count [CBC]), liver function tests (LFTs) and renal profile at weeks 4–6, 4 months and then annually if stable. Further testing may be required according to clinical signs and risks.

USE IN KIDNEY DISEASE

No dose adjustment is needed in patients with mild or moderate renal impairment. Very limited data are available in patients with severe renal impairment and hepatic impairment.

CONTRAINDICATIONS

- Hypersensitivity to dupilumab/tralokinumab or excipients.
- Untreated helminth infection.

CAUTIONS

- Helminth infection: Dupilumab and tralokinumab may impair the immune response against helminths by inhibiting IL-4/IL-13 signalling. Patients with pre-existing helminth infections should be treated before initiation. If patients become infected while receiving treatment and do not respond to anti-helminth treatment, treatment should be discontinued until infection resolves.

TABLE 19.2

Dupilumab/Tralokinumab Baseline Investigations

Consider for All Patients	Where Clinically Indicated
- FBC (CBC) – peripheral blood eosinophils - LFTs - Creatinine, electrolytes - Hepatitis B virus, hepatitis C virus, human immunodeficiency virus (HIV) - *Note*: SmPC does not state a requirement for specific baseline investigations	- Screen for invasive parasites (prolonged travel in areas endemic for parasite infections, particularly helminths) - Chest x-ray - Spirometry (consider in co-morbid asthma)

- Comorbid asthma
  - Dupilumab is also licensed for the treatment of severe asthma.
  - A fatal asthma exacerbation occurred in a patient following cessation of dupilumab treatment in a phase 3 atopic dermatitis (AD) trial. This was due to the patient stopping their regular maintenance inhaled corticosteroid (ICS), since their asthma improved on dupilumab. For patients with comorbid asthma, the supervising respiratory physician should be informed at the time of dupilumab/tralokinumab discontinuation to arrange additional monitoring of asthma.
- Pregnancy and breastfeeding.
- Past or current malignancy or increased future risk of malignancy: Consider possible increased risk of malignancy.
- Infections: Due to the potential of biological therapies to increase the risk of infections and to reactivate latent infections, dupilumab should be used with caution in patients with chronic infection, history of recurrent infection or immunodeficiencies.
- Vaccinations: Flu and pneumococcal vaccination are recommended for people who are on immunosuppressant medication; ideally these inactive vaccines should be administered at least 2 weeks before therapy is started. Prescribers are advised to consult the latest recommendation on COVID-19 vaccine and booster scheduling (see e.g. https://www.nhs.uk/conditions/coronavirus-covid-19/coronavirus-vaccination/health-conditions/).
- COVID-19: Current COVID-19 guidelines should be consulted for dermatology patients with immune-mediated inflammatory disorders (IMID) who are eligible for treatment with neutralizing monoclonal antibodies or antivirals.

IMPORTANT DRUG INTERACTIONS

No drug interactions have been reported to date.

- Systemic, topical or inhaled corticosteroids should not be discontinued abruptly upon initiation of therapy with dupilumab/tralokinumab. Reductions in the corticosteroid dose, if appropriate, should be gradual and performed under the direct supervision of a physician.
- The safety and effectiveness of these drugs in combination with other immunosuppressants, including biologics or phototherapy, have not been evaluated.

ADVERSE EFFECTS AND THEIR MANAGEMENT

- Ocular side effects
  - Eye symptoms are reported as a common side effect of both drugs, including conjunctivitis, blepharitis and pruritus. These are usually mild, and treatment in the majority of cases can be continued.
  - For patients with a known pre-existing ophthalmic condition (e.g. keratoconus or previous corneal grafts), consider an ophthalmology review before starting treatment to ensure optimized eye care.
  - Patients who develop conjunctivitis that does not resolve following simple eye-directed management (e.g. lubricants with or without antihistamine eye drops) or symptoms/signs of keratitis (pain, red eye) should be referred for ophthalmological assessment. Severe keratitis, if left untreated, can lead to permanent visual loss.
- Headache and injection site reactions are common and usually short-lived.
- Eosinophilia has been reported with both drugs. It may resolve with ongoing treatment. Anti-drug antibodies have been detected in a minority of patients, but they do not appear to affect efficacy.

- Infections and reactivation of latent infections: A recent pooled analysis of clinical trial data suggested that dupilumab was not associated with an increased risk of serious/severe infections or non-herpetic skin infections (versus placebo) in patients with AD. This data must be interpreted with caution due to the limited trial duration. Common non-skin infections that were more frequent in the dupilumab groups (combined) than in the placebo group were nasopharyngitis, upper respiratory tract infection, conjunctivitis/bacterial conjunctivitis and oral herpes.
- Serum sickness-like reactions are very rare (<1 in 10,000 patients). Cases of anaphylactic reaction and angioedema have been reported.
- Head and neck dermatitis: Data from real-world use of dupilumab in clinical practice has highlighted other important adverse events, including dupilumab-associated head and neck dermatitis/exacerbation of existing head and neck dermatitis/sebopsoriasis.
- Psoriasis, enthesitis and inflammatory arthritis have also been reported. This may relate to upregulation of Th1/17 cytokines. It is important to ask patients about musculoskeletal symptoms and to seek rheumatology specialist advice if needed.

As dupilumab and tralokinumab are new therapies in AD, it is important that prescribers are vigilant about the possibility of unknown or long-term adverse events. Biological registries have been established in several European countries and should provide increasingly robust data on the safety and effectiveness of these agents. It is strongly recommended that all patients being treated with biological therapy should be enrolled into these registries.

USE IN SPECIAL SITUATIONS

PREGNANCY AND PRE-CONCEPTION

There is very limited data on the use of dupilumab and tralokinumab in pregnancy. The SmPCs state that "animal studies do not indicate direct or indirect harmful effects with respect to reproductive toxicity. However, as IgG can cross the placenta, these drugs should only be used during pregnancy if the potential benefit justifies the potential risk to the fetus."

Pregnancy should be avoided and effective, contraception is strongly recommended during treatment and for at least 12 weeks after cessation. In patients who are planning a pregnancy, dupilumab and tralokinumab should be avoided (and/or stopped in advance) so the fetus is drug-free during the critical developmental period of the first 12 weeks, although trans-placental transfer of monoclonal antibodies is negligible at this stage of pregnancy. If a patient established on therapy discovers they are pregnant, they should be referred urgently to the obstetric medicine service for further assessment.

LACTATION

It is unknown whether dupilumab and tralokinumab are excreted in human breast milk, or, if excreted, whether they would be absorbed by the infant. The SmPCs advise making a decision taking into account the benefit of breastfeeding for the child and the benefit of therapy for the patient.

CHILDREN

The safety profile of dupliumab in children aged 6 and above in AD clinical trials (and in adolescents ages 12–17 in asthma clinical trials) was similar to that seen in adults. There is safety data up to 52 weeks from asthma studies. The safety and efficacy of tralokinumab in children under the age of 18 has not been established.

OLDER PEOPLE

No dose adjustment is recommended for patients over the age of 65. Though no differences in safety or efficacy were observed between older and younger adult patients with atopic dermatitis in clinical trials, relatively few patients were over 65. Due to declining immune function and the increased risk of infections in older people, caution is advised when treating this age group with biological drugs.

ESSENTIAL PATIENT INFORMATION

- Information on the risks of infections and guidance on vaccinations should be provided.
- Due to its earlier licensing, there is more long-term safety data for the use of dupliumab in AD. It is envisaged that the safety and efficacy profile of tralokinumab will be similar, but real-world data is essential for confirmation.

FURTHER READING

Blauvelt A, de Bruin-Weller M, Gooderham M, et al. Long-term management of moderate-to-severe atopic dermatitis with dupilumab and concomitant topical corticosteroids (LIBERTY AD CHRONOS): A 1-year, randomised, double-blinded, placebo-controlled, phase 3 trial. Lancet Lond Engl. 2017;389:2287–303.

de Bruin-Weller M, Thaçi D, Smith CH, et al. Dupilumab with concomitant topical corticosteroid treatment in adults with atopic dermatitis with an inadequate response or intolerance to ciclosporin A or when this treatment is medically inadvisable: A placebo-controlled, randomized phase III clinical trial (LIBERTY AD CAFÉ). Br J Dermatol. 2018;178:1083–101.

Popiela MZ, Ramez B, Turnbull AMJ, et al. Dupilumab-associated ocular surface disease: Presentation, management and long-term sequelae. Eye. 2021;35:3277–84.

Sears AV, Woolf RT, Gribaleva E, et al. Real-world effectiveness and tolerability of dupilumab in adult atopic dermatitis: A single centre, prospective 1-year observational cohort study of the first 100 patients treated. Br J Dermatol. 2021;184(4):755–57.

Wollenberg A, Blauvelt A, Guttman-Yasky E, et al. Tralokinumab for moderate-to-severe atopic dermatitis: Results from two 52-week, randomized, double-blind, multicentre, placebo-controlled phase III trials (ECZTRA 1 and ECZTRA 2). Br J Dermatol. 2021;184(3):437–49.

20 Interleukin (IL)-12/23 and IL-23 Inhibitors

Charles H. Earnshaw and Richard B. Warren

CLASSIFICATION AND MODE OF ACTION

Biologic therapies have transformed the treatment of moderate-to-severe psoriasis. This is a rapidly evolving field, with several new monoclonal antibody medications reaching the market over the last few years. A number of classes of biologic agents now exist, corresponding to the underlying cytokine target of the antibody therapy. The interleukin (IL)-12/23 and IL-23 inhibitors make up two closely related and commonly prescribed classes and are reviewed in this chapter.

Psoriasis is a complex immunopathological disease that results from aberrant activation of pathways in the innate and adaptive arms of the immune system. Interleukins are cytokines that allow communication between different immune cells. In the skin, dendritic cells are the major source of these cytokines. IL-12 signalling leads to the activation of Th1 T-lymphocytes. IL-23 signalling leads to activation of the Th17 arm of the immune system. Altered activities of both arms, but especially the Th17 arm, play major contributory roles in the pathogenesis of psoriasis.

During the development of ustekinumab, a biologic agent designed to target IL-12, it was fortuitously discovered that ustekinumab inhibited both IL-12 and IL-23 due to a common structural subunit, p40. Ustekinumab was shown to be very effective in the treatment of moderate-to-severe psoriasis, partly due to its inhibition of the IL-23 pathway. Subsequent biologic agents were therefore designed to target IL-23 specifically (which they do by binding to the p19 subunit of IL-23). These IL-23 inhibitors specifically inhibit the Th17 pathway. Approved members of this class include guselkumab, risankizumab and tildrakizumab (Figure 20.1).

Therefore, this chapter will review the use of two related groups of biologics: The IL-12/23 inhibitors (led by ustekinumab) and the IL-23 specific inhibitors (guselkumab, risankizumab and tildrakizumab). Together these biologic medications lead to improvements in disease severity in the majority of psoriasis patients for whom they are prescribed.

INDICATIONS AND DERMATOLOGICAL USES

Ustekinumab is licensed for treatment of adults with moderate-to-severe plaque psoriasis, psoriatic arthritis, Crohn disease and ulcerative colitis. Guselkumab, risankizumab and tildrakizumab are licensed for treatment of adults with moderate-to-severe plaque psoriasis and are under investigation for use in inflammatory bowel disease and psoriatic arthritis. Funding criteria in the UK are determined by the National Institute for Health and Care Excellence (NICE) and are shown in Table 20.1.

Initiation and supervision of biologic therapy for people with psoriasis should be undertaken by specialist physicians (dermatologists) experienced in the diagnosis and treatment of psoriasis.

The 2020 British Association of Dermatologists guidelines on the use of biologic therapy in psoriasis recommend any of the licensed biologics as first-line treatment options for patients with psoriasis who meet the criteria for biologic therapy. Of note, the guidelines recommend IL-17 inhibitors or TNF-alpha antagonists as first-line choices in patients with both psoriasis and psoriatic arthritis. Biologics may help, and could be considered early, in cases where psoriasis is severe at localized sites such as the nails, palms and scalp (with the caveat that obtaining drug funding in these scenarios can be challenging). The original reference containing these guidelines can be found at the end of this chapter (Smith CH, et al., Br J Dermatol. 2020).

DOI: 10.1201/9781003016786-20

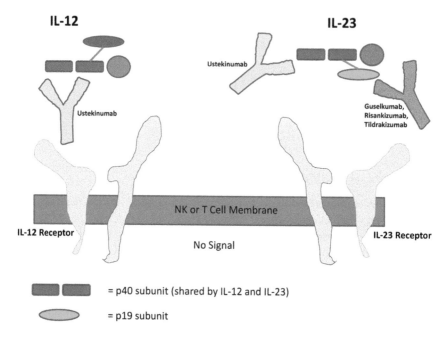

FIGURE 20.1   Mode of action of ustekinumab, guselkumab, risankizumab and tildrakizumab. Ustekinumab binds the p40 subunit shared by IL-12 and IL-23, thereby inhibiting both IL-12 and IL-23 binding to cell surface receptors and subsequent activation of T-lymphocyte subsets. Guselkumab, risankizumab and tildrakizumab bind the p19 subunit of IL-23 and therefore specifically inhibit IL-23 binding to receptors.

TABLE 20.1

NICE Funding Criteria for IL-12/23 and IL-23 Inhibitors

Medication	Requirements	Discontinue
Ustekinumab	Psoriasis Area Severity Index (PASI) score ≥10 and a Dermatology Life Quality Index (DLQI) score ≥10 AND documented failure to and/or unsuitability for other standard systemic treatments, including ciclosporin and methotrexate	Stop 16 weeks after starting treatment if the patient has not shown a 75% reduction in PASI, or 50% reduction in PASI and 5-point reduction in DLQI
Guselkumab	PASI ≥10 and DLQI score ≥10 AND documented failure to and/or unsuitability for other standard systemic treatments, including ciclosporin and methotrexate AND the manufacturer provides the drug according to the commercial arrangement	Stop 16 weeks after starting treatment if the patient has not shown a 75% reduction in PASI, or 50% reduction in PASI and 5-point reduction in DLQI
Risanzkizumab	PASI ≥10 and DLQI score ≥10 AND documented failure to and/or unsuitability for other standard systemic treatments, including ciclosporin and methotrexate AND the manufacturer provides the drug according to the commercial arrangement	Stop 16 weeks after starting treatment if the patient has not shown a 75% reduction in PASI, or 50% reduction in PASI and 5-point reduction in DLQI
Tildrakizumab	PASI ≥10 and DLQI score ≥10 AND documented failure to and/or unsuitability for other standard systemic treatments, including ciclosporin and methotrexate AND the manufacturer provides the drug according to the commercial arrangement	Stop 28 weeks after starting treatment if the patient has not shown a 75% reduction in PASI, or 50% reduction in PASI and 5-point reduction in DLQI

FORMULATIONS/PRESENTATION

Before injection, the pre-filled syringe should be taken out of the refrigerator and left to stand at room temperature for about 30 minutes. This allows the solution to be better-tolerated at injection. Rotation of injection sites (including upper thighs, abdomen and posterior upper arms) can help to reduce pain when injecting. Injection into areas of active psoriasis should be avoided.

USTEKINUMAB

- Ustekinumab 45 mg solution in a 0.5 mL (or 90 mg in 1 mL) pre-filled syringe for s/c injection.
- The pre-filled syringe should be kept in the outer carton in order to protect from light.
- Ustekinumab should be stored in a refrigerator (2–8°C).

GUSELKUMAB

- Guselkumab 100 mg solution in a 1 mL pre-filled syringe for s/c injection.
- The pre-filled syringe should be kept in the outer carton in order to protect it from light.
- Guselkumab should be stored in a refrigerator (2–8°C).

RISANKIZUMAB

- Risankizumab 75 mg solution in a 0.83 mL pre-filled syringe for s/c injection (2 per unit).
- The pre-filled syringe should be kept in the outer carton in order to protect it from light.
- Risankizumab should be stored in a refrigerator (2–8°C).

TILDRAKIZUMAB

- Tildrakizumab 100 mg solution in a 0.5 mL pre-filled syringe for s/c injection.
- The pre-filled syringe should be kept in the outer carton in order to protect it from light.
- Tildrakizumab should be stored in a refrigerator (2–8°C).

DOSAGES AND SUGGESTED REGIMENS

USTEKINUMAB

- Patients ≤100 kg: 45 mg administered s/c at weeks 0 and 4, then every 12 weeks.
- Patients >100 kg: 90 mg administered subcutaneously at weeks 0 and 4, then every 12 weeks.
- Consider dose escalation to 90 mg every 12 weeks if the patient weighs ≤100 kg or 90 mg every 8 weeks if the patient is >100 kg and has only achieved a partial response (ustekinumab high dose is available at the same cost in many parts of the UK, and therefore no specific funding approval may be required for this dose escalation).
- Children and young people <60 kg: 0.75 mg/kg, otherwise dosing as per adults.

Pharmacokinetic data have shown that in patients weighing more than 100 kg there is a 55% greater clearance and a 37% greater volume of distribution. Clinical trials also showed a reduced efficacy in patients >100 kg using a standard 45 mg dose, and this is the rationale for the use of a higher (90 mg) dose in these individuals.

GUSELKUMAB

- 100 mg administered s/c at weeks 0 and 4, then every 8 weeks.

RISANKIZUMAB

- 150 mg administered s/c at weeks 0 and 4, then every 12 weeks.

TILDRAKIZUMAB

- 100 mg administered s/c at weeks 0 and 4, then every 8 weeks.
- Certain subgroups, which may include patients with an elevated BMI or high disease burden, may benefit from an increased dose of 200 mg.

BASELINE INVESTIGATIONS AND CONSIDERATIONS

- Full blood count (FBC) (complete blood count [CBC]), liver function tests (LFTs) and urea, electrolytes and creatinine.
- Tuberculosis (TB) screening, including chest radiograph, and interferon gamma release assay (e.g. QuantiFERON® Gold).
- Human immunodeficiency virus (HIV) serology (HIV-1 and HIV-2 antibodies and HIV-1 antigen).
- Hepatitis B serology (surface antigen and core antibody), hepatitis C serology (IgG).
- Varicella zoster virus serology in people with negative or uncertain chickenpox history.
- Autoantibodies (anti-nuclear antibodies, anti-nuclear double-stranded DNA antibodies).
- Urinalysis.
- Pregnancy test.
- Body weight.
- Patients who begin these therapies should be offered the opportunity to participate in long-term safety registries (BADBIR in the UK and Republic of Ireland: http://badbir.org).

MONITORING

FBC, LFTs, and U&Es (including creatinine) should be performed at 3–4 months and at least every 6 months thereafter and/or as clinically indicated.

Experience to date suggests that both IL-12/23 and IL-23 inhibitors are relatively safe to use in renal disease. U&Es (including creatinine) make up part of the baseline screening for biologic drugs and should be monitored as per the monitoring regime to ensure no significant deterioration in renal function occurs.

CONTRAINDICATIONS

- Hypersensitivity to the biologic medication.
- Significant active infection.

CAUTIONS

- Due to the potential of biological therapies to increase the risk of infections and to reactivate latent infections, biologic treatments should be used with caution in patients with chronic infection or history of recurrent infection, especially TB (see section on TB below).
- Consider risk of malignancy (see Special Point below).
- Use with caution in older people.
- Provide age-appropriate immunizations before initiating therapy.
- See section below for information regarding use of IL-12/23 and IL-23 inhibitors in pregnancy (see Use in Special Situations: Pregnancy and Pre-Conception).

- Vaccinations: Flu and pneumococcal vaccination are recommended for people who are on immunosuppressant medication; ideally, these inactive vaccines should be administered at least 2 weeks before therapy is started. Prescribers are advised to consult the latest recommendation on COVID-19 vaccine and booster scheduling (see e.g. https://www.nhs.uk/conditions/coronavirus-covid-19/coronavirus-vaccination/health-conditions/). Do not give live vaccines to patients concurrently receiving treatment with IL-12/23 or IL-23 inhibitors or infants <6 months old whose mothers received biologic therapy beyond 16 weeks' gestation. Live vaccines should not be given for 6 months following cessation of biologic treatment (12 months for herpes zoster vaccination). Biologic therapy can be commenced 4 weeks after live vaccination.
  - Current COVID-19 guidelines should be consulted for dermatology patients with immune-mediated inflammatory disorders (IMID) who are eligible for treatment with neutralizing monoclonal antibodies or antivirals.

SPECIAL POINTS

Biologic Therapy and Tuberculosis

Screen for latent TB with an interferon gamma release assay and a chest radiograph. In patients requiring treatment for latent TB, complete 2 months of treatment before starting biologic therapy.

The IMMhance clinical trial for Risankizumab included 55 patients with latent TB, 31 of which received no treatment for it. None of these 31 patients went on to develop active TB. Risankizumab is therefore generally considered one of the safer biologic treatment options in this patient population (Blauvelt A, et al., JAMA Dermatol. 2020).

Biologic Therapy and Cancer Risk

Assess patients before and during biologic therapy with respect to the past or current history of cancer and any future risk of cancer. Discussion with the relevant specialist is advised in patients with a history of cancer (especially in the last 5 years) and where the baseline risk of skin cancer is elevated (e.g. previous non-melanoma skin cancer). Patients should be encouraged to enroll in national cancer screening programmes.

IMPORTANT DRUG INTERACTIONS

- No drug interactions have been reported thus far. No studies have identified a significant effect of IL-12/23 or IL-23 inhibitors on cytochrome P450 enzyme activities.
- Ustekinumab has been licensed in combination with methotrexate for the treatment of psoriatic arthritis. However, the use of other immunosuppressants should be stopped for at least 1 month before starting biologic therapy.

ADVERSE EFFECTS AND THEIR MANAGEMENT

- The most common side effects are listed below:
  - Ustekinumab: Headache, upper respiratory tract infection, injection site reaction, nasal congestion, oropharyngeal pain, bronchitis, sinusitis, urinary tract infections, vaginal yeast infections, fever, lethargy, pruritus, nausea and vomiting, diarrhoea and abdominal pain.
  - Guselkumab: Headache, upper respiratory tract infection, injection site reaction, arthralgia, diarrhoea, bronchitis, fungal skin infections and herpes simplex infections.
  - Risankizumab: Headache, upper respiratory tract infection, injection site reaction, lethargy, and fungal skin infections.

- Tildrakizumab: Headache, upper respiratory tract infection, injection site reaction, diarrhoea.
- Headache, upper respiratory tract infection and injection site reactions are usually mild, and treatment can generally be continued after monitoring and discussions with the patient.
- Serious hypersensitivity reactions (including anaphylaxis and angioedema) are rare but have been reported.
- The needle cover on the pre-filled syringe of ustekinumab contains natural rubber (a latex derivative) and should not be handled by individuals with an allergy to latex.
- Infections and reactivation of latent infections, including serious bacterial, fungal and viral infections (such as herpes zoster and viral hepatitis), have been observed in patients receiving biologic treatment. If a patient develops a serious infection, the biologic therapy should be withheld until the infection has resolved.

USE IN SPECIAL SITUATIONS

PREGNANCY AND PRE-CONCEPTION

Females of childbearing potential with psoriasis who are starting biologic therapy should be advised to use effective contraception. Discussions around conception planning should be had with the specialist/consultant responsible for the management of their psoriasis. No interactions between contraceptive methods and biologics are currently known.

Advise pregnant patients that good control of their psoriasis is important to maximize maternal health, and that most pregnancies reported in patients receiving biologic therapy have good outcomes. There is insufficient data to quantify the risk of foetal abnormalities in these patients, however. Pregnant patients should be told that these medications, like maternal IgG, will cross the placenta, and therefore live vaccines must be avoided in infants (up to 6 months of age) born to mothers taking biologic medication beyond 16 weeks' gestation. It is therefore generally recommended that pregnant patients stop their treatment before that point.

LACTATION

The 2020 British Association of Dermatology guidelines on biologic use in psoriasis recommend a discussion with the patient, explaining that biologic therapies are unlikely to be present in large concentrations in breast milk, and the biologic present is unlikely to be absorbed systemically by the infant. The guidelines suggest continuing or restarting biologic therapy in patients wishing to breastfeed.

CHILDREN

Ustekinumab is licensed for use in patients over the age of 12 with moderate-to-severe plaque psoriasis. The recommendations and requirements for cessation are the same as detailed above. Guselkumab, risankizumab and tildrakizumab have not been licensed for use in children. However, clinical trials of the IL-23 inhibitors in children are currently ongoing.

OLDER PEOPLE

No overall significant differences in efficacy or safety of IL-12/23 or IL-23 inhibitors have been observed in patients aged 65 or above compared with younger patients, and no dose adjustment is required. However, due to declining immune function and the increased risk of infections in older people, caution is advised when treating this age group with biologic drugs.

ESSENTIAL PATIENT INFORMATION

- Patients should be offered the opportunity to enroll in long-term safety registries (BADBIR in the UK and Republic of Ireland: http://badbir.org).
- Information on the risks of infections and guidance on vaccinations should be provided.
- Female patients of childbearing potential should use contraception and have discussions with their dermatologist should they be planning for a pregnancy.

FURTHER READING

Blauvelt A, Leonardi CL, Gooderham M, et al. Efficacy and safety of continuous risankizumab therapy vs treatment withdrawal in patients with moderate to severe plaque psoriasis: A phase 3 randomised clinical trial. JAMA Dermatol. 2020;156(6):649–58.

Kimball AB, Papp KA, Wasfi Y, et al. Long-term efficacy of ustekinumab in patients with moderate-to-severe psoriasis treated for up to 5 years in the PHOENIX 1 study. J Eur Acad Dermatol Venereol. 2013;27:1535–45.

Krueger GG, Langley RG, Leonardi C, et al. A human interleukin-12/23 monoclonal antibody for the treatment of psoriasis. N Engl J Med. 2007;356(6):580–92.

Maghfour J, Elliott E, Gill F, et al. Effect of biologic drugs on renal function in psoriasis patients with chronic kidney disease. J Am Acad Dermatol. 2020;82:1249–51.

Smith CH, Yiu ZZ, Bale T, et al. British Association of Dermatologists guidelines for biologic therapy for psoriasis 2020: A rapid update. Br J Dermatol. 2020; doi:10.1111/bjd.19039.

21 Interleukin-17 Inhibitors

Leena Chularojanamontri and Christopher E.M. Griffiths

CLASSIFICATION AND MODE OF ACTION

The cytokine interleukin (IL)-17 is mainly produced by T-helper 17 cells and to a lesser extent by other innate immune cells. By binding to its receptor, IL-17 activates the transcription factor nuclear factor-κB (NF-κB), leading to a pro-inflammatory cascade. Keratinocytes are the principal targets of IL-17 in psoriasis, contributing to epidermal hyperproliferation and skin barrier disruption. The IL-17 family has six known members (termed IL-17A to IL-17F), which function as homodimers or heterodimers. These cytokines play essential roles in the host defence against microbial infections and are implicated in various inflammatory disorders and cancers. IL-17A is a homodimeric glycoprotein with varying homology with other family members (IL-17B to F), ranging from 55% for IL-17F to 17% for IL-17E. The IL-17A/A homodimer (IL-17A) is approximately 10–30 times more potent than the IL-17F/F homodimer (IL-17F). Pathological production of IL-17A leads to excess inflammation and tissue damage. Given its central role in chronic immune-mediated inflammatory disease, inhibitors of IL-17A have been developed for therapeutic use.

IL-17 cytokines act via their receptor family, which is distinct from other known cytokine receptors. The IL-17 receptor (IL-17R) family contains 5 subunits (termed IL-17RA to IL-17RE), each of which contains an extracellular domain, single transmembrane domain and a signalling adaptor protein (proteins that are accessory to main proteins in a signal transduction pathway). IL-17A binds with high affinity to the IL-17RA subunit, which is expressed on a wide range of tissues and cell types. This then forms a complex with IL-17RC, activating downstream signalling pathways. IL-17F also signals through the same receptor subunits with a lower affinity for IL-17RA.

The IL-17A inhibitors currently used in dermatology can be divided into two groups: Monoclonal antibodies targeting IL-17A (secukinumab and ixekizumab) and monoclonal antibodies targeting IL-17RA (brodalumab).

- Secukinumab is a human immunoglobulin (Ig) G1 monoclonal antibody that binds IL-17A.
- Ixekizumab is a humanized IgG4 monoclonal antibody that binds IL-17A.
- Brodalumab is a human monoclonal IgG2 antibody that binds to IL-17RA; it inhibits the activity of IL-17A, IL-17F, IL-17A/F and IL-17E.

INDICATIONS AND DERMATOLOGICAL USES

- Secukinumab was approved by the US Food and Drug Administration (FDA) and European Medicine Agency (EMA) in 2015 for the treatment of moderate-to-severe psoriasis, psoriatic arthritis and ankylosing spondylitis.
- Ixekizumab was approved by the US FDA and EMA in 2016 for the treatment of moderate-to-severe plaque psoriasis. Later on, it was approved for psoriatic arthritis, ankylosing spondylitis and psoriasis in paediatric patients ages 6 years and older.
- Brodalumab was approved by the US FDA and EMA in 2017 for the treatment of moderate-to-severe plaque psoriasis.

DOI: 10.1201/9781003016786-21

The National Institute for Health and Care Excellence (NICE) in the UK recommends IL-17 inhibitors as an option for treating adults with plaque psoriasis only when:

- The disease is severe, as defined by a total Psoriasis Area and Severity Index (PASI) of ≥10 and a Dermatology Life Quality Index (DLQI) of >10; and
- The disease has not responded to conventional systemic therapies, including ciclosporin, methotrexate and psoralen and long-wave ultraviolet A radiation (PUVA), or these options are contraindicated or not tolerated, or phototherapy (PUVA and ultraviolet B radiation) is ineffective, or cannot be used or has resulted in rapid relapse (rapid relapse is defined as greater than 50% of baseline disease severity within 3 months); and
- The manufacturing company provides the drug at a discounted price agreed upon in the patient access scheme.

Both PASI and DLQI should be calculated before and during treatment. The definition of treatment response is either:

- PASI 50: A 50% or greater reduction from baseline PASI or % body surface area where PASI is not applicable and at least a 5-point reduction in DLQI.
- PASI 75: A 75% reduction from baseline PASI.

IL-17 inhibitors should be discontinued if patients do not achieve these response criteria. According to NICE guidelines, the time for reviewing whether to continue therapy with IL-17 inhibitors (secukinumab, ixekizumab and brodalumab) is at 12 weeks.

IL-17A inhibitors are also licensed for treatment of psoriatic arthritis and ankylosing spondylitis. They have been used off-label for several recalcitrant skin diseases. Data are mostly available for secukinumab due to its earlier approval. Evidence from small open studies and case reports suggests benefit in hidradenitis suppurativa, Behçet's syndrome and pityriasis rubra pilaris.

FORMULATIONS/PRESENTATION

- Secukinumab: Preservative-free, lyophilized powder in 150 mg vials for reconstitution with 1 mL of sterile water and a 150 mg/mL solution containing 150 mg (or a 75 mg secukinumab-paediatric dose) in a pre-filled syringe and/or pen (autoinjector) for subcutaneous administration.
- Ixekizumab: 80 mg/mL solution in a pre-filled syringe or autoinjector for subcutaneous administration.
- Brodalumab: 210 mg/1.5 mL solution in a single-dose pre-filled syringe for subcutaneous administration.

All should be stored at 2–8°C and reconstituted before injection.

DOSAGES AND SUGGESTED REGIMENS

Secukinumab

The initial dose is 300 mg by subcutaneous administration at weeks 0, 1, 2, 3 and 4, followed by 300 mg every 4 weeks.

In randomized controlled trials (RCTs), ERASURE and FIXTURE, the percentage of patients who achieved PASI 75 at week 12 was higher with secukinumab than with either the placebo or etanercept. The rates were 81.6% and 71.6% with 300 mg and 150 mg of secukinumab, respectively.

Secukinumab is approved by the EMA for treatment of children aged 6 and older. The recommended dose is 75 mg for children <50 kg and 150 mg for children ≥50 kg, as per the adult schedule.

IXEKIZUMAB

The initial dose of ixekizumab is 160 mg by subcutaneous administration, followed by 80 mg on weeks 2, 4, 6, 8, 10 and 12. The maintenance dose is 80 mg every 4 weeks.

The RCT (UNCOVER-3) study showed that ixekizumab was superior to etanercept and placebo. At week 12, 84.2%, 53.4%, and 7.3% of patients treated with ixekizumab, etanercept and placebo, respectively, achieved a PASI 75.

Ixekizumab is approved by the EMA for treatment in children aged 6 and older. For those weighing >50 kg, the adult dose regime is used, and for children weighing 25–50 kg, dosages are halved.

BRODALUMAB

The dose is 210 mg by subcutaneous administration at weeks 0, 1 and 2, followed by 210 mg every 2 weeks.

The two RCTs (AMAGINE-2 and AMAGINE-3) showed that at week 12, PASI 75 was achieved by 86% and 67% of patients receiving brodalumab in the two studies, respectively.

Intermittent use of IL-17 inhibitors may provide an alternative approach in patients who are unwilling or unable to maintain a continuous regimen, without any apparent loss or efficacy on retreatment or safety issues compared with continuous dosing.

BASELINE INVESTIGATIONS AND CONSIDERATIONS

- Complete blood count (CBC), liver function tests (LFTs), blood urea nitrogen, creatinine, urinalysis, pregnancy test, hepatitis B virus, hepatitis C virus and human immunodeficiency virus (HIV) infection should be performed.
- Tuberculosis (TB) screening using chest x-ray according to local policy, the Mantoux test or interferon gamma release assay (IGRA) is suggested. If the Mantoux test is positive in those in whom the test is less reliable (e.g. BCG-vaccinated people) or in areas where Mantoux testing is impractical, IGRA should be considered.
- A careful personal and family history and gastrointestinal symptoms should be taken for inflammatory bowel disease (IBD) before starting an IL-17 inhibitor. IL-17 inhibitors are contraindicated in patients with active IBD, and alternative biologics are preferable in patients with quiescent disease. Faecal calprotectin measurement may be used to screen for subclinical gut inflammation.

MONITORING

- No routine laboratory monitoring is required for patients on IL-17 inhibitor treatment.
- Measurement of the full blood count (FBC) every 6 months, or it should be carried out if there are signs or symptoms of infection.
- A careful history should be taken at follow-up consultations (every 3–6 months), specifically enquiring about gastrointestinal symptoms and symptoms of infection.
- Annual testing for latent tuberculosis (IGRA testing, Mantoux test) should be done in patients at high risk, such as patients in contact with individuals with active tuberculosis because of travel, work or a family relationship, and patients with selected medical conditions. For patients who are not at high risk, screening should be done according to expertise.
- An annual chest radiograph may be considered according to expertise.

- Enquire about mental health and screen for depression/suicidal thoughts in patients treated with brodalumab.
- Specific assessment for infections at each visit.
- History and physical examination, including screening for non-melanoma skin cancer. It can be undertaken at the same time as the PASI evaluation according to expertise.

SPECIAL POINTS

ASYMPTOMATIC LATENT TB

IL-17 inhibitors do not appear to play a significant downregulatory role in systemic immunity compared with tumour necrosis factor (TNF) antagonists. An in vitro study showed that the use of secukinumab had no effect on Mycobacterium tuberculosis dormancy within granulomas, in contrast to TNF-antagonists. Nevertheless, screening for latent tuberculosis (TB) is recommended before starting treatment with IL-17 inhibitors, though the risk of progression to active TB during therapy appears to be very low. Patients should be instructed to seek medical advice if signs/symptoms suggestive of TB infection (e.g. persistent cough, wasting/weight loss, low-grade fever or listlessness) occur during or after therapy with IL-17 inhibitors.

HEPATITIS VIRUS

Triple serology, including hepatitis B surface antigen (HBsAg), antibodies to HBsAg (anti-HBs), antibodies to hepatitis B core antigens (anti-HBcs) and antibodies to hepatitis C (anti-HCV) are recommended to be screened before initiating an IL-17 inhibitor.

- No conclusive data are available for IL-17 inhibitor use in patients with HBV or HCV infection.
- IL-17 inhibitors appear to have an acceptable safety profile in HCV patients with psoriasis under close monitoring and collaboration with gastroenterologists.
- HBsAg+ psoriasis patients are at higher risk of HBV reactivation than psoriasis patients with HBsAg−/HBc+. Antiviral prophylaxis may be considered in HBsAg+ psoriasis patients. Both groups should be monitored with LFTs and viral load during the treatment with IL-17 inhibitors.

HIV

No conclusive data are available, but IL-17 inhibitors are less likely to be complicated by opportunistic infections than TNF-antagonists are.

MALIGNANCIES

Currently, evidence is not sufficient to draw conclusions on whether there is any increased risk of solid tumour or lymphoreticular malignancy in patients treated with IL-17 inhibitors. However, available data suggest that incidence rates for malignancy during IL-17 inhibitor (secukinumab and ixekizumab) treatment ranged from 0.4 to 0.6 per 100 person-years, which were less than those seen in the psoriasis population (1.14 per 100 person-years) and general population (0.95 per 100 person-years).

ELECTIVE SURGERY

Agents should be discontinued at least four half-lives before major surgery (3–4 months for secukinumab, 6–8 weeks for ixekizumab and brodalumab).

CONTRAINDICATIONS AND CAUTIONS

ABSOLUTE CONTRAINDICATION AND CAUTION

- Hypersensitivity to any component of the formulation.

RELATIVE CONTRAINDICATIONS AND CAUTIONS

- Active IBD.
- Recent suicidal behaviour or history of suicidal ideation (brodalumab).

Patients should not receive live or live-attenuated vaccination within 2–3 half-lives before treatment. Flu and pneumococcal vaccination are recommended for people who are on immunosuppressant medication; ideally, these inactive vaccines should be administered at least 2 weeks before therapy is started. Prescribers are advised to consult the latest recommendation on COVID-19 vaccine and booster scheduling (see e.g. https://www.nhs.uk/conditions/coronavirus-covid-19/coronavirus-vaccination/health-conditions/). COVID vaccines are safe to use in patients on IL-17 inhibitors as long as there are no other contraindications to use.

Current COVID-19 guidelines should be consulted for dermatology patients with immune-mediated inflammatory disorders (IMID) who are eligible for treatment with neutralizing monoclonal antibodies or antivirals.

IMPORTANT DRUG INTERACTIONS

Although there are relatively scarce data on the combination of IL-17 inhibitors with other systemic treatments for psoriasis, there is no reason to consider these to be contraindicated. If the benefits outweigh the risks, combination treatment can be used. However, concomitant use of other immunosuppressive or immunomodulatory drugs can enhance the degree of immunosuppression and thereby increase the risk of infection.

- Immunization: Patients should not receive live or live-attenuated vaccination within 2 IMIDs 3 half-lives before, during and for 6 months after treatment discontinuation. In the case of shingles (herpes zoster) vaccine, a delay in vaccination of 12 months after discontinuation is recommended. Inactivated/killed vaccines may be given during treatment.

ADVERSE EFFECTS AND THEIR MANAGEMENT

The most common adverse effects of IL-17 inhibitors are nasopharyngitis, upper respiratory tract infection and headache. These are usually mild and do not lead to treatment discontinuation.

MUCOCUTANEOUS CANDIDIASIS

IL-17 plays an important role in innate and adaptive responses against Candida species. This explains the increased susceptibility to persistent or recurrent mucocutaneous candidiasis in patients receiving anti–IL-17 therapy. A recent systematic review showed that the frequency of candida infections was 1.7%, 3.3% and 4.0% with secukinumab, ixekizumab and brodalumab treatment, respectively. Infections are mild to moderate in severity and respond well to standard antifungal treatment without the need to discontinue anti–IL-17 therapy. However, this may be a baseline consideration choice of biologic in patients who are prone to recurrent vulvovaginal candidiasis. Disseminated or invasive Candida infections have been reported rarely.

The incidence of neutropenia in patients treated with IL-17 inhibitors is low, but higher than for placebo. Most cases are grade 1 (<2.0–1.5×10^9/L) and grade 2 (<1.5–1.0×10^9/L) neutropenia, which are not usually associated with serious infections and which resolve spontaneously. The incidence of neutropenia in patients treated with secukinumab, ixekizumab and brodalumab is 4.1%, 2.9% and 1.5% per 100 patient-years of exposure, respectively. Periodic monitoring of neutrophil counts is advised every 6 months, or it should be carried out if there are signs or symptoms of infection.

IBD

The frequency of new onset IBD ranged from 0.06%–0.3% in clinical trials of IL-17 inhibitors. IL-17 inhibitors should be stopped in cases of persistent diarrhoea/abdominal pain, and expert gastrointestinal advice should be sought.

Depression and Risk of Suicide during Brodalumab Therapy

An association between brodalumab and suicide has been highlighted, though analysis of psoriasis clinical trials provides no evidence to support this association. However, it is recommended that a risk evaluation and mitigation strategy – the SILIQ risk evaluation and mitigation strategy programme – should be performed, with patients undergoing brodalumab treatment.

Major Adverse Cardiovascular Events (MACE)

The rates of MACE are low and comparable between different treatment groups, with no class effect identified. Several RCTs showed that IL-17 inhibitors did not cause any significant change in the short-term risk of either MACE or congestive heart failure in patients with psoriasis, compared with placebo.

Dermatological Adverse Effects

A new-onset atopic dermatitis-like eruption has been reported, including facial dermatitis. Topical therapy may help.

Although IL-17 inhibitors appear to offer superior efficacy compared to conventional systemic treatments and older biologics (TNF antagonists and ustekinumab), the available safety data are of shorter duration. It is important that prescribers are vigilant for unexpected adverse effects and long-term safety profiles of IL-17 inhibitors. Data from real world registries such as the British Association of Dermatologists Biologics and Immunomodulators Register (BADBIR), the Corona Psoriasis (PSO) Registry and the Psoriasis Longitudinal Assessment and Registry (PSOLAR), among others, are of the utmost importance for pharmacovigilance.

USE IN SPECIAL SITUATIONS

Pregnancy and Pre-Conception

Animal data on secukinumab and brodalumab in pregnancy have not shown embryo-fetal toxicity, but studies on ixekizumab showed an increased risk in neonatal death when it was administered in later pregnancy. Transplacental transfer of IgG antibodies occurs from as early as 13 weeks' gestation, with highest rates in the last month of pregnancy. In line with guidance for other biologic drugs, it is considered reasonable to use IL-17 inhibitors with care up to the end of the second trimester.

LACTATION

No clinical data is available on the use of IL-17 inhibitors during breastfeeding. However, all are large protein molecules with high molecular weight, and levels in breast milk are likely to be very low. Furthermore, absorption is unlikely, as they are probably destroyed in the infant's gastrointestinal tract. Until more data become available, IL-17 inhibitors should be used with caution during breastfeeding, especially while nursing a newborn or preterm infant.

CHILDREN

Ixekizumab and secukinumab have been approved by the EMA and FDA for the treatment of psoriasis in children aged 6 years and above. The published evidence of the safety and efficacy of these drugs in children is currently limited to relatively small clinical trials of up to 1 year.

OLDER PEOPLE

Small studies and trial data in patients aged ≥65 have reported safe and effective use of IL-17 inhibitors with no dose adjustment required, so age should not be a barrier to using these agents.

ESSENTIAL PATIENT INFORMATION

- Instruct patients to seek medical advice if signs and symptoms of infection occur. Treatment should be discontinued until the infection resolves.
- Patients should be managed according to the individual situation.
    - TB or close contact with someone with TB.
    - Hepatitis or an HIV infection.
    - Infection and vaccination history.
    - Crohn disease.
    - Agents should be discontinued at least four half-lives before major surgery (3–4 months for secukinumab, 6–8 weeks for ixekizumab and brodalumab).
    - Where an IL-17 inhibitor therapy is used outside its indication, written consent should be obtained from the patient.

FURTHER READING

Al-Hammadi A, Ruszczak Z, Magariños G, et al. Intermittent use of biologic agents for the treatment of psoriasis in adults. J Eur Acad Dermatol Venereol. 2020;8. doi:10.1111/jdv.16803.
Di Caprio R, Caiazzo G, Cacciapuoti S, et al. Safety concerns with current treatments for psoriasis in the elderly. Expert Opin Drug Saf. 2020;19:523–31.
Kaushik SB, Lebwohl MG. Psoriasis: Which therapy for which patient: Focus on special populations and chronic infections. J Am Acad Dermatol. 2019;80:43–53.
Menter A, Strober BE, Kaplan DH, et al. Joint AAD-NPF guidelines of care for the management and treatment of psoriasis with biologics. J Am Acad Dermatol. 2019;80:1029–72.
Rungapiromnan W, Yiu ZZN, Warren RB, et al. Impact of biologic therapies on risk of major adverse cardiovascular events in patients with psoriasis: Systematic review and meta-analysis of randomized controlled trials. Br J Dermatol. 2017;176:890–901.
Smith CH, Yiu ZZ, Bale T, et al. British Association of Dermatologists guidelines for biologic therapy for psoriasis 2020: A rapid update. Br J Dermatol. 2020;18. doi:10.1111/bjd.19039.
Speeckaert R, Lambert J, van Geel N. Learning from success and failure: Biologics for non-approved skin diseases. Front Immunol. 2019;10:1918. doi:10.3389/fimmu.2019.01918.

22 Isotretinoin

Alison M. Layton

CLASSIFICATION AND MODE OF ACTION

Acne is the commonest inflammatory dermatosis seen worldwide, and the physical and emotional impact of acne can be burdensome. Oral isotretinoin (13-cis-retinoic acid) is a vitamin A derivative, first approved in the United States by the FDA in 1982 for the treatment of severe, recalcitrant acne. Trace amounts of 13-cis-retinoic acid are detectable in normal human plasma, suggesting that it is an endogenous retinoid.

Oral isotretinoin remains to date the only oral monotherapy that targets all the main factors implicated in the pathogenesis of acne, rendering it a highly effective therapy for severe acne. It has effects on cell cycle progression, cellular differentiation, cellular survival and apoptosis, which lead to a decrease in sebum production and comedogenesis, thereby reducing surface and ductal Cutibacterium acnes (C. acnes) and associated inflammatory processes. Isotretinoin has a profound effect on sebaceous gland activity, causing sebocyte apoptosis by inducing the expression of neutrophil gelatinase-associated lipocalin. Isotretinoin also impairs metabolism of androgens within the sebaceous gland, leading to involution and reduced sebum production. It upregulates genes encoding differentiation markers, tumour suppressors, serine proteases and innate immune proteins, with more delayed effects on extracellular matrix genes, and downregulates numerous genes involved in lipid metabolism. Oral isotretinoin renders the microenvironment within the pilosebaceous follicle less favourable to C. acnes by inihibiting sebum excretion and reducing the size of the intrafollicular duct. Isotretinoin also modifies monocyte chemotaxis, which results in anti-inflammatory effects.

Isotretinoin acts as a pro-drug, as it lacks the ability to bind directly to cellular retinol binding proteins or retinoid nuclear receptors (RAR and RXR), but it has at least 5 biologically important metabolites that are agonists for these receptors: 4-oxo-isotretinoin, tretinoin, 4-oxo-tretinoin, 9-cis-retinoic acid and 4-oxo-9-cis-retinoic acid.

INDICATIONS AND DERMATOLOGICAL USES

Oral isotretinoin is licenced for severe acne (conglobate, nodulocystic or at risk of permanent scarring) that has failed to respond to adequate antimicrobial and topical therapies.

Severe acne is a multidimensional entity, and early-onset acne, persistent refractory acne, hyperseborrhoea and a strong family history of acne are relevant factors that may be associated with more severe or recalcitrant disease, which can lead to scarring.

A high proportion of patients who are treated effectively with oral isotretinoin will remain clear of their acne, and early intervention in those who are starting to scar will avoid the permanent sequelae and associated burden of acne scarring. Relapse rates vary according to patient age, sex, dosage regimens and disease type. It has also been used successfully off-licence for the treatment of severe papulopustular rosacea at low dosages and for severe acneiform eruptions induced by epidermal growth factor receptor (EGRF) inhibitors. There are also reports of benefit in hidradenitis suppurativa, cutaneous lupus, pityriasis rubra pilaris, psoriasis, disorders of keratinization (Darier disease, keratodermas), photoaging and in the chemoprevention of non-melanoma skin cancer in naevoid basal cell carcinoma syndrome and xeroderma pigmentosum.

The manufacturers advise that oral isotretinoin should not be used in pre-pubertal children or children under 12 years; however, in severe cases, it has been used in this context.

DOI: 10.1201/9781003016786-22

FORMULATIONS/PRESENTATION

The dosage of medication and formulation can vary according to the manufacturer but can be summarized as follows:

- Soft capsules containing 5 mg, 10 mg, 20 mg or 40 mg isotretinoin, depending on the manufacturers.
- Excipients may include soya bean oil (refined, hydrogenated and partially hydrogenated), gelatine, beeswax and sorbitol (E420). Various colourants are present in the capsule shell. There is a rare possibility that some patients who are allergic to peanuts may suffer cross-reactivity to products containing soya protein. Therefore, it is important to assess whether the patient is tolerating soya in their diet and to consider testing them for a soya allergy if there is any doubt before starting oral isotretinoin.

DOSAGES AND SUGGESTED REGIMENS

It has been suggested that oral isotretinoin for acne at a dose of 1 mg/kg/day achieves a better clearance than 0.5 mg/kg/day over a 4-month period but leads to increased mucocutaneous effects that may not be tolerated. The European Directive therefore recommends a starting dose of 0.3–0.5 mg/kg/day, with subsequent dose adjustment according to clinical response and side effects. The use of lower dosages at the onset of treatment reduces the likelihood of an acne flare.

Clinical improvement is usually evident by 6–8 weeks, with continued improvement over several months and beyond completion of treatment. Early studies suggest that the cumulative dose is important in preventing relapse in patients with severe disease, and a cumulative dose of 120–150 mg/kg has been indicated in this context. Severe nodulocystic acne or truncal acne in males may require more prolonged therapy and daily doses above 1 mg/kg.

Alternative regimens including intermittent (1 week per month) low-to-moderate dose (0.25–0.4 mg/kg/day) have been described in the literature. These may reduce side effects and the overall cost of therapy, but drawbacks include concerns about increased durations of exposure and therefore teratogenic risk in fertile females, as well as possible increased frequency of relapse. This approach is not included in the product license.

Acne often worsens after starting oral isotretinoin and can occasionally lead to a severe flare, including acne fulminans in rare cases. If a severe flare occurs, isotretinoin should be stopped or the dose reduced, and oral prednisolone/prednisone (0.5–1 mg/kg/day) given, then tapered over 4–6 weeks. Isolated large nodules can be treated with topical or intralesional steroids. Macrocomedones should ideally be treated with cautery or hyfrecation before isotretinoin is commenced, to reduce the risk of a flare which is more likely to occur if these lesions are evident at the start of treatment.

Isotretinoin is highly lipophilic (fat-soluble) and should be taken with food (preferably food containing some fat) or a glass of milk to maximize bioavailability. A novel hard-gelatin capsule, lipid-rich formulation is available in the United States and this has demonstrated good bioavailability independent of whether it is taken with food.

Suggested treatment schedules for unusual forms of acne are listed in Table 22.1.

SYSTEMIC DISEASE

Low starting doses (0.25–0.5 mg/kg/day) and modest increases at 2-month intervals if required for a treatment duration of 24 weeks may be considered for patients with underlying medical illnesses, such as multiple sclerosis, motor neuron disease or chronic renal failure/dialysis. For those with rare diseases where there is a paucity of information, one suggested regimen is to commence isotretinoin at a dose of 20 mg per week and to increase the dose by 20 mg every subsequent week, so that the patient is taking 20 mg daily by the 7th week. The cycle can then be repeated with a twice-daily dose so that by the 14th week patients are taking 20 mg twice a day.

TABLE 22.1

Suggested Treatment Schedules for Unusual Forms of Acne

Acne fulminans	Oral prednisolone 0.5–1 mg/kg/day for 4–6 weeks
	Introduce isotretinoin 0.3–0.5 mg/kg/day after 3–4 weeks
	Continue isotretinoin for 6–8 months to reach a cumulative dose of 120 mg/kg
Pyoderma faciale	Oral prednisolone 0.5–1 mg/kg/day for 4–6 weeks
	Daily application of a very potent topical corticosteroid for 1 week
	Introduce isotretinoin 0.3–0.5 mg/kg/day after 1 week
	Continue isotretinoin for 4–6 months
Gram-negative folliculitis	Isotretinoin 0.3–0.5–1 mg/kg/day for 4–8 months

BASELINE INVESTIGATIONS AND CONSIDERATIONS

The pregnancy prevention programme (PPP) for all systemic retinoids includes:

- Pregnancy testing for all females of childbearing potential (see below).
- Establishment of effective contraception.
- Counselling regarding teratogenicity for all females.

The following are recommended in all patients:

- Full blood count (FBC) (complete blood count [CBC]).
- Liver function tests (LFTs).
- Renal indices (urea, electrolytes and creatinine).
- Fasting lipids.
- Fasting glucose or HbA1C (if family history or known diabetes).
- Assessment of mood/mental health state (see below).

SPECIAL POINT

Oral isotretinoin is a potent teratogen (see Adverse Effects and Their Management). The European Medicines Agency (EMA) has introduced a PPP to reduce the risk of pregnancy in females of childbearing potential who receive oral isotretinoin. A more stringent system (iPLEDGE) has been introduced in the United States.

All females should be carefully counselled about the risk of severe birth deformity associated with oral isotretinoin.

European guidelines stipulate effective contraception for all sexually active females, and the manufacturers specify use of one or preferably two effective contraceptive methods, including condoms or a cap plus spermicide. The effectiveness of the contraception depends on if it is user-independent, therefore considered 'highly effective,' or if it is a user-dependent form considered 'effective.' If the latter, then two forms are recommended to align with the PPP. The classification is based upon the products' 'typical-use failure rate,' which occurs due to user error, e.g. missed pills. Progesterone-only pills (POPs) are referred to as 'effective' because they have a typical-use failure rate of 9%. Parenteral progesterone-only contraception (e.g. depot injections or implants) is preferable for the PPP and classed as highly effective. They have a reported typical-use failure rate of less than 1%.

Appropriate contraception must be started at least 4 weeks before treatment, continued throughout treatment and for at least 4 weeks following cessation. The ultimate choice of specific contraceptive method is a decision made between the patient (and the parent/guardian if relevant) and their consulting physician.

US recommendations include mandatory simultaneous use of two forms of contraception, at least one of which must be highly effective (tubal ligation, partner's vasectomy, intrauterine device or implant).

A negative baseline pregnancy test should ideally be obtained within 2–3 days before menstruation, and the drug should then be started on the 2nd or 3rd day of the menstrual cycle. Due to irregular menses, this is not always possible, but a negative pregnancy test should be documented before starting isotretinoin in this situation. In Europe, no particular form of testing is specified, although any test should meet established standards, and if a home test is used, it should be CE-marked, while the US license stipulates that a negative serum or urine pregnancy test with a sensitivity of at least 25 MIU/mL must be performed within the week before starting therapy.

US monitoring requirements stipulate 2 negative pregnancy tests 30 days apart before starting therapy. Prescriptions for females who are at risk of pregnancy are limited to 30 days and are only valid for 7 days. A negative pregnancy test should be obtained before each repeat prescription, and a post-treatment pregnancy test should be performed 5 weeks after completing therapy to exclude pregnancy.

MONITORING

- Pregnancy testing (in females of childbearing potential at risk of pregnancy).
- Fasting lipids and LFTs: Serum lipids and LFTs should be checked 1 month after the start of treatment and subsequently at 3-month intervals unless more frequent monitoring is clinically indicated.
- HbA1C or blood glucose monitoring in patients with diabetes or impaired glucose tolerance should be considered.

CONTRAINDICATIONS

- Pregnancy (see below).
- Lactation.
- Uncontrolled severe hyperlipidaemia.
- Hypersensitivity to retinoids or excipients.

Patients taking isotretinoin should not donate blood during treatment and for at least 1 month after stopping therapy.

CAUTIONS

- Liver disease.
- Severe renal impairment (elimination reduced).
- Inflammatory bowel disease (IBD) (see Adverse Effects and Their Management).
- Diabetes.
- Hyperlipidaemia.
- Obesity.
- Alcohol intake and/or excess.
- Mental health issues (see Adverse Effects and Their Management).

Lower doses or more frequent monitoring may be indicated in these situations.

IMPORTANT DRUG INTERACTIONS

- Methotrexate may increase the risk of retinoid hepatotoxicity, so careful monitoring is required.
- Carbamazepine levels are reduced by concurrent intake of isotretinoin, which may lead to loss of seizure control, so carbamazepine levels need close monitoring when both drugs are taken. Isotretinoin does not interact with phenytoin.
- Heavy intake of alcohol has been noted to reduce the efficacy of isotretinoin and may increase the risk of hepatotoxicity.
- Tetracyclines should be avoided during isotretinoin therapy, as both drugs have been associated with idiopathic (benign) intracranial hypertension (formerly referred to as pseudo-tumor cerebri).
- Vitamin A intake should not exceed the recommended dietary allowance (4,000–5,000 units/d). Supplements are contraindicated due to the risk of hypervitaminosis/retinoid toxicity.
- St John's wort for depression may reduce the effectiveness of hormonal contraception and should be avoided in females who are reliant on this form of birth control.

ADVERSE EFFECTS AND THEIR MANAGEMENT

While it is highly efficacious for acne, oral isotretinoin is associated with a number of adverse effects which prescribers should be vigilant about and ensure people taking oral isotretinoin are fully informed.

- Teratogenicity: It is established that systemic isotretinoin use in early pregnancy commonly results in fetal abnormalities, including craniofacial, cardiac, thymic and CNS problems. Studies of human exposure to isotretinoin demonstrate that about 30% of infants will have major malformations. It is therefore essential that all females are carefully counseled about this risk and that the PPP is followed with adequate contraception before, during and after therapy.
- Hyperlipidaemia is common, affecting 30–40% of patients, but drug-induced increases in cholesterol or triglycerides do not usually require treatment and are dose-related, resolving within 4–8 weeks of stopping therapy. Retinoid-induced hyperlipidaemia occurs more frequently in patients with underlying predisposing factors, e.g. obesity, alcohol excess, diabetes, familial hyperlipidaemia and concomitant oral contraceptive use. It may be a predictor of idiopathic hyperlipidaemia in later life. The increased low-density (LDL) cholesterol and decreased high-density (HDL) cholesterol in patients receiving retinoids theoretically increases the possibility of accelerated atherosclerosis and ischaemic heart disease. This is a consideration in patients undergoing long-term therapy or those with pre-existing coronary artery disease.

  In the first instance, retinoid-induced increased levels of triglycerides and cholesterol can be managed by an appropriate diet and supplementation with fish oil capsules (omega-3 fatty acids). Lipid-lowering drugs may be indicated in severe hyperlipidaemia. Triglyceride levels >8 mmol/L may be associated with eruptive xanthomas and acute haemorrhagic pancreatitis. There have been isolated reports of these events in patients receiving isotretinoin, but all have occurred in the context of predisposing underlying medical problems.
- Neuropsychiatric issues: Mood changes, depression, suicidal ideation and suicide have been reported as possible adverse effects of isotretinoin. Acne itself is often associated with anxiety and depression, and it is recognised that the population being treated is vulnerable to psychosocial issues and an increasing prevalence of mental health problems. To date, no

causal relationship or mechanism of action has been firmly established to account for any neuropsychiatric changes as a result of oral isotretinoin; however, concerns have been raised that there is a possibility that in rare cases neuropsychiatric issues may arise as an idiosyncratic reaction to the drug and neurobiologists have provided hypoptheses to explain how this may occur. However, recent large populations studies deconstruct the view that a rare idiosyncratic neuropsychiatric reaction could be implicated. Patients with a history of bipolar disorder or family history of psychiatric disorders may be at increased risk. Pre-existing depression and a history of attempted suicide are not contraindications to isotretinoin, but it is important to monitor such patients carefully and to provide additional psychological or psychiatric support when required. The possibility of adverse psychiatric events should be discussed with patients and, where possible and relevant, their family. It is sensible to obtain the patient's signature to a statement in their records that they understand and have had the opportunity to discuss and consider these problems.

An inquiry about psychological symptoms, change in mood and suicidal ideation should be made at each visit. The most commonly described symptoms include fatigue, irritability, poor concentration, tearfulness, apathy and forgetfulness. The following simple screening questions can be asked. Over the past 2 weeks have you consistently:

- Felt unusually sad or fed up?
- Lost interest in things that used to interest you or gave you pleasure?
- Felt more short-tempered, agitated or irritable than previously?
- Had any abnormal thoughts of self harm, suicide or ending your life?

A number of questionnaires to assess depression are available, although not currently mandated. The PHQ-9 is a useful screening tool that asks specifically about suicidal ideation. It has had some validation in adolescents although there is no one tool that is currently recommended in this vulnerable age group. If significant depression is identified, then a psychiatric referral is indicated. Increased aggression has been identified in some male patients, and the FDA in the United States has advised clinicians to warn potential patients about this side effect. If there is any doubt, the drug must be stopped.

- Idiopathic (benign) intracranial hypertension is a rare complication of retinoid therapy. Symptoms include a persistent headache that is unresponsive to simple analgesia, nausea, vomiting and visual disturbance. Patients with these symptoms should be examined for papilloedema, and if present, they should discontinue the drug immediately and be referred for urgent neurological advice. Mild headache in the absence of other symptoms is common on starting retinoid therapy.
- Hepatotoxicity: A transient modest rise in liver transaminases is not unusual, but acute hepatitis and jaundice are rare. Abnormalities are most likely to occur in the context of heavy alcohol intake, and alcohol consumption should be minimized or stopped during isotretinoin therapy. Elevation of liver enzymes above twice the upper limit of normal should lead to discontinuation of treatment. If the elevation of liver enzymes is less than twice the upper limit of normal, the patient can be managed by more frequent monitoring, e.g. every 2 weeks.
- Mucocutaneous adverse effects, especially cheilitis and dryness of the skin and mucous membranes, affect almost all patients receiving isotretinoin and are dose-related and easily manageable with lip salves and emollients. An increase in epidermal fragility may occur, so patients should avoid wax epilation. Due to atrophy of the pilosebaceous apparatus, there is delayed wound healing, and it is advised that dermabrasion or laser resurfacing are deferred until at least 6 months after stopping isotretinoin.

Facial erythema is also common during treatment, and increased sensitivity to sunlight may occur so adequate photoprotection is required. Uncommon cutaneous effects include development of pyogenic granulomas, paronychia and diffuse alopecia. Severe skin reactions (erythema multiforme, Stevens–Johnson syndrome and toxic epidermal necrolysis) have been reported in patients taking isotretinoin, but a causal link is not established.

- Epistaxis may occur occasionally due to drying of the nasal mucosa. Petrolatum can relieve dryness, and topical anti-staphylococcal agents may also be of benefit.
- Impaired hearing has very rarely been reported in association with isotretinoin.
- Ocular adverse effects include conjunctivitis, dry eyes and decreased tolerance of contact lenses. These may be secondary to meibomian gland dysfunction and can usually be alleviated by eye drops ('artificial tears') and use of spectacles rather than lenses. A decrease in night vision has occasionally been reported and may be persistent, which is an important consideration in those whose employment is dependent on good night vision. Affected individuals should stop isotretinoin and have their serum retinol levels checked, with vitamin A supplements given if required. Pilots should not take isotretinoin and if exposed, can only return to flying after a satisfactory eye examination. Refractive eye surgery should not be undertaken within 6 months of treatment with isotretinoin, as this can result in serious sequelae such as corneal ulceration infection and loss of vision.
- Myalgia and muscle stiffness occur in a minority of patients, especially those undertaking strenuous exercise. Mildly elevated creatine phosphokinase levels have been documented in asymptomatic patients, but routine monitoring is not currently considered necessary. Patients should be advised to avoid strenuous exercise or starting fitness training while taking isotretinoin. For keen athletes, a treatment course is best started 'out of season.'
- Skeletal changes: There are reports to suggest children exposed to very high doses of isotretinoin are at risk of premature epiphyseal closure, and adults on long-term therapy (>2 years) may have an increased tendency to develop hyperostosis and other skeletal changes, including calcification of extraspinal tendons and ligaments, especially ankles, pelvis and knees and diffuse idiopathic skeletal hyperostosis (DISH)-like changes in the spine. However, the absolute risk of this is not clearly established. Further investigation with targeted x-rays may be indicated for persistent atypical musculoskeletal pain.
- Gastrointestinal: An association between isotretinoin and IBD (ulcerative colitis) has been proposed, and this has been the subject of malpractice lawsuits in the United States. However, a recent population-based French case-control study reported that isotretinoin was not associated with any increased risk of ulcerative colitis and was associated with a decreased risk of Crohn disease. Until clarified, careful counseling and collaboration with GI physicians is advised for patients with IBD before starting therapy. Patients should be advised to stop treatment immediately and seek urgent medical attention if they develop severe GI symptoms.
- Sexual dysfunction: Recent concerns have been raised about sexual dysfunction occurring during and after treatment with oral isotretinoin. A routine EU review in 2017 showed that some patients taking isotretinoin had reported sexual dysfunction/adverse effects, including erectile dysfunction and decreased libido. One possible mechanism for this effect may be through a reduction in plasma testosterone levels. Advice to healthcare professionals following the review was to be aware of reports of sexual side effects, including erectile dysfunction and decreased libido, in patients taking oral isotretinoin. The exact incidence of these adverse reactions is unknown, but considering the number of patients taking oral isotretinoin, the review suggested that reports are understood to be rare.

USE IN SPECIAL SITUATIONS

PREGNANCY AND PRE-CONCEPTION

Isotretinoin was formerly FDA Category X and is absolutely contraindicated in pregnancy. In addition, females should not become pregnant within at least 1 month of discontinuing treatment (see Special Point). There is no known effect on fertility. There is no evidence of impaired fertility or mutagenic risk in males who receive isotretinoin.

LACTATION

Isotretinoin is excreted in breast milk and should not be taken by females who are breastfeeding.

CHILDREN

Isotretinoin does not have a license for use in children under the age of 12 years. However, it has been used in severe nodular acne in early childhood (infantile acne) in cases that are unresponsive to conventional therapy, and there is a risk of scarring. In addition, some patients in the early stages of puberty with marked seborrhoea may fail to respond to conventional therapy, and isotretinoin may be considered particularly if the patient is at risk of scarring.

ESSENTIAL PATIENT INFORMATION

Patients should be warned of the possible side effects and given an up-to-date patient information leaflet. The British Association of Dermatologists has a comprehensive patient information leaflet available for use, and when the medication is prescribed and dispensed, the patient and family should be encouraged to read the package insert as provided by the drug manufacturer.

Females should be provided with specific information on teratogenicity and contraception and the requirements of the PPP. Information should be provided on the usual frequency of follow-up visits, monitoring requirements and the contact details of relevant nursing or medical staff, should patients or their family have concerns about serious adverse effects.

FURTHER READING

Eichenfield LF, Krakowski AC, Piggott C, Del Rosso J, Baldwin H, Friedlander SF, Levy M, Lucky A, Mancini AJ, Orlow SJ, Yan AC, Vaux KK, Webster G, Zaenglein AL, Thiboutot DM; American Acne and Rosacea Society. Evidence-based recommendations for the diagnosis and treatment of pediatric acne. Pediatrics. 2013 May;131 Suppl 3:S163–86. doi: 10.1542/peds.2013-0490B. PMID: 23637225.

EMA/254364/2018. Pharmacovigilance Risk Assessment Committee (PRAC). Assessment report. Referral under Article 31 of Directive 2001/83/EC.

Goodfield MJD, Cox NH, Bowser A, et al. Advice on the safe introduction and continued use of isotretinoin in acne in the UK 2010. Br J Dermatol. 2010;162:1172–9.

Lee SY, Jamal MM, Nguyen ET, et al. Does exposure to isotretinoin increase the risk for the development of inflammatory bowel disease? A meta-analysis. Eur J Gastroenterol Hepatol. 2016 Feb.;28(2):210–6.

Nast A, Dréno B, Bettoli V, et al. European evidence-based (S3) guideline for the treatment of acne – update 2016 – short version. J Eur Acad Dermatol Venereol. 2016 Aug;30(8):1261–8. doi: 10.1111/jdv.13776. PMID: 27514932.

Thiboutot D, Golnick H, Bettoli V, et al. New insights into management of acne: An update from the Global Alliance to Improve Outcomes in Acne group. J Am Acad Dermatol. 2009;20(7):773–6.

23 Ivermectin

Jonathan Kentley and L. Claire Fuller

CLASSIFICATION AND MODE OF ACTION

Ivermectin is a semisynthetic derivative of the avermectins, a class of broad-spectrum anti-parasitic macrocyclic lactones isolated from Streptomyces avermitili. It has a similar chemical structure to macrolide antibiotics. Ivermectin selectively binds to γ-aminobutyric acid (GABA)-gated chloride channels found in the invertebrate nerve and muscle cells, resulting in paralysis and death of arthropods and insects. This action is specific to invertebrates, as GABA is not involved in human peripheral neurotransmission. At therapeutic doses, ivermectin does not penetrate the blood–brain barrier of vertebrates, and therefore does not enter the central nervous system (CNS) due to the presence of P-glycoprotein (except in collie dogs, which have a variant of P-glycoprotein). This explains the drug's high efficacy and tolerability in humans. High concentrations of ivermectin can overcome the blood–brain barrier and bind to GABA receptors, causing toxicity with hypotension, respiratory failure, coma and death. Following absorption, the drug undergoes hepatic metabolism via cytochrome P450 3A4, and metabolites are slowly excreted in the faeces.

Ivermectin has been a game changer for global health. Seven of the World Health Organization (WHO)-classified neglected tropical diseases are controlled by a single intervention with ivermectin, costing around US $0.5.

INDICATIONS AND DERMATOLOGICAL USES

Ivermectin is an effective treatment for a range of parasitic infections affecting the skin, as well as other organ systems. Oral ivermectin is licensed in the United States for the treatment of strongyloidiasis and onchocerciasis, and in France for strongyloidiasis and scabies. It is not licensed in the UK but may be used for the above infections, and efficacy has also been reported in the treatment of pediculosis, demodicosis, cutaneous larva migrans, myiasis and Toxocara, with reduction of the parasite burden in Loiasis. It has attracted wider attention recently as a potential treatment or prophylactic agent for COVID-19 infection.

LARVA MIGRANS

Cutaneous larva migrans (creeping eruption), caused by epidermal penetration and migration of the larvae of animal hookworms, occurs most commonly in tropical and subtropical regions. The rash manifests as an intensely pruritic erythematous, serpiginous, migratory eruption. Infection is self-limiting and will usually resolve without treatment.

SCABIES

Scabies is a major public health problem worldwide. Poor hygiene, overcrowding and poverty are major factors in treatment failure and reinfestation. Secondary impetiginization can lead to glomerulonephritis, with long-term morbidity, especially in poor communities. Severe, crusted or resistant scabies and institutional outbreaks are the main indication for oral ivermectin in developed countries.

DOI: 10.1201/9781003016786-23

STRONGYLOIDIASIS

Strongyloidiasis, caused by the intestinal nematode Strongyloides stercoralis, is prevalent in tropical and subtropical countries. In the UK, it is predominantly seen in migrants and returning travellers. Positive serology has been documented in between 23–65% of individuals migrating from Africa and southeast Asia to North America. Chronic infection is often asymptomatic, but patients may present with gastrointestinal disturbance, and severe disseminated disease may follow immunosuppression, such as systemic corticosteroid therapy. In patients with a history of travel to areas endemic for strongyloidiasis and a peripheral eosinophilia, screening investigation with three stool samples and S. sterocoralis enzyme-linked immunosorbent assay should be considered before starting oral corticosteroids.

LYMPHATIC FILARIASIS

Ivermectin is the drug of choice for lymphatic filariasis. Wucheria bancrofti causes 90% of infections in tropical regions. Chronic infection of the lymphatic system, especially in the extremities or male genitalia, may lead to severe lymphoedema and hydrocele with major long-term disability. WHO launched a Global Elimination Programme in 2000 involving annual preventative chemotherapy (mass drug administration [MDA]) in at-risk populations for at least 5 years in order to break community transmission cycles.

ONCHOCERCIASIS

Ivermectin is also the drug of choice for onchocerciasis caused by the parasitic worm Onchocerca volvulus, which is endemic in sub-Saharan Africa. Symptoms including severe pruritus, dermatitis, lichenification, depigmentation (leopard skin) and severe visual impairment, including blindness ('African river blindness'). Diagnosis is historically made with small biopsies (skin snips) and clinical assessment.

FORMULATIONS/PRESENTATION

- Ivermectin 3 mg tablets – may be cut or crushed. (Other tablet sizes are available globally.) As ivermectin is an unlicensed medical product in the UK, it is only available on a named-patient basis from 'special order' manufacturers or imported. If ivermectin is not already available on the NHS Trust's formulary, a request and authorisation application may be required, with references supporting its use in the condition being treated. The UK's Medicines and Healthcare Products Regulatory Agency (MHRA) website provides details of manufacturers and wholesalers licensed to distribute medicines. Quality assurance protocols followed by UK NHS Trusts may prolong the time for procurement.
    The cost of oral ivermectin varies considerably (more than 100-fold) from one country to another according to licensing regulations.
- A 1% cream formulation of Ivermectin is approved for treatment of papulopustular rosacea.

DOSAGES AND SUGGESTED REGIMENS

Ivermectin is usually taken as a single oral dose of 200 micrograms/kg. Repeat dosing may be required in some instances. Bioavailability is increased when consumed with a high-fat meal.
    The dosage guidelines according to body weight are shown in Table 23.1.

LARVA MIGRANS

A single dose of ivermectin 200 μg/kg is highly effective for treatment.

TABLE 23.1

Dosage Guidelines for Ivermectin

Body Weight (kg)	Single Oral Dose
15–24	1 × 3 mg tablet
25–35	2 × 3 mg tablets
36–50	3 × 3 mg tablets
51–65	4 × 3 mg tablets
66–79	5 × 3 mg tablets
≥=80	Calculate as 200 µg/kg

SCABIES

An initial dose of 200 µg/kg should be followed with a second dose after 7–14 days due to ivermectin's limited ovicidal activity. Use of an additional topical agent may improve clearance.

Public Health England advises that the health protection team is informed of institutional outbreaks to ensure a timely, coordinated response. Clothes, towel and linens should be laundered, and soft furnishings should be kept out of use for 24 hours following treatment. Residents with crusted scabies are highly contagious and require isolation. Synchronous treatment of all exposed cases with permethrin 5% cream on day 0 and repeated treatment of proven and doubtful cases on days 1 and 14 have been shown to be effective, with oral ivermectin used in the treatment of selected cases (such as crusted scabies).

WHO recommends oral ivermectin 200 µg/kg, repeated after 7 days for treatment and prophylaxis during institutional outbreaks. Multiple doses may be required to treat crusted scabies, e.g. 3 doses (days 1, 2 and 8), 5 doses (days 1, 2, 8, 9 and 15) or 7 doses (days 1, 2, 8, 9, 15, 22 and 29) depending on the severity of infection.

STRONGYLOIDIASIS

The suggested dosing of ivermectin is 200 µg/kg daily for 2 consecutive days.

A 2016 Cochrane review concluded that treatment of patients with ivermectin was more effective than treatment with albendazole and equally efficacious as thiabendazole. This study also found that treatment with two 200 µg/kg doses was not associated with higher cure rates than a single dose.

LYMPHATIC FILARIASIS

Treatment is with 1 dose of ivermectin 200 µg/kg. When given as part of MDA, ivermectin 150 µg/kg is given with 6 mg/kg diethylcarbamazine citrate (DEC) +/– 400 mg albendazole in areas that are also endemic for onchocerciasis.

ONCHOCERCIASIS

Treatment is with a single dose of 150 µg/kg, repeated at intervals of 6–12 months. Ivermectin does not kill adult worms, and prolonged treatment may be required until the transmission chain is interrupted. WHO currently recommends treatment at least annually for between 10–15 years.

BASELINE INVESTIGATIONS AND CONSIDERATIONS

Relevant diagnostic investigations should be performed. For further advice, the reader is advised to consult texts on tropical medicine.

MONITORING

- No routine blood monitoring is required.
- Treatment response is usually assessed clinically.

CONTRAINDICATION

- Pregnancy (see Use in Special Situations).

CAUTIONS

- Caution is advised in severe hepatic disease.
- See Neurotoxicity.

IMPORTANT DRUG INTERACTIONS

As ivermectin is typically administered as a single dose, interactions are unlikely to be clinically relevant. However, ivermectin may interact with coumarin anticoagulants. Rifampicin and phenobarbital enhance CYP3A4 activity and so may reduce efficacy.

ADVERSE EFFECTS AND THEIR MANAGEMENT

Ivermectin is widely used globally and is well-tolerated, with few reported significant adverse effects. Gastrointestinal symptoms and headaches are infrequent and self-limiting.

Pruritus may worsen temporarily following treatment of scabies. This should not be confused with treatment failure or an adverse reaction to the drug.

Systemic inflammatory and anaphylactoid reactions with fever, myalgia, malaise and hypotension have occasionally been reported in patients with helminth infection. Lethargy, confusion and coma have been reported in patients treated for Loa loa. Systemic inflammatory reactions consisting of fever, urticaria, lymphadenopathy, arthralgia and cardiovascular instability have been reported rarely in patients treated for onchocerciasis ('Mazzoti reactions'). These occur most frequently in patients with a high microfilarial load following treatment with DEC but have also been observed with ivermectin. In all of these cases, reactions have been attributed to the release of parasite antigens following their death, rather than ivermectin itself.

Neurotoxicity appears to be very rare except when ivermectin is used for treatment of Loiasis. Clinicians may be reluctant to treat certain patient groups, especially older people and young children, with oral ivermectin due to concerns about CNS toxicity, but this has never been fully substantiated in human studies or extensive post-marketing surveillance. It has been speculated that CNS toxicity may occur due to polymorphisms in the MDR1 gene, which encodes P-glycoprotein.

USE IN SPECIAL SITUATIONS

PREGNANCY AND PRE-CONCEPTION

Ivermectin was formerly FDA Category C and is not recommended in pregnancy due to toxicity observed in animal studies. A meta-analysis of 899 pregnancy outcomes did not identify any neonatal or maternal harm, but it remained unclear whether ivermectin during pregnancy affected the rate of spontaneous abortions, stillbirths or congenital abnormalities.

Although limited data show that excretion of ivermectin is at low levels in breast milk (<1% of the weight-adjusted maternal dose), it is not recommended during lactation.

Historically, treatment with oral ivermectin has not been recommended in children under the age of 5 or those weighing under 15 kg. However, a recent study of 170 children weighing <15 kg observed only 7 mild adverse events, suggesting that ivermectin is safe to use in this situation. It has also been reported to be a safe and effective treatment in infants with recalcitrant or relapsing scabies.

ESSENTIAL PATIENT INFORMATION

The unlicensed nature of ivermectin should be explained to the patient with information about risks and benefits in order to obtain their informed consent to treatment. This should be documented in their medical records.

FURTHER READING

Campillo JT, Boussinesq M, Bertout S, et al. Serious adverse reactions associated with ivermectin: A systematic pharmacovigilance study in sub-Saharan Africa and in the rest of the world. PLOS Negl Trop Dis 2021;15(4):e0009354.

Dhana A, Yen H, Okhovat JP, et al. Ivermectin versus permethrin in the treatment of scabies: A systematic review and meta-analysis of randomized controlled trials. J Am Acad Dermatol. 2018;78(1):194–8.

Dourmishev AL, Dourmishev LA, Schwartz RA. Ivermectin: Pharmacology and application in dermatology. Int J Dermatol. 2005;44(12):981–8.

Nicolas P, Maia MF, Bassat Q, et al. Safety of oral ivermectin during pregnancy: A systematic review and meta-analysis. Lancet Glob Health. 2020 Jan;8(1):e92–e100.

Pion SD, Tchatchueng-Mbougua JB, Chesnais CB, et al. Effect of a single standard dose (150–200 mug/kg) of ivermectin on Loa loa microfilaremia: Systematic review and meta-analysis. Open Forum Infect Dis. 2019;6(4):ofz019.

Taylor MJ, Hoerauf A, Bockarie M. Lymphatic filariasis and onchocerciasis. Lancet. 2010;376(9747):1175–85.

24 Intravenous Immunoglobulin

Derrick Phillips

CLASSIFICATION AND MODE OF ACTION

Immunoglobulin (Ig) preparations, derived from human blood, are important biological agents. They were first used to treat immune deficiency states in 1952. Intravenous immunoglobulin (IVIg) is purified from the pooled human plasma of 3,000–10,000 healthy donors. Pooling provides the entire array of antibodies normally present in healthy immunocompetent individuals. Since there are large numbers of donors, there is a possibility of diluting rare antibodies that may be present in low concentration.

The manufacturing process is complex and includes important steps such as careful donor selection, screening of plasma samples for infectious agents and the use of modern viral inactivation techniques in order to optimize safety. Standards are set by various regulatory agencies, including the Food and Drug Administration (FDA), European Medicines Agency (EMA) and the World Health Organization (WHO).

Various modifications have been applied to the original technique of obtaining purified commercial IVIg by ethanolic fractionation of plasma.

A novel purification process combining caprylate precipitation, viral inactivation and double anion exchange chromatography has been developed. This procedure yields a highly purified product in a shorter time and with minimal protein denaturation.

A single donation of whole blood (500 mL) yields approximately 15 mL of plasma proteins, of which only 2–3 mL is highly concentrated pure gammaglobulin. IVIg contains relatively pure concentrate of IgG with a distribution of IgG subclasses corresponding to that of normal serum. The product may also contain variable amounts of albumin, IgA, IgM, IgE, sugars, salts, solvents, detergents and buffers. These may affect the tolerability of IVIg infusions, especially the sugar, salt and/or IgA content. The powder product that has a longer shelf life is dissolved in sucrose. The sucrose content affects the osmotic load of the preparation and can increase the risk of acute renal failure in predisposed individuals.

Within human antibody classes, IgG antibodies have the most potent proinflammatory potential. They play a critical role in driving autoimmune diseases but, paradoxically, can also effectively treat them. The exact mechanism of action of IVIg is unclear and may differ in different diseases. Proposed actions include functional blockade of Fc receptors, complement inhibition, enhanced steroid sensitivity, modulation of dendritic cell properties, autoantibody neutralization and inhibition of autoantibody production, modulation of cytokine and cytokine antagonist production, signalling through the inhibitory Fc receptor (Fc gamma RIIB) and inhibition of keratinocyte apoptosis due to blockade of the Fas death receptor (CD95) by anti-Fas antibodies (the suspected mechanism of action in Kawasaki disease). In treating any disease, more than one mechanism may operate. It is possible that in diseases that have multiple stages, different mechanisms may play an important role at different stages.

INDICATIONS AND DERMATOLOGICAL USES

Human normal immunoglobulin (HNIG) is given IM as protection against viral infections (hepatitis A, measles and rubella). HNIG is also used as replacement therapy for patients with congenital agammaglobulinaemia/hypogammaglobulinaemia, and for the prophylaxis of infection following bone marrow transplantation and in children with human immunodeficiency virus (HIV) infection.

IVIg is used to treat various autoimmune and infectious diseases, e.g. idiopathic (immune) thrombocytopenic purpura (ITP) and Kawasaki disease. Other indications include chronic inflammatory demyelinating polyneuropathy (CIDP) and the acute form of the disease, Guillan–Barré

 DOI: 10.1201/9781003016786-24

syndrome. More recently, IVIg was investigated as a therapeutic option for treating severe acute respiratory syndrome coronavirus 2 (SARS-CoV-2). In dermatology, high-dose IVIg has been used with promising results for the treatment of multiple conditions. However, adult dermatomyositis is the only indication approved by the FDA.

DERMATOMYOSITIS

This is the dermatological disease with the highest level of evidence for treatment with IVIg. Multiple case reports, case series and, recently, a double-blind, randomized, placebo-controlled phase III study have demonstrated the efficacy of high-dose IVIg in patients with dermatomyositis. This has culminated in FDA approval of OCTAGAM® 10% for this indication. All severe forms of dermatomyositis and/or polymyositis represent potential indications for the use of IVIg. However, it is not effective as monotherapy and should be used as adjuvant therapy (together with corticosteroids with or without immunosuppressants). IVIg therapy is usually considered as a second-line therapy when steroids have failed or are contraindicated. However, in patients with a severe progressive course, severe myolysis or paralysis, initial treatment with IVIg may be justified. Treatment should be administered for a 6-month period in order to determine efficacy. A total dose of 2 g/kg/month is generally recommended and should be infused over a period of 2–5 days. Usually, about 3–4 treatment cycles are required at monthly intervals before achieving a significant improvement.

AUTOIMMUNE BLISTERING DISEASES

Adjuvant therapy with IVIg may be considered for all severe, treatment-resistant forms of autoimmune blistering disease. Good results have been reported for the treatment of pemphigus vulgaris, pemphigus foliaceus, mucous membrane pemphigoid and epidermolysis bullosa acquisita; IVIg may warrant consideration in severe bullous pemphigoid, linear IgA disease and paraneoplastic pemphigus. In all these cases, IVIg therapy should be used as a second-line agent after an adequate trial of systemic steroids and other immunosuppressive agents, such as azathioprine or mycophenolate mofetil. As for dermatomyositis, IVIg appears to have greater efficacy as adjunctive therapy rather than monotherapy, and treatment should therefore be combined with systemic corticosteroids with or without other immunosuppressive agents. IVIg may be used in combination with Rituximab (anti-CD20 biologic) in severe cases of pemphigus vulgaris. IVIg should be administered for a period of 3–6 months in order to assess its efficacy. A total dose of 2 g/kg/month is generally recommended. It could be infused over a period of 2–5 days or 2–3 days, depending on total dose required and the general health of the patient. Slow infusion of 4–5 hours or longer reduces the incidence of infusion-related side effects.

Guidelines for the indications, dosage, frequency of administration and monitoring of IVIg were established by a large panel of experts on blistering diseases from the United States, Canada and Europe, in a consensus statement.

TOXIC EPIDERMAL NECROLYSIS

Although the early administration of IVIg in toxic epidermal necrolysis (TEN) was reported to reverse the progression of skin disease with a favourable (potentially life-saving) outcome, some controversy remains about its effectiveness. Randomized controlled trials are needed to provide a definitive answer. A systematic review and meta-analysis in 2021 found that the combination of IVIg and corticosteroids resulted in fewer deaths than predicted by the SCORTEN. However, the strength of the evidence was not sufficient to recommend widespread use.

In the treatment of TEN, IVIg may be given as monotherapy or in combination with systemic corticosteroids. A total dose of 3–4 g/kg is generally recommended and should be infused in divided doses over a period of 3–5 days.

SYSTEMIC VASCULITIS

Initial treatment usually consists of high-dose corticosteroids with or without immunosuppressive agents such as cyclophosphamide. In patients who fail to respond, IVIg may be included as a therapeutic option. Benefit has been reported in Wegener's granulomatosis, Churg–Strauss vasculitis, polyarteritis nodosa, microscopic polyangitis, IgA-associated vasculitis and catastrophic antiphospholipid syndrome. Only in Kawasaki syndrome is the use of IVIg recommended as first-line treatment. However, the early use of IVIg in Wegener's granulomatosis or in haemorrhagic necrotizing vasculitis of the skin may prevent massive tissue destruction. The recommended dose for the treatment of Kawasaki syndrome in children is 2 g/kg (as a bolus infusion) in combination with anti-inflammatory doses of acetylsalicylic acid (aspirin).

Other dermatoses that have been reported to improve with the use of IVIg include autoimmune chronic urticaria, severe atopic dermatitis, pyoderma gangrenosum, systemic lupus erythematosus (SLE) and other collagen vascular diseases, pretibial myxedema and scleromyxedema. The role of IVIg in the management of these diseases (with the exception of dermatomyositis) awaits clarification by double-blind, placebo-controlled trials. Although relatively safe compared with immunosuppressive agents, the high cost, combined with the logistical issues involved in its administration, has limited the use of IVIg in dermatological diseases.

FORMULATIONS/PRESENTATION

Different preparations of IVIg for IV administration exist, depending on the manufacturer. Lyophilized formulations have to be reconstituted with normal saline, water for injection or 5% dextrose in water just before treatment to achieve concentrations of 3–12%. Liquid preparations are also available, reducing the time required for reconstitution and limiting the risk of error. Most liquid preparations are available in concentrations of 5% (0.05 g/mL or 1 g/20 mL) or 10% (0.1 g/mL or 1 g/10 mL).

The sugar, sodium, IgA, osmolarity and pH of IVIg vary according to manufacturer and may influence the rate of adverse effects.

In the United Kingdom, it is becoming increasingly difficult to prescribe IVIg in the National Health Service (NHS). The number of conditions for which treatment with IVIg will be funded has reduced. At the time of publication, IVIg will no longer be available for treatment of pyoderma gangrenosum or Stevens Johnson Syndrome/TEN in the NHS.

DOSAGES AND SUGGESTED REGIMENS

The doses and regimens of high-dose IVIg have varied in different studies. A total dose of 2 g/kg body weight at monthly intervals given over 2, 3 or 5 consecutive days is recommended. The recommended total dose for treatment of TEN is 3–4 g/kg administered on 3–5 consecutive days. The speed of the infusion is carefully monitored and adjusted to reduce the risk of adverse events. As the half-life of IVIg after IV infusion is approximately 2–3 weeks, infusions are initially administered at monthly intervals. After 6 months, a gradual increase to 6-week intervals can be considered if there is a satisfactory response. It is usual to prescribe only one treatment cycle of IVIg for TEN and Kawasaki disease.

BASELINE INVESTIGATIONS AND CONSIDERATIONS

- Full blood count (FBC) (complete blood count [CBC]).
- Urea, electrolytes and creatinine.
- Liver function tests (LFTs).
- Hepatitis B and C serology.
- Antinuclear antibody, rheumatoid factor +/– cryoglobulins.
- Quantitative serum immunoglobulins (IgG, IgM and IgA; if IgA is low or absent, measure anti-IgA antibodies).

MONITORING

- During infusion, vital signs (blood pressure [BP], heart rate and temperature) should be monitored every 15–30 minutes, particularly during the initial infusion and throughout the first course of therapy.
- Post-infusion, FBC should be measured frequently (daily at first, then at least at monthly intervals) for the rare occurrence of Coombs-positive haemolytic anaemia (reticulocyte count, haptoglobin) and neutropenia. Renal indices and LFTs should be checked on day 2 or 3 of treatment.

CONTRAINDICATIONS

- Previous anaphylaxis or severe systemic response to Ig preparations.
- Rapidly progressive renal failure.
- Selective IgA deficiency with antibodies to IgA is cited by most manufacturers as a contraindication to their product. However, an IgA depleted preparation of IVIg may be used with caution. Selective IgA deficiency occurs in approximately 1 in 700 of the population, so IgA should be measured before therapy.
- Recent or imminent live virus vaccination (relative contraindication) as the immune response may be affected.

CAUTIONS

- Impaired renal function or concurrent nephrotoxic drug therapy.
- Patients at increased risk of thromboembolism (including obesity, prolonged immobilization, hyperviscosity, cryoglobulinaemia or impaired cardiac function).
- History of SLE and rheumatoid arthritis.
- History of migraine, as IVIg may trigger a migraine attack.
- Diabetes mellitus.
- Sepsis.
- Older individuals; in patients over 65 years of age, the recommended dose should not be exceeded. The infusions should be administered at a very slow rate.

IMPORTANT DRUG INTERACTIONS

No drug interactions have been reported to date with IVIg products.

- Nephrotoxic drugs should be used with great caution and in consultation with the treating physician during IVIg therapy. This is emphasized to minimize the risk of causing acute renal failure.
- Live virus vaccines, such as measles, mumps and rubella, should not be given for 12 days before or 3 months after IVIg, as the product may contain antibodies which can interact with these vaccines.

ADVERSE EFFECTS AND THEIR MANAGEMENT

With the current careful selection of plasma donors and advances in the manufacturing and purification of IVIg products, the rate of adverse events associated with IVIg infusion has decreased considerably. Most reactions are mild and self-limiting or easy to treat. Frequently, they occur during the first cycle and often during the first few hours of the infusion.

- Headache, fever, chills, nausea, vomiting, dizziness, flu-like symptoms, arthralgia, migraine, hypotension and urticarial rash are some of the most common side effects.

These can usually be overcome by reducing the rate of infusion, administering non-steroidal anti-inflammatory drugs (NSAIDs), acetaminophen, corticosteroids and/or antihistamines before beginning the infusion.

The incidence of adverse events is reported by the manufacturers to be in the range of 1–15% and is usually less than 5% but may be higher in hypogammaglobulinaemic patients. The management of specific adverse events is shown in Table 24.1.

- Although rare, severe adverse events can also occur, especially in patients with co-morbidities or risk factors. Therefore, it is important to obtain a complete medical history and to perform a thorough medical evaluation before initiation of IVIg therapy. Adverse events include aseptic meningitis, acute renal failure, deep venous thrombosis and/or pulmonary embolism, myocardial infarction, stroke and anaphylactic shock.

In practice, when prescribing IVIg, it is important to consider underlying risk factors and choose a brand of IVIg with a suitable composition. For example, in older patients or those with renal dysfunction, use a sugar-free preparation. Despite the absence of comparative data regarding the

---

TABLE 24.1
Adverse Effects of IVIg Therapy and Their Management

Minor Adverse Events	Management
Headache	Paracetamol (acetaminophen)/codeine
	Slow rate of infusion
Fever, chills, nausea, vomiting, dizziness, flu-like symptoms, arthralgias, sore throat	Paracetamol (acetaminophen)
	Slow rate of infusion
Migraine	Bed rest
	Consider prophylaxis 2 days prior, during and 2 days post-therapy with propranolol, or
	Whichever drug has worked in the past, for future infusions
Hypotension/hypertension	Slow rate of infusion
Phlebitis at infusion site	Change infusion site
Transient elevation of serum creatinine	Observe
Transient elevation of liver enzymes	Observe
Transient urticarial eruption	Oral antihistamines
Vesicular hand/foot and generalized eczema	Topical corticosteroids

Severe Adverse Events (Rare)	Management
Aseptic meningitis	Bed rest
	Paracetamol (acetaminophen)/codeine/stronger analgesia. For future infusions: Pre-medicate with cetirizine, encourage high oral intake of fluids, infuse at a slow rate and the most dilute solution available
	Check if patient or family has a history of migraines
Acute renal failure	Slow rate, low IVIg concentration, sucrose-free preparations
	Supportive haemodialysis
Anaphylactic shock	Intravenous hydrocortisone + antihistamines, intravenous fluids +/– adrenaline
Deep venous thrombosis (DVT)/pulmonary embolism (PE)	Stop infusion
	Specific treatment of DVT or PE
	Consult vascular surgeon to prevent a future recurrence
Myocardial infarction (MI)	Stop infusion
	Specific treatment of MI
Transfusion-related acute lung injury (TRALI)	Stop infusion
	Ventilatory support

incidence of side effects among different IVIg brands, the variable content of sugar, sodium, IgA, pH and osmolarity may influence the occurrence of side effects. Moreover, the rate of infusion, concentration and total volume infused are important contributing factors.

USE IN SPECIAL SITUATIONS

PREGNANCY

There are no animal data regarding the use of IVIg in pregnancy. Manufacturers recommend that IVIg be administered in pregnancy only if clearly needed. IVIg has been safely used in pregnant patients with pemphigus vulgaris, with positive outcomes. Benefits have been shown in a number of other conditions in pregnancy, including antiphospholipid syndrome with recurrent spontaneous abortions, ITP and pemphigus gestationis. However, IVIg crosses the placenta, and there have been isolated reports of neonatal haemolysis. The potential for transmission of infectious agents remains a concern.

LACTATION

The proteins in IVIg are likely to be excreted in breast milk without having an adverse effect on the breastfed infant. However, there is no information regarding the safety of IVIg during lactation.

CHILDREN

High-dose IVIg has been used for non-dermatological diseases in children, such as ITP and Kawasaki syndrome.

ESSENTIAL PATIENT INFORMATION

Patients should be informed that the product is prepared from human blood or plasma, and the transmission of infectious agents (in particular, currently unrecognized ones) cannot be excluded.

With acknowledgement to Francisco Kerdel and Luis Dehesa, who contributed this chapter to the previous edition.

FURTHER READING

Aggarwal R, Charles-Schoeman C, Schessl J, et al. Prospective, double blind, randomized, placebo-controlled, phase III study evaluating efficacy and safety of OCTAGAM 10% in patients with dermatomyositis ('ProDERM study'). Medicine. 2021;100(1):e23677.

Ahmed AR, Dahl MV. Consensus statement on the use of intravenous immunoglobulin therapy in the treatment of autoimmune mucocutaneous blistering diseases. Arch Dermatol. 2003;139:1051–9.

Eleftheriou D, Levin M, Shingadia D, et al. Management of Kawasaki disease. Arch Dis Child. 2014;99(1):74–83.

Guo Y, Tian X, Wang X, Xiao Z. Adverse effects of immunoglobulin therapy. Front Immuno. 2018;9:1299.

Harman KE, Brown D, Exton LS, et al. British Association of Dermatologists' guidelines for the management of pemphigus vulgaris 2017. Brit J Dermatol. 2017;177:1170–1201.

Huang YC, Li YC, Chen TJ. The efficacy of intravenous immunoblobulin for the treatment of toxic epidermal necrolysis: A systematic review and meta-analysis. Brit J Dermatol. 2012;167:424–32.

Torres-Navarro I, Briz-Redón Á, Botella-Estrada R. Systemic therapies for Stevens-Johnson syndrome and toxic epidermal necrolysis: A SCORTEN-based systematic review and meta-analysis. J Eur Acad Dermatol Venereol. 2021;35(1):159–71.

25 Janus Kinase (JAK) Inhibitors

Courtney E. Heron, Lindsay C. Strowd and Steven R. Feldman

CLASSIFICATION AND MODE OF ACTION

Abrocitinib, baricitinib and upadacitinib are orally available reversible inhibitors of tyrosine protein kinases within the Janus kinase (JAK) pathway, a pathway involved in the growth, development, differentiation and survival of immune and hematopoietic cells. Oral JAK inhibitors have so far been most commonly used for the treatment of rheumatoid arthritis (RA). Baricitinib has been approved for this indication internationally.

Baricitinib potently blocks JAK1 and JAK2 (Figure 25.1), resulting in a modification of gene transcription via alteration of the signal transducers and activators of the transcription (STAT) pathway and downstream cytokine signalling, ultimately decreasing inflammation via inhibition of inflammatory cytokines and potentially reducing proliferation of neoplastic cells. Inhibition of JAK1 and JAK2 decreases the proinflammatory signalling associated with interleukin (IL)-6, IL-12, IL-23, and interferon gamma (IFN-γ). Abrocitinib and upadacitinib have increased selectivity for JAK1 vs. JAK2, JAK3 and tyrosine kinase 2, with the intention of increased safety and efficacy.

Recent clinical trials have evaluated the use of these drugs for the treatment of atopic dermatitis (AD), with promising results.

INDICATIONS AND DERMATOLOGICAL USES

- In 2020, the European Medicines Agency (EMA) recommended approval of baricitinib for adult patients with moderate-to-severe AD. Approval by the National Institute for Health and Care Excellence (NICE) followed in 2021 for patients who had failed to respond to at least one systemic immunosuppressant, such as ciclosporin, methotrexate, azathioprine or mycophenolate mofetil, or those not suitable to take those medications.
- Upadacitinib was approved by the EMA in 2021 for treatment of moderate-to-severe AD in adults and children aged 12 and over who were candidates for systemic therapy. Abrocitinib was subsequently approved by the EMA in late 2021 for use in adults.
- In January 2022, the FDA approved abrocitinib for moderate-to-severe AD in adults and upadacitinib for this indication in adults and children aged 12 and above.
- Baricitinib, used alone or in combination with topical corticosteroids, is an efficacious therapy for AD treatment; nearly two thirds of patients being treated with baricitinib in combination with topical corticosteroids achieve 50% lesion clearance after 16 weeks of treatment, and the addition of baricitinib to topical corticosteroids increases treatment efficacy by over 20% compared with treatment with topical corticosteroids alone. Abrocitinib and upadacitinib are also efficacious and work quickly; 200 mg dosing of abrocitinib was superior to dupilumab in itch reduction at two weeks, with no significant difference in efficacy between either 100 or 200 mg abrocitinib and dupilumab at 16 weeks.
- The US FDA approved Olumiant (baricitinib) oral tablets to treat adult patients with severe alopecia areata in June 2022. There has also been good clinical evidence of efficacy in psoriasis.
- Other JAK inhibitors, including tofacitinib, ruxolitinib, itacitinib and solcitinib, have been studied in a variety of dermatological conditions and systemic conditions with dermatological manifestations, including alopecia areata, AD, dermatomyositis, graft versus host disease, lupus erythematosus with skin involvement, lichen planopilaris, psoriasis, psoriatic arthritis, Sjogren syndrome, systemic sclerosis, sarcoidosis and vitiligo.

DOI: 10.1201/9781003016786-25

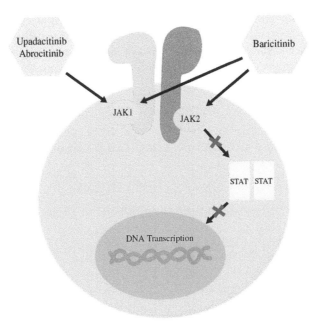

FIGURE 25.1   Baricitinib inhibits JAK1 and JAK2. Abrocitinib and upadacitinib have increased selectivity for JAK1. JAK inhibition prevents the phosphorylation and subsequent activation of STATs, ultimately hindering DNA transcription and decreasing the proinflammatory cytokine signalling associated with IL-6, IL-12, IL-23 and IFN-γ. DNA, deoxyribonucleic acid; IFN-γ, interferon gamma; IL, interleukin; JAK, Janus kinase.

FORMULATIONS/PRESENTATION

- Baricitinib is available as 1 mg, 2 mg and 4 mg (Europe only) tablets for oral use.
- Upadacitinib is available as 15 mg and 30 mg prolonged-release tablets in both the United States and Europe.
- Abrocitinib is available as 50 mg, 100 mg and 200 mg tablets in both the United States and Europe.

DOSAGES AND SUGGESTED REGIMENS

Oral JAK inhibitors elicit a dose-dependent response and are more efficacious at higher doses.

- Baricitinib: While 2 mg once-daily dosing is recommended by the FDA for treatment of RA, 4 mg dosing has been used commonly for the treatment of AD in clinical trials and is the recommended dose by the EMA. Lower (2 mg) dosing may be appropriate for certain patient populations, including patients over 75 years old, patients with active infections or a history of long-standing or recurring infections and patients with renal impairment and a creatinine clearance between 30 and 60 mL/min.
- Upadacitinib: For adolescents (from 12 to 17 years of age) weighing at least 30 kg and adults ≥65, the recommended dose is 15 mg once daily. For other adults, initiate 15 mg/day; higher dosing of 30 mg daily can be considered in those who do not achieve adequate response, with the lowest effective dose used for maintenance.
- Abrocitinib: For adolescents (from 12 to 17 years of age) and adults, 100 mg once daily is the recommended starting dose, with 200 mg once daily recommended for patients not responding to 100 mg daily dosing. Dosing with 50 mg once daily is recommended for patients with moderate renal impairment or for patients who are receiving treatment with cytochrome P450 2C19 (CYP2C19) inhibitors or are known or anticipated to be poor metabolizers of CYP2C19.

JAK inhibitors are rapidly absorbed, reaching peak plasma concentrations approximately one hour after ingestion. They may be taken with or without food. Therapeutic benefit is expected by 8 weeks of treatment and is often apparent within a few weeks of initiation, with improvement in itch occurring in as little as one to two weeks. If an adequate treatment response has not been achieved at 16 weeks, treatment should be discontinued.

NICE defines an adequate response (to baricitinib) as a reduction of at least:

- 50% in the Eczema Area and Severity Index score (EASI 50), and
- 4 points in the Dermatology Life Quality Index (DLQI) from baseline.

BASELINE INVESTIGATIONS AND CONSIDERATIONS

- Full blood count (FBC) (complete blood count [CBC]).
- Liver function tests (LFTs).
- Screening for tuberculosis (TB).
- Viral hepatitis screening for hepatitis B and C in accordance with community guidelines.
- Oral JAK inhibitors, which should be used cautiously in patients with a personal or family history of deep vein thrombosis (DVT)/pulmonary embolus (PE) or with risk factors for venous thromboembolism, such as patients who are current or past smokers.
- Baseline EASI score, taking into account how this may be affected by skin colour and DLQI to fulfil NICE guidelines.

MONITORING

- Fasting lipid profile should be assessed 12 weeks after treatment initiation and afterwards according to clinical guidelines for hyperlipidaemia management.
- Absolute neutrophil count (ANC), absolute lymphocyte count (ALC) and other blood counts should be monitored according to routine patient management. Treatment should be temporarily halted if haemoglobin is less than 80 g/L (8 g/dL), platelet count is less is than 50,000 cells/mm³, ALC is less than 500 cells/mm³ and/or ANC is less than 1000 cells/mm³.
- Hepatic transaminases should be monitored according to routine patient management while taking oral JAK inhibitors. Treatment should be temporarily halted if drug-induced hepatotoxicity is suspected.
- EASI and DLQI should be done to assess efficacy at 8 weeks and 16 weeks.

CONTRAINDICATIONS AND CAUTIONS

- Oral JAK inhibitors are contraindicated during pregnancy and should not be used during breastfeeding.
- The FDA has called for additional 'black box' warnings on oral JAK inhibitors to include serious heart-related events, cancer, blood clots and death.
- Serious and sometimes fatal infections have been reported with the use of oral JAK inhibitors, including active tuberculosis, invasive fungal infections such as candidiasis and pneumocystosis and other bacterial and viral opportunistic infections. Reactivation of viral infections, such as herpes simplex virus, has also been reported. Lymphoma and non-melanoma skin cancers (NMSCs) have also been reported in clinical studies. Patients should be tested for latent TB before initiating treatment and monitored for active TB during treatment, even if the initial latent testing was negative.
- DVTs and PEs have been reported in patients taking oral JAK inhibitors, and some of these events have resulted in death.

TABLE 25.1
Prescribing Considerations Related to the Black Box Warnings for Oral JAK Inhibitors

Serious infections	Treatment should be stopped or otherwise not initiated in patients with any of the following laboratory abnormalities: • Anaemia with a haemoglobin less than 8 g/dL • Lymphocytopenia with an ALC less than 500 cells/mm^3 • Neutropoenia with an ANC less than 1000 cells/mm^3
Malignancy	Regular skin checks should be performed in patients at an increased risk for skin cancer
Thrombosis	Use caution when prescribing these agents in patients predisposed to thromboses, as arterial thrombosis, DVT and pulmonary embolisms have occurred in patients with inflammatory conditions being treated by JAK inhibitors

Abbreviations: ALC, absolute lymphocyte count; ANC, absolute neutrophil count; g/dL, grams per decilitre; JAK, Janus kinase; mm, millimetre.

• Arterial thromboses in the extremities have also been reported. Given the risk of these serious adverse events, certain considerations should be taken when considering appropriate patients for treatment with oral JAK inhibitors and while prescribing these drugs (Table 25.1). Other considerations and concerns related to the prescription of JAK inhibitors include their use with live vaccines and in patients with renal and/or hepatic impairment (Table 25.2); flu and pneumococcal vaccination is recommended for people who are on immunosuppressant medication, so ideally these inactive vaccines should be administered at least two weeks before therapy is started. Prescribers are advised to consult the latest recommendation on COVID-19 vaccine and booster scheduling (see e.g. https://www.nhs.uk/conditions/coronavirus-covid-19/coronavirus-vaccination/health-conditions/).

IMPORTANT DRUG INTERACTIONS

• Strong organic anion transporter 3 (OAT3) inhibitors, such as probenecid, may increase total systemic exposure of baricitinib. Use of baricitinib is cautioned and may not be recommended in patients taking these medications. If used concurrently with OAT3 inhibitors, baricitinib daily dosing should not exceed 2 mg.

TABLE 25.2
Other Considerations and Concerns Related to the Prescription of JAK Inhibitors

Paediatric populations	Upadacitinib is licensed for use in children aged 12 and above
Live vaccines	Live vaccines should not be given to patients taking oral JAK inhibitors
Gastrointestinal perforations	Use of baricitinib or upadacitinib is cautioned in patients at an increased risk for gastrointestinal perforation, such as patients with a history of diverticulitis or gastrointestinal ulcers
Renal impairment	Avoid treatment in patients with renal impairment resulting in a creatinine clearance of less than 30 mL/min. For patients with a creatinine clearance of less than 60 mL/min, use a reduced dose (50 mg once daily) of abrocitinib
Alterations in blood lipid parameters	Levels of total, HDL, and LDL cholesterol may increase
Hepatic impairment	Levels of AST and ALT may increase. These medications are not recommended for use in patients with severe hepatic impairment

Abbreviations: ALT, alanine transaminase; AST, aspartate transaminase; HDL, high-density lipoprotein; LDL, low density lipoprotein; mL/min, millilitres per minute.

- Upadacitinib is primarily metabolized by CYP3A4. Co-administration of upadacitinib with other medicinal products that either inhibit or induce CYP3A4 can respectively increase or decrease upadacitinib plasma exposures.
- Abrocitinib is metabolized by multiple CYP enzymes, including CYP2C19, CYP2C9, CYP3A4 and CYP2B6. Avoid concomitant use of abrocitinib with moderate-to-strong inhibitors of both CYP2C19 and CYP2C9, or strong CYP2C19 or CYP2C9 inducers.
- Abrocitinib is an inhibitor of P glycoprotein (P-gp). Caution should be exercised with co-administration of abrocitinib with drugs that function as P-gp substrates, such as dabigatran.
- Combining these medications with biological (biologic) therapies or other biologic immunomodulators is not recommended due to the potential risk of additive immunosuppression.
- Combining potent immunosuppressives such as azathioprine, tacrolimus and ciclosporin with oral JAK inhibitors may cause additive immunosuppression and is not recommended.
- Non-steroidal anti-inflammatory medications, corticosteroids and opioids may increase the risk of diverticulitis and subsequent gastrointestinal perforation in patients simultaneously taking baricitinib or upadacitinib.

ADVERSE EFFECTS AND THEIR MANAGEMENT

Prevalence of adverse events varies by agent (Table 25.3). Different adverse event profiles may be preferred depending on individual patient characteristics.

- Infections and infestations: Upper respiratory infections are one of the most common adverse effects associated with oral JAK inhibitor use in patients with AD and RA. Other infections include reactivation of herpes zoster virus, herpes simplex virus, gastroenteritis, urinary tract infections, influenza, cellulitis and pneumonia; the frequency of each of these adverse events varies slightly between agents. Serious and sometimes fatal opportunistic infections have been reported in patients receiving oral JAK inhibitors; although rare overall, the likelihood of these infections presenting with disseminated rather than localized disease may be increased in patients taking concomitant immunosuppressants such as methotrexate. Use of these agents should be paused in patients who develop a serious or opportunistic infection, and treatment should be catered according to infectious species.
- Changes in lipid parameters: Hypercholesterolaemia and hypertriglyceridemia are associated with oral JAK inhibitor use; hypercholesterolaemia may be less likely with abrocitinib use. In clinical trials, patients with increased levels of LDL cholesterol were responsive to statin therapy and returned to pre-treatment levels.
- Haematological and vascular disorders: Possible changes in haematologic parameters include thrombocytosis, neutropenia, anaemia and thrombocytopenia. Treatment should be temporarily interrupted in patients experiencing these laboratory changes. Patients experiencing clinical features of DVT/PE should promptly discontinue treatment and be treated appropriately.
- Gastrointestinal complaints: Abdominal pain, nausea and vomiting are adverse events associated with oral JAK inhibitors used in RA and AD patients. Mild cases of abdominal pain and nausea do not require treatment interruption. Patients presenting with signs and symptoms concerning for diverticulitis should be evaluated promptly, given the possibility of gastrointestinal perforation.
- Hepatobiliary disorders: Elevated liver transaminases may be seen in patients using oral JAK inhibitors. In clinical trials, most incidences of elevations in hepatic transaminases were transient and self-resolving. If a drug-induced liver injury is suspected, treatment should be interrupted.
- Malignancy and lymphoproliferative disorders: Risk of lymphoma and other cancers may be increased in patients taking oral JAK inhibitors for RA, although this risk is likely lower in patients with AD.

TABLE 25.3

Differences in the Frequency of Adverse Events by Oral JAK Inhibitor

	Very Common (May Affect More Than 1 in 10 Patients)	Common (May Affect up to 1 in 10 Patients)	Uncommon (May Affect up to 1 in 100 Patients)
Abrocitinib	• Nausea	• Abdominal pain • Acne • Dizziness • Headache • Increased CPK • Infections and infestations (herpes simplex, herpes zoster) • Vomiting	• DVT/PE • Hyperlipidaemia (dyslipidaemia, hypercholesterolaemia) • Lymphopenia • Pneumonia • Thrombocytopenia
Baricitinib	• Hypercholesterolaemia • Upper respiratory tract infections	• Abdominal pain • Acne • Headache • Increased ALT • Increased CPK • Infections and infestations (herpes zoster, herpes simplex, gastroenteritis, UTI, pneumonia) • Nausea • Thrombocytosis • Rash	• Diverticulitis • DVT/PE • Facial swelling • Hypertriglyceridemia • Increased AST • Increased weight • Neutropoenia • Urticaria
Upadacitinib	• Acne • Upper respiratory infections	• Abdominal pain • Anaemia • Cough • Fatigue • Headache • Hypercholesterolaemia • Increased AST and ALT • Increased CPK • Increased weight • Infections and infestations (bronchitis, herpes zoster, herpes simplex, folliculitis, influenza) • Neutropoenia • Pyrexia • Urticaria	• Diverticulitis • Hypertriglyceridemia • Oral candidiasis • Pneumonia

Abbreviations: ALT, alanine transaminase; AST, aspartate transaminase; CPK, creatine phosphokinase; DVT, deep vein thrombosis; HDL, high-density lipoprotein; LDL, low density lipoprotein; PE, pulmonary embolism; UTI, urinary tract infection.

• Variation in adverse effects: Adverse events experienced by AD patients receiving treatment with other oral JAK inhibitors are similar to those experienced by patients receiving treatment with baricitinib, although gastrointestinal adverse events such as nausea and vomiting may be especially common in patients receiving abrocitinib. Upadacitinib and abrocitinib preferably inhibit JAK1 while minimally inhibiting JAK2; this theoretically decreases the risk of unwanted haematological adverse events, such as anaemia and neutropenia, as compared to the risk with therapeutic agents with increased inhibition of JAK2.

USE IN SPECIAL SITUATIONS

PREGNANCY

Oral JAK inhibitors should not be used during pregnancy. The JAK pathway is involved in cell adhesion and polarity; thus, use during pregnancy could potentially impact embryonic development. Studies in animals have shown reproductive toxicity and teratogenicity. Females of childbearing potential should use effective contraception during treatment. This should be continued for at least 1 week after discontinuing baricitinib and 4 weeks after discontinuing upadacitinib and abrocitinib.

LACTATION

It is not known if JAK inhibitors or their metabolites are excreted in human breast milk; thus, use while breastfeeding is not recommended.

CHILDREN

Upadacitinib is approved for use in adolescents with AD aged 12 and older by the EMA and FDA.

OLDER PEOPLE

JAK inhibitors are largely excreted by the kidneys; thus, older adults, who are more likely to have impaired renal function, may be more likely to experience adverse events. Low dosing should be used, and monitoring of renal function considered in patients at risk of impairment.

ESSENTIAL PATIENT INFORMATION

Dermatologists should inform their patients of the need for laboratory testing before initiation of therapy, and during therapy to monitor for adverse events, including increases in levels of cholesterol and decreases in haematological parameters. Patients should be aware of their increased risk for serious and potentially fatal infections while taking oral JAK inhibitors. Patients should report symptoms of infection such as fever, diarrhoea and stomach pains and shortness of breath to their healthcare provider immediately if these symptoms occur during treatment. Patients should also be informed of an increased risk of thrombosis during treatment and that they should immediately report symptoms of thrombosis, such as lower extremity swelling, pain, tenderness or sudden onset shortness of breath or chest pain to their healthcare provider.

FURTHER READING

Bieber T, Simpson EL, Silverberg JI, et al. Abrocitinib versus placebo or dupilumab for atopic dermatitis. N Engl J Med. 2021;384(12):1101–12. doi:10.1056/NEJMoa2019380.

Papp KA, Menter MA, Raman M, et al. A randomized phase 2b trial of baricitinib, an oral Janus kinase (JAK) 1/JAK2 inhibitor, in patients with moderate-to-severe psoriasis. Br J Dermatol. 2016;174(6):1266–76.

Singh R, Heron CE, Ghamrawi RI, et al. Emerging role of Janus kinase inhibitors for the treatment of atopic dermatitis. Immunotargets Ther. 2020;9:255–72.

Solimani F, Meier K, Ghoreschi K. Emerging topical and systemic JAK inhibitors in dermatology. Front Immunol. 2019;10:2847.

26 Malignant Melanoma Drug Treatments

Charlotte L. Edwards and Louise A. Fearfield

Treatment of malignant melanoma (MM) is dependent on the stage at presentation. The Union of International Cancer Control (UICC) Tumour, Node, Metastases (TNM) staging, linked to the eighth edition of the American Joint Committee on Cancer (AJCC) staging, is the preferred classification system. Changes from the seventh-edition staging system include a move away from the use of tumour mitotic rate as a staging criterion for T1 tumours; instead, tumour thickness and ulceration are used alone. Breslow thickness should now be recorded to the nearest 0.1 mm and not 0.01 mm, and sentinel lymph node staging is now included.

Mutation testing for actionable mutations for patients with resectable or unresectable stage III or IV disease is essential to aid decision-making regarding further treatment where necessary. It is also recommended in high-risk resected stage IIC disease. BRAF mutation testing is mandatory and, to confirm wild-type status, testing for NRAS and c-KIT are also recommended. Sentinel lymph node biopsy (SLNB) is recommended for precise staging in melanoma of the UICC and AJCC eighth-edition stage pT1b or higher. The Multicentre Selective Lymphadenectomy Trial I (MSLT-1) validated the staging potential of SLNB but did not show any survival benefit. Complete lymph node dissection (CLND) is no longer recommended for SLNB-positive patients. In the case of isolated locoregional clinically detectable (i.e. macroscopic, non-sentinel node) LN metastases, CLND is indicated, as removal of only the tumour-bearing lymph node is insufficient. Patients with fully resected stage III and IV melanoma with no evidence of on going metastatic disease should be evaluated for adjuvant therapy with checkpoint inhibitor therapies (CPI), anti-PD-1 (nivolumab/pembrolizumab) (all patients) or BRAF/MEK inhibitor combination (only for patients with BRAF-mutated melanoma).

For metastatic disease, surgical removal of locoregional recurrence or single distant metastases should be considered in fit patients as a therapeutic option offering potential for long-term disease control. Options for first-line and second-line treatments include CPI, anti-PD-1 (nivolumab/pembrolizumab) and anti-CTLA-4 (ipilimumab) in all patients and a BRAF inhibitor/MEK inhibitor combination for patients with BRAF-mutated melanoma. For unresectable stage IIIB/C, IVM1a – Talimogene laherparepevec (T-VEC) is also an option. The current first-line standard of care treatment, regardless of BRAF status, for unresectable stage III/IV melanoma is CPI including a PD-1 blockade or a PD-1 blockade combined with a CTLA-4 blockade (ipilimumab).

For BRAF wild-type disease, second-line options are very limited, and inclusion in clinical trials/personalized approaches may be considered. If the first-line treatment was anti-PD-1 alone, then ipilimumab or ipilimumab/nivolumab are options. For BRAF-mutated disease, all the options available for WT melanoma are still valid with the addition of BRAF inhibitors/MEK inhibitors, if not used in the first-line setting. For NRAS-mutated melanoma, due to the limited efficacy of MEK inhibitors, first-line CPI options identical to those of WT melanoma are first choice. For management of brain metastases, ipilimumab/nivolumab combination therapy is the preferred first-line treatment. For small numbers of metastases, stereotactic radiosurgery can be considered upfront or reserved for non-responding lesions.

DOI: 10.1201/9781003016786-26

CHECKPOINT INHIBITOR THERAPY FOR MELANOMA

INDICATIONS AND DERMATOLOGICAL USES

TREATMENT OF ADVANCED (STAGE IV) MELANOMA

CPI has significantly improved overall survival for several cancers, including melanoma. The European Medicines Agency (EMA) approved the use of ipilimumab (anti CTLA-4) monotherapy in advanced melanoma in 2012. Nivolumab and pembrolizumab (anti-PD-1) monotherapy followed in 2015, and ipilimumab and nivolumab combination therapy was approved for use in 2016. The expectation for survival in patients with advanced melanoma now exceeds 50% at 5 years in patients treated with first-line combination ipilimumab and nivolumab.

The current first-line standard of care treatment, regardless of BRAF status, for unresectable stage III/IV melanoma is a PD-1 blockade or a PD-1 blockade combined with CTLA-4 blockade.

ADJUVANT THERAPY OF MALIGNANT MELANOMA

The cure rate following surgical removal of early melanoma is high, but patients with more advanced disease (stage III) are at higher risk of recurrence and should be considered for adjuvant therapy. In 2018, the EMA extended approval for use of both nivolumab and pembrolizumab to include adjuvant treatment of melanoma. In the adjuvant setting recurrence, free survival is 70% at 12 months and 58% at 36 months for stage IIIB/C or IV melanoma. Adjuvant treatment of stage III melanoma with a BRAF V600 mutation following complete resection can also include a BRAF/MEK inhibition.

CLASSIFICATION AND MODE OF ACTION

ANTI-PD-1

- Nivolumab
  - A human immunoglobulin G4 monoclonal antibody which binds to the programmed cell death-1 (PD-1) receptor, thereby potentiating an immune response to tumour cells.
  - Other uses include: In advanced renal cell carcinoma, as monotherapy or in combination with ipilimumab, non-small cell lung cancer, urothelial carcinoma, squamous cell cancer of the head and neck and classical Hodgkin lymphoma.
- Pembrolizumab
  - A monoclonal antibody which binds to the PD-1 receptor, thereby potentiating an immune response to tumour cells.
  - Other uses include: Non-small cell lung cancer, urothelial carcinoma, squamous cell cancer of the head and neck and classical Hodgkin lymphoma.

ANTI-CTLA-4

- Ipilimumab
  - A monoclonal antibody which causes T-cell activation, resulting in tumour cell death.
  - Other uses include: Advanced renal cell carcinoma and metastatic colorectal cancer with MMR/MSI-H aberrations in combination with nivolumab.

DOSAGES AND SUGGESTED REGIMENS FOR MELANOMA

- Nivolumab given by intravenous infusion 240 mg every 2 weeks, alternatively 480 mg every 4 weeks.
- Pembrolizumab given by intravenous infusion 200 mg every 3 weeks, alternatively 400 mg every 6 weeks.

- Ipilimumab given by intravenous infusion 3 mg/kg every 3 weeks for 4 doses.
- Adjuvant therapy for melanoma: A combination of either Nivolumab or Pembrolizumab for 12 months.
- Metastatic melanoma: A combination of nivolumab and ipilimumab (4 doses) with nivolumab continued for up to 24 months, or single-agent nivolumab or pembrolizumab for 24 months.

FORMULATION/PRESENTATION

- Nivolumab is available as 4 mL, 10 mL and 24 mL vials. Each mL of concentrate for solution for infusion contains 10 mg of nivolumab, 4 mL contains 40 mg of nivolumab, 10 mL contains 100 mg of nivolumab and 24 mL contains 240 mg of nivolumab.
- Pembrolizumab is available in 4 mL vials of concentrate containing 100 mg of pembrolizumab. Each mL of concentrate contains 25 mg of pembrolizumab.
- Ipilimumab is available as 10 mL and 40 mL vials. Each mL of concentrate contains 5 mg ipilimumab. One 10 mL vial contains 50 mg of ipilimumab. One 40 mL vial contains 200 mg of ipilimumab.

BASELINE INVESTIGATIONS AND CONSIDERATIONS

- Full blood count (FBC) (complete blood count [CBC]).
- Urea, electrolytes and creatinine.
- Liver function tests (LFTs).
- Glucose.
- Thyroid function.
- Urinalysis.
- Echocardiogram (ECG) if there are pre-existing cardiac abnormalities.

MONITORING

Monitoring should be done for signs and symptoms of infusion and immune-related reactions, cardiac and pulmonary reactions, thyroid funtion, glucose and electrolyte disturbances, before and periodically during treatment. Patients should be monitored for adverse reactions for at least 5 months after the last dose.

CONTRAINDICATIONS

For detailed advice, the individual product literature should be consulted.

CAUTIONS

- Caution is advised in moderate-to-severe hepatic impairment.
- Anti-PD-1 therapy may increase the risk of severe graft versus host reaction in patients who have had prior a haematopoietic stem cell transplant; patients may need pre-medication to minimize the development of infusion-related reactions.
- There is a risk of organ rejection in organ transplant recipients receiving anti-PD-1 therapy or anti CTLA-4 therapy.

IMPORTANT DRUG INTERACTIONS

- Hydrocortisone, betamethasone, prednisolone, methylprednisolone and dexamethasone are predicted to decrease the efficacy of checkpoint inhibitors.
- Live vaccines, e.g. BCG, influenza, MMR, rotavirus, typhoid, VZV and yellow fever, should be avoided as they are predicted to increase the risk of generalized infection.

- Trimethoprim, mycophenolate, methotrexate, fluorouracil, vismodegib and valganciclovir can increase the risk of myelosuppression with nivolumab therapy.

ADVERSE EFFECTS AND THEIR MANAGEMENT

Modulating the immune system is recognized to cause immune-related adverse events. These effects may target any organ; however, the skin is most commonly affected, occurring in 50% of those on ipilimumab and 40% on anti-programmed cell death-1 inhibitors. The majority of cutaneous toxicities are mild; however, severe reactions are reported. The benefit of adding ipilimumab to nivolumab has been shown with higher response rates, durations and progression-free survival, but is associated with more toxicities.

- Dermatological: Maculopapular eruptions and pruritus most commonly, lichenoid eruptions, bullous pemphigoid, alopecia and vitiligo.
- Gastrointestinal (GI) adverse effects: Diarrhoea and colitis.
- Hepatic: Hepatitis.
- Respiratory: Pneumonitis.
- Cardiovascular: Arrhythmias, pericarditis and myocarditis.
- Haematological: Anaemia and thrombocytopenia.
- Metabolic adverse effects: Thyroiditis, hypophysitis and diabetes mellitus.
- Rheumatological: Arthritis.
- Renal: Nephritis.
- Neurological: Encephalopathy and neuropathy.
- Ophthalmologic: Uveitis and episcleritis.
- CMV GI infection or reactivation. (For corticosteroid-refractory immune related colitis, use of an additional immunosuppressive agent should only be considered if other causes are excluded using viral PCR on biopsy and eliminating other viral, bacterial and parasitic causes.)

Most immune-related adverse reactions improve or resolve with appropriate management, including initiation of corticosteroids and treatment modifications.

Patients with mild/moderate infusion reactions may continue treatment with close monitoring and use of pre-medication. Severe reactions will necessitate the discontinuation of treatment.

USE IN SPECIAL SITUATIONS

PREGNANCY AND PRE-CONCEPTION

- Effective contraception is required during treatment and for 5 months after treatment in females of childbearing potential.
- Avoid in pregnancy unless potential benefit outweighs risk – toxicity in animal studies have been seen.

LACTATION

- Avoid in breastfeeding.

CHILDREN

- Unlicensed – only used in trial settings.

ESSENTIAL PATIENT INFORMATION

Patients should be advised of the common side effects and should be provided with a patient alert card with each prescription.

Further information can be obtained from www.macmillan.org.uk.

TARGETED TREATMENTS

BRAF AND MEK INHIBITORS

For BRAF V600-mutated melanoma, additional first-line options are provided by BRAF and MEK inhibition. BRAF inhibition (vemurafenib, dabrafenib and encorafenib) combined with MEK inhibition (cobimetinib, trametinib and binimetinib) can be used. BRAF/MEK double inhibition is superior to single-agent BRAF in terms of response rates, progression-free survival and overall survival.

BRAF INHIBITORS (VEMURAFENIB, DABRAFENIB AND ENCORAFENIB)

CLASSIFICATION AND MODE OF ACTION

- BRAF kinase inhibitors.

VEMURAFENIB

INDICATIONS AND DERMATOLOGICAL USES

- Monotherapy for the treatment of BRAF V600 mutation-positive unresectable or metastatic melanoma.

DOSAGES AND SUGGESTED REGIMENS

- For adults, orally 960 mg Bd – for dose adjustment due to side effects.

FORMULATIONS/PRESENTATION

- Available as 240 mg coated tablets.

BASELINE INVESTIGATIONS AND CONSIDERATIONS

- ECG and electrolytes before treatment; treatment is not recommended if the QT interval is greater than 500 milliseconds at baseline.
- LFTs.
- Skin check.

MONITORING

- ECG and electrolytes monthly during the first 3 months of treatment, followed by 3 monthly thereafter – risk of prolonged QTc.
- LFTs.
- Monitor for uveitis, iritis and retinal vein occlusion.
- Monitor for cutaneous and non-cutaneous squamous cell carcinoma and new primary melanoma before, during and up to 6 months after treatment.

CONTRAINDICATION

- Wild-type BRAF malignant melanoma.

CAUTIONS

- Electrolyte disturbances.
- Susceptibility to QT prolongation.
- Prior or concurrent cancer associated with RAS mutation – increased risk of tumour progression.
- Moderate-to-severe hepatic impairment.
- Severe renal impairment.

IMPORTANT DRUG INTERACTIONS

- Avoid any other medication that is known to prolong the QTc interval or cause hypokalaemia.
- Itraconazole, ketoconazole and voriconazole are predicted to increase exposure to vemurafenib.

ADVERSE EFFECTS AND THEIR MANAGEMENT

- Dermatological: Rash, alopecia, folliculitis, panniculitis, photosensitivity and DRESS (drug rash with eosinophilia and systemic symptoms).
- Renal: Nephritis, acute tubular necrosis and acute kidney injury.
- Hepatic: Liver injury.
- Ophthalmological: Retinal occlusion, uveitis and iritis.
- Rheumatological: Arthritis, arthralgia, myalgia, asthenia, connective tissue disorders and vasculitis.
- Neurological: Headaches, dizziness, 7th nerve paralysis, altered taste and peripheral neuropathy.
- GI: Vomiting, constipation, diarrhoea, nausea and pancreatitis.
- Other: Fever.

There is a risk of potentiation of radiation toxicity in patients treated with vemurafenib before, during or after radiotherapy.

USE IN SPECIAL SITUATIONS

Pregnancy and Pre-Conception

- Effective contraception required during and for at least 6 months after treatment.
- Avoid unless potential benefit outweighs risk in pregnancy.

Lactation

- Avoid – no information available.

Children

- Unlicensed.

ESSENTIAL PATIENT INFORMATION

Patients should be advised of the common side effects.
  Further information can be obtained from www.macmillan.org.uk.

DABRAFENIB

INDICATIONS AND DERMATOLOGICAL USES

- Unresectable or metastatic melanoma with a BRAF V600 mutation (as monotherapy or in combination with trametinib). Also licensed for use in advanced non-small cell lung cancer with a BRAF V600 mutation (in combination with trametinib).
- Adjuvant treatment of stage III melanoma with a BRAF V600 mutation following complete resection (in combination with trametinib).
- Monotherapy for the treatment of BRAF V600 mutation-positive unresectable or metastatic melanoma.

DOSAGES AND SUGGESTED REGIMENS

- For adults, 150 mg every 12 hours, for dose adjustments due to side effects, consult product literature.
- For adjuvant therapy for adults, 150 mg every 12 hours for 12 months (in combination with trametinib), for dose adjustments due to side effects consult product literature.

FORMULATIONS/PRESENTATION

- Available as 50 mg and 75 mg hard capsules.

BASELINE INVESTIGATIONS AND CONSIDERATIONS

- Skin check.
- Full blood count (FBC) (complete blood count [CBC]).
- Renal indices.
- LFTs.

MONITORING

- Monitoring for cutaneous and non-cutaneous squamous cell carcinoma and new primary melanoma before, during and up to 6 months after treatment.
- Full blood count (FBC) (complete blood count [CBC]).
- Renal indices.
- LFTs.
- Monitor for ophthalmologic reactions.

CONTRAINDICATIONS

- Wild-type BRAF malignant melanoma.

CAUTIONS

- Prior or concurrent cancer associated with RAS mutation – increased risk of tumour progression.
- Older people (more frequent dose adjustments may be required).
- Moderate-to-severe hepatic impairment.
- Severe renal impairment.

IMPORTANT DRUG INTERACTIONS

- Mycophenolate and methotrexate can increase the risk of myelosuppression; other agents that increase the chances of myelosuppression should be avoided.
- Dabrafenib can increase the anticoagulant effect of warfarin.
- Clarithromycin can increase the exposure to dabrafenib.

ADVERSE EFFECTS AND THEIR MANAGEMENT

- Dermatological: Skin reactions, alopecia, photosensitivity and panniculitis, risk of new squamous cell carcinoma and primary melanoma.
- Rheumatological: Arthralgia, myalgia and asthenia.
- GI: Decreased appetite, nausea, vomiting, constipation and diarrhoea.
- Renal: Nephritis and renal impairment.
- Ophthalmological: Uveitis.
- Others: Flu-like symptoms, fever and chills, hyperglycaemia, hypophosphatemia, pain in extremities and pancreatitis.

Additional side effects when used in combination with trametinib:

- Dizziness, hypotension, hyperhidrosis, hyponatraemia, leukopenia, neutropenia and thrombo-cytopenia, muscle spasms, myocarditis and night sweats.

USE IN SPECIAL SITUATIONS

PREGNANCY AND PRE-CONCEPTION

- Females of childbearing potential should use effective non-hormonal contraception during and for 4 weeks after stopping treatment.
- Dabrafenib should be avoided in pregnancy unless potential benefit outweighs risk. There is toxicity in animal studies.

LACTATION

- Avoid – no information available.

CHILDREN

- Unlicensed.

ESSENTIAL PATIENT INFORMATION

Patients should be advised of the common side effects and to immediately report new skin lesions – there is a risk of squamous cell carcinoma and new primary melanoma.

Patients should be counselled about the effects on driving and performance of skilled tasks – there is increased risk of ocular adverse events.

Further information can be obtained from www.macmillan.org.uk.

ENCORAFENIB

INDICATIONS AND DERMATOLOGICAL USES

- Unresectable or metastatic melanoma with a BRAF V600 mutation (in combination with binimetinib).

DOSAGES AND SUGGESTED REGIMENS

- For adult, orally 450 mg once daily; for dose adjustments due to side effects, consult product literature.

FORMULATIONS/PRESENTATION

- Available as 50 mg and 75 mg hard capsules.

BASELINE INVESTIGATIONS AND CONSIDERATIONS

- ECG.
- Skin check.
- Full blood count (FBC) (complete blood count [CBC]).
- LFTs.
- Renal indices.

MONITORING

- Monitoring for cutaneous and non-cutaneous squamous cell carcinoma and new primary melanoma before, during and up to 6 months after treatment.
- ECG.
- LFTs.
- Renal indices.
- Monitoring for ophthalmologic reactions.

CONTRAINDICATION

- Wild-type BRAF malignant melanoma.

CAUTIONS

- Prior or concurrent cancer associated with RAS mutation – there is an increased risk of tumour progression.
- Susceptibility to QT prolongation.
- Avoid in moderate-to-severe hepatic impairment, caution in mild hepatitis impairment – reducing dose to 300 mg od in mild impairment.
- Avoid in severe renal impairment.

IMPORTANT DRUG INTERACTIONS

- Avoid any other medication that is known to prolong the QTc interval or cause hypokalaemia.
- Grapefruit juice, azoles and clarithromycin will increase exposure to encorafenib.
- St John's wort will decrease exposure to encorafenib.

ADVERSE EFFECTS AND THEIR MANAGEMENT

- Dermatological: Rash, alopecia, panniculitis, photosensitivity and neoplasms (e.g. squamous cell carcinoma).
- Cardiac: Arrhythmia, QT prolongation, left ventricular dysfunction, heart failure and hypertension.
- Ophthalmological: Eye inflammation and detachment of retinal pigment epithelium.
- GI: Diarrhoea, vomiting, constipation and ulcerative colitis.

- Haematological: Embolism, thrombosis and intracranial haemorrhage.
- Renal: Renal impairment.
- Neurological: Headache, nerve disorders and paresis.
- Other: Arthritis, arthralgia, pancreatitis and fatigue.

USE IN SPECIAL SITUATIONS

PREGNANCY AND PRE-CONCEPTION

- Females of childbearing potential should use effective non-hormonal contraception during and for 4 weeks after stopping treatment.

LACTATION

- Avoid – no information available.

CHILDREN

- Unlicensed.

ESSENTIAL PATIENT INFORMATION

Patients should be advised of the common side effects and should be advised immediately to report new skin lesions – there is a risk of squamous cell carcinoma and new primary melanoma.

Patients should be counselled in the effects on driving and performance of skilled tasks – there is an increased risk of ocular adverse events.

Further information can be obtained from www.macmillan.org.uk.

MEK INHIBITORS (COBIMETINIB, TRAMETINIB AND BINIMETINIB)

CLASSIFICATION AND MODE OF ACTION

- A mitogen-activated protein kinase (MAPK) inhibitor.

COBIMETINIB

INDICATIONS AND DERMATOLOGICAL USES

- Treatment of BRAF V600 mutation-positive melanoma in combination with vemurafenib.

DOSAGES AND SUGGESTED REGIMENS

- For adults, given orally 60 mg once daily for 21 days – subsequent cycles repeated after a 7-day interval – for dose adjustment due to side effects.

FORMULATIONS/PRESENTATION

- Available as 20 mg film-coated tablets.

BASELINE INVESTIGATIONS AND CONSIDERATIONS

- Creatinine kinase and creatinine.
- Ejection fraction, which should be evaluated before initiation of treatment.
- LFTs.

MONITORING

- Monthly creatinine kinase and creatinine.
- Ejection fraction, which should be evaluated after the first month then at 3-monthly intervals.
- LFTs monthly.
- Assessment for new or worsening visual disturbances.

CAUTIONS

- Left ventricular dysfunction.
- Risk factors for bleeding.
- Hepatic impairment.
- Severe renal impairment.

IMPORTANT DRUG INTERACTIONS

- Grapefruit juice and azoles increase exposure to cobimetinib.
- St John's wort decreases the exposure to cobimetinib.

ADVERSE EFFECTS AND THEIR MANAGEMENT

- Dermatological: Rashes, photosensitivity and basal cell carcinoma.
- Haematological: Anaemia and haemorrhage.
- Respiratory: Pneumonitis.
- Ophthalmological: Retinopathy and visual disorders.
- GI: Vomiting and diarrhoea.
- Other: Electrolyte imbalance, rhabdomyolysis, hyperglycaemia, fever and hypertension.

USE IN SPECIAL SITUATIONS

PREGNANCY AND PRE-CONCEPTION

- Two forms of effective contraception advised for treatment and 3 months afterwards.
- Use in pregnancy should be avoided unless essential – toxicity on animal studies.

LACTATION

- Avoid – no information available.

CHILDREN

- Unlicensed.

ESSENTIAL PATIENT INFORMATION

Patients should be advised of the common side effects and effects on driving and performing skilled tasks due to visual disturbances.

Further information can be obtained from www.macmillan.org.uk.

TRAMETINIB

INDICATIONS AND DERMATOLOGICAL USES

- Treatment of BRAF V600 mutation-positive unresectable or metastatic melanoma as monotherapy or in combination with dabrafenib.

- Adjuvant treatment of stage III melanoma following complete resection, with a BRAF V600 mutation.
- Also used in advanced non-small cell lung cancer with a BRAF V600 mutation-positive melanoma in combination with dabrafenib.

DOSAGES AND SUGGESTED REGIMENS

- For adults, given orally 2 mg once daily, the dose should be taken at the same time each day with either the morning or evening dose of dabrafenib, for dose adjustment due to side effects.
- For adults, given orally 2 mg once daily for 12 months, the dose should be taken at the same time each day with either the morning or evening dose of dabrafenib; for dose adjustments due to side effects, consult product literature.

FORMULATIONS/PRESENTATION

- Available as 0.5 mg or 2 mg film-coated tablets.
- Manufacturer advises storage in a refrigerator (2–8°C); once opened, the bottle may be stored for 30 days at no more than 30°C.

BASELINE INVESTIGATIONS AND CONSIDERATIONS

- Blood pressure.
- Creatinine kinase and creatinine.
- Left ventricular ejection fraction, which should be evaluated before initiation of treatment.
- LFTs.

MONITORING

- Blood pressure.
- Monthly creatinine kinase and creatinine.
- Ejection fraction, which should be evaluated after the first month, then 3-monthly.
- LFTs monthly for 6 months.
- Assessment for new or worsening visual disturbances.

CONTRAINDICATION

- History of retinal vein occlusion.

CAUTIONS

- Patients with risk factors for GI perforation or on other medications that can cause GI perforation.
- Concomitant antiplatelet or anticoagulant therapy – increased risk of haemorrhage.
- Impaired left ventricular function.
- Predisposing factors for retinal vein occlusion.
- Moderate-to-severe hepatic impairment.
- Severe renal impairment.

IMPORTANT DRUG INTERACTIONS

- Clarithromycin, erythromycin, ciclosporin, azoles and vemurafenib are known to increase concentration of trametinib.

ADVERSE EFFECTS AND THEIR MANAGEMENT

- Dermatological: Rashes and alopecia.
- Ophthalmological: Eye inflammation, retinal detachment, retinal occlusion, chorioretinopathy and visual disorders.
- GI: Abdominal pain, vomiting, diarrhoea and constipation.
- Haematological: Anaemia, haemorrhage and intracranial haemorrhage.
- Respiratory: Dry mouth, dyspnoea and respiratory disorder.
- Cardiac: Left ventricular dysfunction, heart failure and bradycardia.
- Other: Electrolyte imbalance, rhabdomyolysis, lymphoedema, fever, hypertension and increased risk of infection.

Additional side effects reported when used in combination with dabrafenib:

- Leukopenia, thrombocytopenia, neutropenia, muscle spasms, myocarditis, dizziness, hypotension, hyponatraemia and night sweats.

USE IN SPECIAL SITUATIONS

PREGNANCY AND PRE-CONCEPTION

- Effective non-hormonal contraception is advised during treatment and for 4 months afterwards.
- Use in pregnancy should be avoided unless essential – toxicity on animal studies.

LACTATION

- Avoid – no information available.

CHILDREN

- Unlicensed.

ESSENTIAL PATIENT INFORMATION

Patients should be advised of the common side effects and the signs and symptoms of gastric perforation. Further information can be obtained from www.macmillan.org.uk.

BINIMETINIB

INDICATIONS AND DERMATOLOGICAL USES

- Treatment of BRAF V600 mutation-positive unresectable or metastatic melanoma in combination with encorafenib.

DOSAGES AND SUGGESTED REGIMENS

- For adults, given orally 45 mg twice daily, for dose adjustment due to side effects.

FORMULATIONS/PRESENTATION

- Available as 15 mg film-coated tablets.

BASELINE INVESTIGATIONS AND CONSIDERATIONS

- LFTs.
- Left ventricular ejection fraction, which should be evaluated before initiation of treatment.
- Blood pressure.
- Creatinine kinase and creatinine.

MONITORING

- LFTs monthly for 6 months.
- Ejection fraction, which should be evaluated after first month then 3-monthly.
- Assessment for new or worsening visual disturbances.
- Blood pressure.
- Monthly creatinine kinase and creatinine during first 6 months and as clinically indicated.

CONTRAINDICATION

- History of retinal vein occlusion.

CAUTIONS

- Left ventricular dysfunction – ejection fraction below 50%.
- Risk factors for retinal vein occlusion.
- Risk factors for venous thromboembolism.
- Neuromuscular conditions associated with elevated creatinine kinase and rhabdomyolysis.
- Moderate-to-severe hepatic impairment.

IMPORTANT DRUG INTERACTIONS

- None.

ADVERSE EFFECTS AND THEIR MANAGEMENT

- Dermatological: Rashes, alopecia, panniculitis and photosensitivity.
- Ophthalmological: Eye inflammation, retinal detachment, retinal occlusion and visual disorders.
- GI: GI discomfort/disorders, nausea, diarrhoea, constipation and ulcerative colitis.
- Haematological: Anaemia, embolism and thrombosis, haemorrhage and intracranial haemorrhage.
- Respiratory: Respiratory disorders.
- Cardiac: Left ventricular dysfunction, heart failure and oedema.
- Renal: Renal failure.
- Neurological: Headache, nerve disorders, altered taste, paresis and facial paralysis.
- Other: Arthralgia, angioedema, dizziness, fatigue, fever, hypersensitivity, vasculitis, hypertension, lip squamous carcinoma, muscle complaints, muscle weakness, myopathy, neoplasms and pancreatitis.

USE IN SPECIAL SITUATIONS

PREGNANCY AND PRE-CONCEPTION

- Effective contraception advised during treatment and for at least 1 month afterwards.
- Use in pregnancy should be avoided unless essential – toxicity on animal studies.

- Avoid – no information available.

CHILDREN

- Unlicensed.

ESSENTIAL PATIENT INFORMATION

Patients should be advised of the common side effects and the effects on driving and performance of skilled tasks.

Further information can be obtained from www.macmillan.org.uk.

INTERFERONS

CLASSIFICATION AND MODE OF ACTION

Interferons (IFNs) are glycoprotein cytokines, first discovered in the 1950s by Alick Isaacs and Jean Lindeman. They have immunomodulatory, antiproliferative and anti-infective actions and are released by host cells in response to pathogens or tumour cells. They are especially important in protection against viral infection. Three classes of IFNs are recognized (Types I–III IFN), and these differ in the protein sequence, receptors, genetic loci and cell types responsible for their production.

Type I IFNs have an alpha α-helical structure and include IFNs-α2 and -beta (β). There are many subtypes of IFN-α, but only one form of IFN-β. Type II IFN in humans is IFN-gamma (IFN-γ), and Type III IFNs (IFN-λ, IFN-ι) have only recently been described.

INDICATIONS AND DERMATOLOGICAL USES

Various formulations of IFN-α are commercially available and differ in their individual product licenses. Indications include the treatment of chronic viral hepatitis, various haematological malignancies, renal cancer, carcinoid, malignant melanoma, Kaposi sarcoma and cutaneous T-cell lymphoma.

INTERFERON USE IN MALIGNANT MELANOMA

Adjuvant IFN-α has been used for over 10 years at various regimens (low-, medium- and high-dose >10 MU/dose). High-dose IFN-α2b (HDI) has been shown to prolong disease-free survival, but its effects on overall survival are unclear, and treatment is associated with significant toxicity. IFN-α is licensed as an adjuvant therapy in patients who are disease-free after surgery but are at high risk of systemic recurrence. European consensus guidelines from 2012 concluded that IFN-α may be offered to patients with stage II and III melanoma as an adjuvant therapy, as it increases disease-free survival. However, the 2010 British Association of Dermatology melanoma guidelines do not recommend its routine use for primary or stage III melanoma, due to the lack of clear evidence for overall survival benefit. Moreover, with the advent of immunotherapy and targeted therapy in the adjuvant treatment of MM, interferon is no longer recommended.

FORMULATIONS/PRESENTATION

- IFN-α2b is available in 1 mL and 2.5 mL vials containing 10 million units/mL ready for injection and in pre-filled syringes and injection pen devices.
- All preparations should be stored at 2–8°C.

DOSAGES AND SUGGESTED REGIMENS

- There are a few standardized regimens for treatment of dermatological disease with IFNs, though doses have varied between different clinical trials.

BASELINE INVESTIGATIONS AND CONSIDERATIONS

- Full blood count (FBC) (complete blood count [CBC]).
- Urea, electrolytes and creatinine.
- LFTs.
- Glucose.
- Lipids.
- Thyroid-stimulating hormone (TSH).
- Urinalysis.
- ECG if there are pre-existing cardiac abnormalities.

MONITORING

IFN-α (and IFN-β):

- FBC with differential white cell count (WCC) and LFTs weekly during induction phase, then monthly throughout therapy.
- Urea, electrolytes and creatinine and lipids every 1–3 months.

CONTRAINDICATIONS

For detailed advice, the individual product literature should be consulted. General contraindications to IFN therapy include:

- Hypersensitivity to specific interferons.
- Severe cardiac, renal or hepatic dysfunction.

CAUTIONS

- Use with caution in patients with seizure disorders, depression and older people.

IMPORTANT DRUG INTERACTIONS

- Metronidazole and atorvastatin: Increased risk of peripheral neuropathy and neurotoxic effects.
- Theophylline: Associated with decreases in clearance and increases in plasma concentration and elimination of the half-life of theophylline.
- Zidovudine (AZT): May result in severe bone marrow toxicity, most often manifested as granulocytopenia and/or thrombocytopenia.

ADVERSE EFFECTS AND THEIR MANAGEMENT

- Flu-like symptoms such as fatigue, fever myalgia, arthralgia, headache, sweating and chills affect most patients during the first weeks of treatment with all IFNs. They are usually manageable with simple analgesics and by administering IFN injections in the evening. Symptoms may improve with continued therapy as tolerance develops.

- Psychiatric (all IFNs but predominantly IFN-α): Side effects are common, especially depression, and more rarely, suicidal ideation and attempted suicide. Irritability, anxiety, insomnia and other behavioural disturbances have also been reported, and additional adverse effects of IFN-α include mood and personality change. Development of the IFN-α-induced depressive symptoms may arise through depletion of central and peripheral 5-hydroxytryptamine (serotonin, 5-HT) and reduction of tryptophan plasma levels. Psychiatric advice should be obtained if severe symptoms develop.
- GI adverse effects are common and include nausea, anorexia, vomiting and diarrhoea, and they may result in weight loss. Gingival bleeding and GI haemorrhage have been reported more rarely. Antiemetic medication and adequate hydration may improve nausea, especially during IV administration. Pancreatitis has been reported rarely.
- Neurological (all IFNs but predominantly IFN-α): Headache and dizziness are very common, and other neurological effects include impaired concentration, lethargy, sleep disturbance, confusion, paraesthesia, resting and action tremor and involuntary movements. Most of the CNS adverse effects are mild and reversible within a few days to 3 weeks after dose reduction or discontinuation of therapy. Seizures may occur in up to 1% of patients and are reversible on discontinuation of therapy.
- Dermatological (predominantly IFN-α and IFN-β): Injection site reactions are common, and various rashes have been reported, including psoriasiform, eczematous and pemphigus-like eruptions. Seborrhoea, dry skin, pruritus and alopecia may occur.
- Respiratory (all IFNs): Common flu-like adverse effects include cough, throat irritation and rhinosinusitis. Dyspnoea and pneumonia may occur.
- Cardiovascular (all IFNs): Cardiovascular adverse effects may include hypertension and hypotension, cardiac failure and rarely, myocardial infarction. Cardiomyopathy has also been reported rarely in patients treated with IFN-α.
- Hepatic (all IFNs): Adverse effects have included transient increases of liver transaminase or alkaline phosphatase and the development of autoimmune hepatitis.
- Haematological (all IFNs): Myelosuppression may occur, particularly a reduction in granulocytes, so regular monitoring of the FBC is required throughout therapy.
- Rhabdomyolysis and multiorgan failure have been reported shortly after starting high-dose IFN.
- Metabolic adverse effects include hypertriglyceridemia and hyperglycaemia. Thyroid function may become abnormal (hypo- or hyperthyroidism).
- Autoimmune abnormalities have been reported, including vasculitis, lupus and vitiligo.

USE IN SPECIAL SITUATIONS

Pregnancy and Pre-Conception

- IFNs are contraindicated during pregnancy unless absolutely necessary.
- Fertility may be impaired by IFN-α, which is known to cause miscarriages in primates.
- Contraception is recommended for both males and females during treatment.
- Spontaneous abortions have been reported in females taking IFN-β for multiple sclerosis.

Lactation

- IFNs should be avoided, as there are insufficient data regarding safety in lactation.

Children

- IFN-α has been used safely in children in doses of up to 10 mLU/m^2.
- IFN-γ has been used in children, but the safety and efficacy in infants under 6 months is not known.

ESSENTIAL PATIENT INFORMATION

Patients should be advised of the common side effects of flu-like symptoms and fatigue.
Further information can be obtained from www.macmillan.org.uk.

FURTHER READING

Belum VR, Benhuri B, Postow MA, et al. Characterisation and management of dermatologic adverse events to agents targeting the PD-1 receptor. Eur J Cancer. 2016;60:12–25.

Chan L, Hwang SJE, Byth K, et al. Survival and prognosis of individuals receiving programmed cell death 1 inhibitor with and without immunologic cutaneous adverse events. J Am Acad Dermatol. 2020;82(2):311–6.

Edwards CL, Comito F, Agraso Busto S, et al. Cutaneous toxicities in patients with melanoma receiving checkpoint inhibitor therapy: A retrospective review. The experience of a single large specialist institution. Clin Exp Dermatol. 2021 Mar;46(2):338–41.

Gershenwald JE, Scolyer RA, Hess KR, et al. Melanoma of the skin. Amin M, Edge SB, Greene FL, et al. eds. AJCC Cancer Staging Manual. 8th ed. Switzerland: Springer; 2017:563–85.

Larkin J, Chiarion-Sileni V, Gonzalez R, et al. Five-year survival with combined nivolumab and ipilimumab in advanced melanoma. N Engl J Med. 2019;381(16):1535–46.

Michielin O, van Akkooi ACJ, Ascierto PA, et al. Cutaneous melanoma: ESMO clinical practice guidelines for diagnosis, treatment and follow up. Ann Oncol. 2019;30:1884–901. doi:10.1093/annonc/mdz411.

27 Methotrexate

Richard Woolf and Catherine Smith

CLASSIFICATION AND MODE OF ACTION

Methotrexate (MTX) is an analogue and antagonist of folic acid. It is classified as an antimetabolite cytotoxic agent. MTX is used to treat a range of malignant diseases and immune-mediated inflammatory diseases.

The bioavailability of oral MTX is high but can vary widely between individuals (64–90%) and plateau at doses above 15 mg/week, suggesting saturation of the intestinal transporters. Subcutaneous (SC) MTX injection leads to a linear, dose-proportional increase in the blood circulation and no plateau, indicating better bioavailability than oral administration. MTX is a pro-drug that is actively transported into cells as MTX-monoglutamate. Within the cell, further glutamic acid residues are added to form biologically active MTX polyglutamates (Figure 27.1). These cannot be transported extracellularly unless hydrolysed back to MTX monoglutamate, thereby leading to intracellular accumulation of the MTX polyglutamates. Free MTX is rapidly cleared from the serum by renal tubular filtration, which is the primary mode of drug elimination.

In malignant disease, high-dose MTX acts as a folate antagonist, competitively inhibiting dihydrofolate reductase, thymidylate synthase and other enzymes involved in de novo purine synthesis. Purines are a key component of nucleic acids, and this in turn inhibits cell replication. At low doses, MTX has anti-inflammatory actions, the mechanisms of action being complex and not clearly understood. These include the inhibition of pro-inflammatory cytokine signalling through inhibition of Janus kinases, the accumulation of extracellular adenosine and the selective generation of reactive oxygen species in dysregulated inflammatory lymphocytes. The mechanism of action of the adverse events (AE) seen with MTX is not clear, but it is likely due to both folate deficiency (gastrointestinal and haematological AEs) and folate-independent mechanisms (hepatic and pulmonary fibrosis).

INDICATIONS AND DERMATOLOGICAL USES

Licensed dermatological indications (adults):

- Psoriasis: MTX is licensed for the treatment of severe, uncontrolled psoriasis. In practice, it is recommended as a first-line systemic therapy for psoriasis and historically has been considered the gold standard comparator for newer interventions, such as biologics. MTX is a well-established treatment for different variants of psoriasis, including chronic plaque disease, pustular psoriasis, erythrodermic psoriasis and psoriatic arthritis. Published studies indicate that MTX reduces plaque-type psoriasis severity by at least 50% in approximately two-thirds of patients.

Unlicensed dermatological indications (adults):

- MTX has been reported to be beneficial in the unlicensed treatment of a variety of inflammatory skin conditions. Patients should be counselled that they are being prescribed MTX outside of the terms of its license, and the rationale for prescribing should be explained. Such conditions include:
  - Alopecia areata.
  - Atopic eczema (atopic dermatitis).

DOI: 10.1201/9781003016786-27

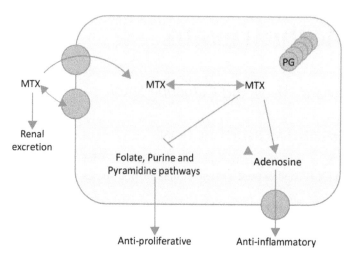

FIGURE 27.1   Methotrexate metabolism in the target cell.

- Bullous pemphigoid.
- Chronic spontaneous/idiopathic urticaria.
- Cutaneous small vessel vasculitis (including cutaneous polyarteritis nodosa, Behçet's disease and erythema elevatum diutinum).
- Dermatomyositis.
- Granuloma annulare.
- Hailey–Hailey disease.
- Langerhans cell histiocytosis.
- Lymphoproliferative disorders (including CTCL, mycoses fungoides, lymphomatoid papulosis and pityriasis lichenoides).
- Lupus erythematosus, systemic and cutaneous (DLE, SCLE, chilblain lupus, lupus profundus).
- Necrobiosis lipoidica.
- Oral lichen planus.
- Pemphigus.
- Pyoderma gangrenosum.
- Sarcoidosis.
- Systemic sclerosis (including limited systemic sclerosis)/localized scleroderma (morphoea).

MTX is also licensed in the treatment of rheumatoid arthritis, Crohn disease and, at higher doses, for certain malignancies, such as leukaemia, non-Hodgkin lymphoma and certain solid tumours.

FORMULATIONS/PRESENTATION

- Scored tablets containing 2.5 mg or 10 mg MTX. (NB: Different tablet strengths may be a source of confusion for patients and increase the risk of an inadvertent overdose; many dermatologists restrict prescribing to 2.5 mg tablets only to avoid patient error.)
- Pre-filled pen devices are available for SC administration that contain 7.5 mg to 30 mg MTX. With appropriate training these can be self-administered by patients.

DOSAGES AND SUGGESTED REGIMENS

MTX should be given as a once-weekly single dose with explicit verbal and written instructions to the patient. A divided dose regimen (e.g. 3 12-hourly doses) should be avoided unless there is significant nausea, as this can significantly increase the risk of dosing error by the patient.

Oral administration is convenient and preferable, with the starting dose dependent on the renal function, age of the patient and associated comorbidities.

In normal, healthy adults, consider starting at a therapeutic dose of 15 mg weekly with full blood count (FBC) (complete blood count [CBC]) measured at 1 week. However, it is common practice to begin with a smaller dose, e.g. 7.5 mg weekly. In older people and those with renal impairment, an initial test dose of 2.5–5 mg should be given and FBC (CBC) measured at 1 week. This should detect those that are unduly sensitive to the drug. If the FBC remains stable, the dose can be increased in increments of 2.5 mg a week. More cautious dosing is due to the increased risk of MTX accumulation and toxicity.

The maintenance dose should be adjusted according to disease response and kept as low as possible. MTX is a slow-acting drug, and the complete clinical response for a given dose may take up to 8 weeks to achieve. The maximum licensed dose in psoriasis is 30 mg/wk. However, disease control is usually achieved at a lower dose.

If bioavailability or patient compliance is of concern, SC administration may be appropriate. When switching from oral to parenteral administration, be aware that there may be enhanced bioavailability, so consider a modest dose reduction, particularly if the oral dose >5 mg weekly, and re-check blood monitoring for 2 weeks after the switch.

Following a treatment break of several weeks, MTX should be reintroduced as at first initiation (with a potential lower dose and subsequent titration to a higher therapeutic dose) with appropriate monitoring.

BASELINE INVESTIGATIONS AND CONSIDERATIONS

Baseline investigations:

- Full blood count (FBC) (complete blood count [CBC]), red cell folate.
- Serum electrolytes and renal indices.
- Consider glomerular filtration rate (GFR) or creatinine clearance in patients over the age of 60 years, with a raised serum creatinine level, low eGFR (<50 mL/min) or history that indicates potential renal impairment.

Baseline liver assessment:

- Liver function tests (LFTs), including AST and gamma-GT.
- Hepatitis B and C virus.
- Non-invasive assessment for liver fibrosis using serum biomarkers (e.g enhanced liver fibrosis [ELF], Fibrosis-4 (FIB-4), pro-collagen III) or imaging (transient elastography [Fibroscan]) (see also Special Point).
- Consider serum ferritin (male patients) to exclude hemochromatosis and antimitochondrial autoantibodies (female patients) to exclude primary biliary cirrhosis.
- Consider liver ultrasound to exclude gross liver pathology.

Special Point: Hepatotoxicity

Long-term use of MTX can be associated with hepatotoxicity, including the development of liver fibrosis. MTX hepatotoxicity is an important cause of treatment withdrawal but rarely leads to cirrhosis and liver failure. Proactive monitoring can limit this risk. The pathogenesis of MTX-associated liver fibrosis is not clear and may be multifactorial. Patients on MTX for rheumatoid arthritis appear to be less at risk of liver toxicity. In patients with psoriasis, a high cumulative MTX dose (>1.5 g), type 2 diabetes mellitus, high alcohol intake, obesity and viral hepatitis B or C infections are considered risk factors for hepatotoxicity. These factors can be independently associated with an increased risk of chronic liver disease (fibrosis and cirrhosis) and may confound the risk of MTX hepatotoxicity. Therefore, these factors should be considered as cautions when initiating MTX, and advice should be offered on modifiable risk factors before initiating MTX.

Although abnormal LFTs may indicate underlying liver disease, they are unreliable in detecting chronic MTX hepatotoxicity, as there is poor correlation with histological changes. Percutaneous liver biopsy is the gold standard for the detection of liver fibrosis/cirrhosis, but its disadvantages include non-diagnostic results due to sampling error and a small but significant risk of serious complications, including bleeding and death. Additional non-invasive serum and imaging tests have been developed to aid the diagnosis of liver fibrosis, which include serum pro-collagen III peptide (PIIINP), additional composite scores of serum biomarkers (such as the ELF score and FIB-4 index) and liver transient elastography (such as FibroScan). Generally, non-invasive tests can be used to identify patients before or during MTX therapy who are at high risk of liver fibrosis and who need further assessment by a relevant specialist in hepatology.

Factors associated with false-positive PIIINP results include young age, smoking, non-steroidal anti-inflammatory drugs (NSAIDs) and active arthritis. Local guidelines and access to non-invasive screening tools may vary, with local hepatologists recommending alternative serial measures, such as Fibroscan or composite serum markers (although not validated in populations with psoriasis). If in doubt, specialist hepatological advice should be sought.

Other baseline investigations/assessments:

- Pregnancy test (urine/serum) in females of childbearing potential.
- Human immunodeficiency virus (HIV) testing.
- Assessment of disease severity (e.g. Psoriasis Area and Severity Index [PASI], Body Surface Area [BSA], Physician's Global Assessment [PGA]) and health-related quality of life (e.g. Dermatology Life Quality Index [DLQI]).
- Consider chest x-ray: Useful if significant pulmonary symptoms or risk of prior tuberculosis exposure (to exclude foci of old tuberculosis that may become reactivated as a result of the immunosuppressive effect of MTX therapy).

MONITORING

- Full blood count (FBC), serum electrolytes, renal indices and liver function tests (LFTs):
  - Consider weekly for 4 weeks at initiation.
  - Weekly for 2 weeks after each dose increase.
  - 8–12-weekly once dose stabilized.
- Red cell folate annually or if MCV increases.
- Serum biomarkers for fibrosis (e.g. PIIINP or ELF/FIB-4) at 3-monthly intervals or annual transient elastography (FibroScan).
- Refer to a specialist in hepatology if non-invasive markers indicate possible liver fibrosis to consider need for liver biopsy (see Special Point).
- Assessment of disease severity to monitor MTX efficacy.

CONTRAINDICATIONS

- Severe haematological abnormality – severe anaemia, leukopenia or thrombocytopenia.
- Severe liver disease (fibrosis or cirrhosis).
- Severe renal insufficiency (eGFR <20 mL/min) or renal replacement therapy (dialysis).

- Pregnancy or breastfeeding.
- Severe and/or active infectious disease (such as tuberculosis, viral hepatitis or uncontrolled HIV).
- Immunodeficiency.
- Active peptic ulcer disease.
- Significantly reduced lung function.
- Alcoholism.
- Patient unreliability.
- Hypersensitivity to MTX.
- Concurrent anti-folate medication.

CAUTIONS

- Renal impairment, i.e. GFR <50 mL/min: Since MTX is eliminated by renal excretion, toxic levels may rapidly accumulate in the presence of renal impairment, increasing the risk of myelosuppression. This is particularly liable to occur in older people during episodes of dehydration, or as a result of concomitant drug administration, e.g. NSAIDs.
- Pre-existing liver disease or current high alcohol intake may predispose to hepatotoxic effects of MTX.
- Previous hepatitis B or C infection (untreated).
- Controlled HIV infection.
- Gastritis.
- History of malignancy.
- Flu and pneumococcal vaccination are recommended for people who are on immunosuppressant medication; ideally these inactive vaccines should be administered at least 2 weeks before therapy is started. Prescribers are advised to consult the latest recommendation on COVID-19 vaccine and booster scheduling (see e.g. https://www.nhs.uk/conditions/coronavirus-covid-19/coronavirus-vaccination/health-conditions/). In patients that are stable and well-controlled on MTX, consider a 2-week pause in treatment following inactive vaccine doses (primary or booster) as studies have shown this leads to augmented antibody responses. Live vaccines are contraindicated on theoretical grounds once patients commence taking MTX.
- Current COVID-19 guidelines should be consulted for dermatology patients with immune-mediated inflammatory disorders (IMID) who are eligible for treatment with neutralizing monoclonal antibodies or antivirals.

IMPORTANT DRUG INTERACTIONS

- Ciclosporin, leflunomide, azathioprine and sulfasalazine: Concomitant use with nephrotoxic, myelotoxic or hepatotoxic drugs is not recommended.
- NSAIDs, penicillin, colchicine and probenecid may reduce MTX elimination, leading to increased risk of MTX toxicity. Where NSAIDs are considered essential, the lower starting dose of 2.5 mg MTX is indicated with monitoring of renal function after 1 week and at further weekly intervals after dose increases or changes in NSAID therapy. Ideally, NSAIDs should not be taken on a sporadic basis, as the effects on MTX levels can be difficult to predict.
- Penicillin, ciprofloxacin, tetracyclines and chloramphenicol may increase risk of MTX toxicity.
- Trimethoprim, sulphonamides and phenytoin are folate antagonists and may increase risk of MTX toxicity.
- Retinoids may increase risk of MTX hepatotoxicity.
- Radiotherapy: Radiation recall (burns) may occur at sites of prior irradiation.
- St John's wort may increase the risk of MTX toxicity.

ADVERSE EFFECTS AND THEIR MANAGEMENT

- Folic acid deficiency may arise in patients on MTX and is often identified by a rise in mean corpuscular volume (MCV). This may be exacerbated by concomitant medications that have antifolate activity (see Important Drug Interactions). If suspected, patients should receive folic acid supplementation for the duration of MTX therapy. Some physicians recommend routine folic acid supplementation to reduce the gastrointestinal or hepatic adverse effects of MTX. Different folic acid dosing regimens have been proposed, including 1–5 mg daily, 1–5 mg daily except for days of MTX and 2.5–5 mg once weekly 24 hours or more following THE MTX dose. There is no convincing evidence that concomitant folic acid administration reduces MTX efficacy. It is essential that the regimen for folic acid replacement is clearly explained to the patient to avoid confusion with MTX dosing. If the MCV continues to rise (>106 fL) despite folic acid supplementation and other causes are excluded (B12 deficiency or alcohol excess), MTX should be discontinued.
- Gastrointestinal: Nausea/vomiting affects about 10% of patients, usually occurring 12 hours after ingestion and persisting up to 3 days after therapy. Possible (although unproven) solutions include reducing the dose, adding folic acid, taking MTX with food and administering MTX SC.
- Myelosuppression may affect up to 20% of patients on long-term therapy for psoriasis, manifesting as leukopenia, thrombocytopenia, anaemia or pancytopenia. Myelosuppression can be severe and lead to fatal complications. The risk is increased in those with renal impairment, especially in older people, those taking concomitant drugs that reduce MTX excretion and in folate deficiency. MTX should be discontinued if severe leukopenia, thrombocytopenia or anaemia occur.
  - Hepatotoxicity: MTX has been associated with both acute and chronic hepatotoxicity (see Special Point). Acute elevation in serum aminotransferase concentrations frequently occurs 1–3 days after a dose of MTX. These changes are usually transient and asymptomatic. Long-term use of MTX is associated with fibrosis and/or cirrhosis. The absolute risk of developing liver fibrosis specifically attributable to MTX has not been robustly established, but this is, nevertheless, a reason for treatment withdrawal. If transaminases (ALT, AST) rise above 3 times the upper limit of normal, then MTX should be discontinued. For mild rises in LFTs, a minor dose reduction may be considered with close monitoring of LFTs to ensure normalization. Referral to a hepatologist and liver biopsy should be considered if there is persistent elevation of liver enzymes and/or non-invasive assessment reaches the threshold for further investigation (e.g. at least three PIIINP results >4.2 mg/L or two consecutive results >8.0 mg/L within a 12-month period or an abnormal FibroScan).
- Pulmonary toxicity appears to be more common in patients given MTX for rheumatoid disease and is an idiosyncratic adverse effect. If respiratory symptoms develop, such as a dry persistent cough, MTX should be stopped until MTX-induced pulmonary toxicity has been excluded.
- Carcinogenicity: There is no clear evidence that long-term MTX therapy is associated with increased risk of cancer. If a patient develops a cancer on MTX therapy, the decision to continue systemic immunosuppressive treatment should be made with the cancer specialist and patient.
- MTX overdose: Expert advice should be sought in the event of an MTX overdose.

Clinical manifestations of acute toxicity include myelosuppression, mucosal ulceration (particularly oral ulcers) and rarely acute skin ulceration. This latter complication is occasionally seen in patients with active extensive psoriasis if the dose of MTX is increased too rapidly. Toxicity can also be precipitated by factors that interfere with either the renal excretion of the drug, such as dehydration, or drug interactions. Folinic acid (calcium leucovorin) is a fully reduced folate coenzyme that can bypass the metabolic effects of MTX. Folinic acid should be prescribed without delay, ideally within 4 hours of MTX administration, as its efficacy decreases with time. An initial dose of 20 mg of folinic acid should be given IV or IM, followed by measurement of serum MTX levels if available. Further doses of folinic acid can be titrated accordingly. If MTX levels cannot be measured, 20 mg of folinic acid should continue to be given every 6 hours until the blood count has normalized and mucosae healed.

USE IN SPECIAL SITUATIONS

PREGNANCY AND PRE-CONCEPTION

MTX is strictly contraindicated during pregnancy, and patients must not become pregnant while taking MTX. MTX is both an abortifacient and a teratogen. The current EMA license advises that MTX therapy should be stopped at 6 months before conception by both males and females. However, controversy exists around the necessity for this precaution in males taking low-dose MTX, and it is advised that men planning on conceiving should talk to their healthcare team as soon as possible. In the event of an unplanned pregnancy, expert advice should be sought.

LACTATION

MTX is contraindicated in lactation, as it is excreted in breast milk.

CHILDREN

MTX may be used under specialist supervision for children (2–18 years old) with severe psoriasis, atopic dermatitis, localized scleroderma, pityriasis lichenoides et varioliformis acuta and dermatomyositis. However, it is not licensed for these indications in this age group. MTX is given as a once-weekly dose, usually initiated at 0.2 mg/kg, which can be increased to 0.5 mg/kg (max. 25 mg) as guided by clinical response. The lowest possible dose required to maintain disease control should be prescribed. The safety profile is relatively favourable in terms of known long-term oncogenic risk. Normal serum PIIINP levels are much higher in children and are therefore of little value in monitoring for hepatotoxicity.

ESSENTIAL PATIENT INFORMATION

- The patient must understand and be able to comply with regular blood test monitoring.
- Patients should be counselled about the weekly MTX dosing schedule with clear prescribing information, especially when folic acid is co-prescribed, to avoid confusion between these drugs.
- Patients should seek urgent medical attention if they develop symptoms of serious infection, including fever, sore throat, breathlessness or unexplained bleeding or bruising.
- Patients should be aware that MTX is an immunosuppressant and that they may need to stop treatment (usually temporarily) if they develop an infection that fails to improve after a few days or respond to initial conventional treatment.
- Patients should consider receiving any planned live vaccinations before starting MTX, as these will be contraindicated once MTX is started.
- Patients who have not had chickenpox and come into contact with either chickenpox or shingles should seek urgent medical advice.
- Patients should inform their doctor/pharmacist that they are taking MTX before starting any new medication.

- Patients should be advised to significantly limit their alcohol intake and to avoid conception/ pregnancy.
- To help improve the safety of MTX prescribing, an MTX treatment booklet is recommended for patients to keep a record of any dose changes and the results of monitoring investigations.

FURTHER READING

Chalmers RJ, Kirby B, Smith A, et al. Replacement of routine liver biopsy by procollagen III aminopeptide for monitoring patients with psoriasis receiving long-term methotrexate: A multicentre audit and health economic analysis. Br J Dermatol. 2005;152:444–50.

Maybury CM, Samarasekera E, Douiri A, et al. Diagnostic accuracy of noninvasive markers of liver fibrosis in patients with psoriasis taking methotrexate: A systematic review and meta-analysis. Br J Dermatol. 2014;170(6):1237–47.

National Institute for Health and Clinical Excellence. Psoriasis: The assessment and clinical management of psoriasis. Clinical guidelines CG153. October 2012. http://guidance.nice.org.uk/CG153.

Warren RB, Weatherhead SC, Smith CH, et al. British Association of Dermatologists' guidelines for the safe and effective prescribing of methotrexate for skin disease 2016. Br J Dermatol. 2016;175(1):23–44.

28 Mycophenolate Mofetil

Joey E. Lai-Cheong and Jane Setterfield

CLASSIFICATION AND MODE OF ACTION

Mycophenolate mofetil (MMF) is a lymphocyte selective immunosuppressive agent. It inhibits de novo purine synthesis via its active metabolite, mycophenolic acid, a potent selective and reversible inhibitor of inosine monophosphate dehydrogenase. Lymphocytes are critically dependent for their proliferation on de novo synthesis of purines, whereas other cell types can use salvage pathways. MMF thereby prevents the proliferation of T-cells and the formation of antibodies by B-cells. It may also inhibit leukocyte recruitment to inflammatory sites.

MMF is used for the prophylaxis of acute organ transplant rejection, and like several other immunosuppressive agents developed for this use, it has been found to be an effective treatment for various inflammatory dermatoses. The appeal of MMF in dermatology is related to both its potential steroid-sparing effects and its relative lack of toxicity.

INDICATIONS AND DERMATOLOGICAL USES

MMF is licensed for use in combination with prednisolone or ciclosporin for the prevention of acute kidney, heart and liver transplant rejection.

It has been demonstrated to be of benefit in the treatment of many inflammatory skin diseases, but it is used off-license. It may be used either as a monotherapy or as a steroid-sparing agent and is generally well-tolerated. Examples include:

- Autoimmune blistering diseases: Bullous pemphigoid, mucous membrane pemphigoid, epidermolysis bullosa acquisita, paraneoplastic pemphigus, pemphigus foliaceus and pemphigus vulgaris.
- Dermatitis: Actinic dermatitis, atopic dermatitis and psoriasis.
- Connective tissue disorders: Dermatomyositis, lupus erythematosus, scleroderma.
- Vasculitides: Pyoderma gangrenosum, Churg–Strauss syndrome, hypocomplementemia urticarial vasculitis, microscopic polyangiitis and granulomatosis with polyangiitis (GPA).
- Graft-versus-host disease: Acute and chronic variants.
- Granulomatous disorders: Cutaneous Crohn disease and sarcoidosis.
- Others: Lichen planus, relapsing idiopathic nodular panniculitis.

FORMULATIONS/PRESENTATION

- 250 mg capsules and 500 mg tablets of MMF.
- Oral suspension (1 g/5 mL) and 500 mg vials of MMF for IV injection.
- Mycophenolic acid 180 mg and 360 mg delayed-release tablets.

In patients who are unable to tolerate the gastrointestinal side effects of MMF, mycophenolic acid delayed-release tablets may be an alternative. Mycophenolic acid 720 mg is approximately equivalent to 1 g of MMF, but unnecessary switching should be avoided due to pharmacokinetic differences.

DOI: 10.1201/9781003016786-28

DOSAGES AND SUGGESTED REGIMENS

The usual starting dose of MMF in dermatological disease is 500 mg Bd. If there is no improvement after 1 month, doses are typically increased in 500 mg increments. The usual maintenance dose is 1 g Bd, increased to a maximum of 1.5 g Bd if required.

Dose adjustment is required for patients with renal insufficiency. In those with a glomerular filtration rate (GFR) of less than 25 mL/min, the maximum dose is 1 g twice a day.

BASELINE INVESTIGATIONS AND CONSIDERATIONS

- Full blood count (FBC) (complete blood count [CBC]) and differential white blood count (WBC).
- Urea, electrolytes and creatinine.
- Liver function tests (LFTs).
- Hepatitis B and C serology.
- Human immunodeficiency virus (HIV) testing.
- Chest x-ray.
- Pregnancy testing and effective contraception for females of childbearing potential.
- Thorough examination of skin to exclude malignancy and clinical examination to detect lymphadenopathy, breast lumps or organomegaly.
- Up-to-date cervical screening.

MMF may be used with caution in patients with HIV and hepatitis B and C virus infection, under close collaboration with other specialist medical practitioners. The immunosuppressant action of MMF can reactivate hepatitis B and C as well as worsen the immunosuppressive status of patients with HIV. Other serious viral infections reported include:

- Polyomavirus-associated nephropathy (PVAN), especially due to BK virus infection, is associated with deteriorating renal function and renal graft loss.
- John Cunningham virus-associated progressive multifocal leukoencephalopathy (PML), which can be fatal, commonly presents with hemiparesis, apathy, confusion, impaired cognition and ataxia.
- Cytomegalovirus (CMV) acquired from a seropositive transplant donor is associated with a high risk of CMV viraemia and CMV disease.

Varicella zoster virus (VZV) vaccine (live attenuated) should be given to non-immune patients several weeks before starting MMF if treatment can safely be delayed.

MONITORING

FBC, urea, electrolytes and creatinine and LFTs should be monitored weekly for 4 weeks, then twice a month for 2 months and then monthly for the first year. Thereafter, most clinicians would advise monitoring every 3 months, provided the patient has been stabilized on MMF. It may take up to 3 months for the therapeutic effect to be observed.

It is recommended to stop or withhold treatment and contact an initiating specialist in the following situations:

- Total white cell count $<4 \times 10^9$/L.
- Neutrophil count $<2 \times 10^9$/L.
- Platelet count $<150 \times 10^9$/L.
- Aspartate or alanine aminotransferase $>2 \times$ the upper normal limit.
- Hypogammaglobulinemia.

CONTRAINDICATIONS

- Hypersensitivity to MMF or mycophenolic acid.
- Pregnancy and lactation.
- Rare inherited deficiencies of the enzyme hypoxanthine-guanine phosphoribosyl-transferase, such as Lesch–Nyhan and Kelley–Seegmiller syndrome, as MMF exacerbates the underlying abnormality of uric acid metabolism.

CAUTIONS

- Peptic ulcer disease (active or past history) and other inflammatory gastrointestinal (GI) diseases may be associated with an increased risk of GI haemorrhage, ulceration and perforation.
- HIV and hepatitis B or C.
- There is an increased risk of hypogammaglobulinemia and bronchiectasis, especially in patients who are taking concomitant immunosuppressive treatments. It is advised to check immunoglobulin levels in cases of recurrent infection, cough or persistent respiratory infections.
- Flu and pneumococcal vaccination are recommended for people who are on immuno-suppressant medication; ideally these inactive vaccines should be administered at least 2 weeks before therapy is started. Prescribers are advised to consult the latest recommendations on COVID-19 vaccine and booster scheduling (see e.g. https://www.nhs.uk/conditions/coronavirus-covid-19/coronavirus-vaccination/health-conditions/).
- Current COVID-19 guidelines should be consulted for dermatology patients with immune-mediated inflammatory disorders (IMID) who are eligible for treatment with neutralizing monoclonal antibodies or antivirals.

IMPORTANT DRUG INTERACTIONS

Patients should be advised to check with pharmacists and treating physicians before taking any prescribed or over-the-counter medication while on MMF.

- Antacids with magnesium and aluminium hydroxides: May impair MMF absorption.
- Cholestyramine and bile acid sequestrants: May reduce the enterohepatic circulation and efficacy of MMF.
- Rifampicin: May decrease MMF efficacy.
- Broad-spectrum antibiotics such as ciprofloxacin and amoxicillin plus clavulanic acid: May reduce the efficacy of MMF due to the alteration of GI flora and reduced enterohepatic drug recirculation.
- Azathioprine: Also inhibits purine metabolism with potential enhanced toxicity.
- Acyclovir, valaciclovir and related anti-viral drugs: May increase mycophenolic acid plasma concentration, as they compete for renal tubular secretion, so closer monitoring of blood counts is needed.
- Hormonal contraceptive efficacy may be reduced.

ADVERSE EFFECTS AND THEIR MANAGEMENT

MMF is generally well-tolerated with fewer nephrotoxic, hepatotoxic and neurotoxic side effects than other immunosuppressive agents.

- Gastrointestinal: The most commonly reported side effects are GI and are dose-dependent, occurring in up to 20% of patients at doses of 2 g daily. They include diarrhoea, nausea, vomiting, abdominal pain, anal tenderness and constipation. These are usually mild and rarely severe enough to result in discontinuation of therapy. Diarrhoea and nausea may be reduced by increasing the dose frequency of MMF. Serious adverse effects include GI haemorrhage, perforation and peptic ulceration.

- Myelosuppression: These are mostly anaemia and neutropenia and are usually mild, dose-related and reversible with discontinuation of therapy or dose reduction. Abnormal neutrophil morphology may occur with a left shift phenotype in the absence of infection.
- Urinary: These include dysuria, urgency, frequency and sterile pyuria, as well as haematuria and urinary tract infection.
- Infection: The risk of common and opportunistic infections is increased, especially at high doses. This includes herpes simplex, herpes zoster and staphylococcal skin infections in patients with atopic dermatitis, tuberculosis, atypical mycobacterial infections and lower respiratory tract infection/pneumonia. Recurrent infections indicate the need for immunoglobulin levels to be checked, as MMF can lead to hypogammaglobulinemia.
- Carcinogenicity: Animal studies have shown an increase in lymphoma; use of MMF in transplant recipients is associated with an increased risk of malignancy, especially lymphoma and lymphoproliferative disorders and non-melanoma skin cancer. These are generally considered to be related to the duration and intensity of immunosuppression rather than an MMF-specific effect. However, MMF may also impair UVB-induced DNA damage repair and apoptosis by immunosuppression-independent mechanisms. There have been reports of malignancy in dermatology patients. Patients should be advised to minimize exposure to sunlight by wearing protective clothing and high-SPF sunscreens. Rare cases of primary CNS lymphoma and Epstein–Barr virus (EBV)-related B-cell lymphoma of the CNS have also been reported in non-transplant patients.

USE IN SPECIAL SITUATIONS

PREGNANCY

MMF should be avoided in pregnancy due to an increased rate of first-trimester foetal loss (45–49%) and severe birth defects (23–27%). Congenital malformations include anomalies of the ears, eyes, cleft lip and palate, development of the fingers, heart, oesophagus, kidneys and nervous system.

Animal studies have shown reproductive toxicity at doses equivalent to and less than clinical doses. Females of childbearing potential should be established on effective contraception before starting MMF, during therapy and for 6 weeks following discontinuation of treatment. Two methods of effective contraception are recommended. Patients should consult their physician immediately should pregnancy occur.

Although there is no clinical evidence of an increased risk of malformations or miscarriage in pregnancies where the father was taking MMF, the MHRA has recommended that male patients and their female partners should use effective contraception during treatment and for 90 days following discontinuation, as the genotoxic risk cannot be excluded.

LACTATION

Mothers who are taking MMF should not breastfeed. Animal studies have shown that MMF is excreted in milk, and although it is not known whether this applies to humans, breastfeeding should be discontinued because of the potential risk to the infant.

CHILDREN

MMF is licensed for use in children of 2 years and above after renal transplantation, at doses of 600 mg/m^2 twice daily (maximum 2 g daily). There are very few reports of its use for skin disease in children. There is limited safety and efficacy data for the use of MMF in infants under 2 years, and therefore use in this age group is not recommended. Treatment is not appropriate in children with a body surface area less than 1.5 m^2.

Older People

Older patients (>65 years) may generally be at increased risk of adverse reactions due to immuno-suppression, especially infection and possibly GI disease.

ESSENTIAL PATIENT INFORMATION

- Patients should be fully informed of the indications for therapy and the unlicensed use of the drug.
- The need for close monitoring with blood tests, especially during the initiation phase of treatment, should be emphasized.
- Patients should be informed of the increased risk of common and unusual infections and the need to seek urgent medical attention if they become unwell with a high fever.
- The increased risk of skin cancer and the potential risk of lymphoma must be discussed. Use of sun protection is recommended.
- Females of childbearing potential should be given advice on the teratogenic risk in pregnancy and effective contraception should be advised before treatment is commenced.
- Patients on MMF should not give blood during treatment and for 6 weeks after stopping the medication. In addition, men should not donate semen during therapy and for 90 days following discontinuation of MMF.

FURTHER READING

Strathie Page SJ, Tait CP. Mycophenolic acid in dermatology a century after its discovery. Australas J Dermatol. 2015;56(1):77–83.

29 Omalizumab

Chris Rutkowski, Annette Wagner and Clive Grattan

CLASSIFICATION AND MODE OF ACTION

Omalizumab is a recombinant humanized (95%) murine monoclonal immunoglobulin (Ig) G1-kappa antibody against the Cϵ3 domain on the Fc region of immunoglobulin E (IgE). This is the same domain that binds to the high-affinity IgE receptor (FcϵRI) on mast cells and basophils as well as the low-affinity receptor (FcϵRII; CD23) on monocytes, macrophages, B and T lymphocytes, dendritic and epithelial cells. IgE that is bound to omalizumab is unable to bind to either the FcϵRI or FcϵRII. This leads to a reduction in receptor expression and, in the case of FcϵRI, the capacity of mast cells and basophils to degranulate and release mediators such as histamine and leukotrienes. A reduction in free IgE and receptor expression leads to a reduction in the inflammatory response in both the early and late phase of allergic reactions. This is considered relevant to its actions in allergic asthma. The reduction in free IgE serum levels occurs rapidly after administration of omalizumab, and the magnitude of this effect is dependent on the ratio of omalizumab to total serum IgE before treatment. The peak reduction is reached on average 7 days after administration.

The mechanism of action of omalizumab in chronic urticaria is not fully understood and may involve reduction of FcϵRI density with reduced mast cell releasability, capture of IgE autoantibodies against autoantigens (type I autoimmune urticaria), improvement in secondary basopenia and normalization of increased blood coagulation markers. Once IgE is bound to extracellular receptors (high- or low-affinity), omalizumab is no longer able to bind to IgE, and it therefore has no intrinsic cross-linking (anaphylactogenic) activity.

Omalizumab's half-life varies from 1 to 4 weeks (average 26 days). Immune complexes with IgE are removed by liver elimination and excretion into bile. Omalizumab is not disease-modifying, and in most patients, CSU relapses within 4–6 weeks of stopping treatment. Repeat 6-month courses can be given for many years (until spontaneous remission occurs) with no loss of response or development of clinically relevant anti-omalizumab antibodies.

INDICATIONS AND DERMATOLOGICAL USE

In the UK, omalizumab has been approved for use in the treatment of patients age ≥ 6 years with persistent, moderately severe and severe allergic asthma since 2003 and as an add-on therapy in patients ≥ 12 with chronic spontaneous urticaria (CSU) not adequately controlled with H$_1$ antihistamines since 2014. It can be used for CSU presenting as urticaria, urticaria and angioedema and angioedema only.

The 2015 UK National Institute of Health and Care Excellence (NICE) technology appraisal recommended the use of omalizumab as additional therapy for CSU in patients aged ≥ 12 years if:

- CSU has not responded to standard treatment with (up-dosed) H$_1$ antihistamines and leukotriene receptor antagonists (LTRA).
- CSU severity is assessed objectively, e.g. a weekly Urticaria Activity Score (UAS7) ≥ 28.

Omalizumab is stopped at or before the 4th dose if the condition has not responded. It is stopped at the end of a course of 6 doses if the condition has responded to check if spontaneous remission occurred and restarted only if the condition relapses. NICE requires that this agent is administered

DOI: 10.1201/9781003016786-29

by a secondary care specialist in allergy, dermatology or immunology (self-administration – see below).

Although off-license, there is increasing evidence for its use in chronic inducible urticarias (CIU) (solar, cholinergic, symptomatic dermographism, cold and heat contact, delayed pressure and aquagenic) as well as normocomplementaemic urticarial vasculitis. It has also been used off-license (small trials and case reports) in atopic dermatitis with some clinical benefit, but the lack of large randomized controlled trials and the availability of new licensed and more effective treatments limit its usefulness. Omalizumab can reduce mast cell mediator symptoms in systemic mastocytosis, especially in the context of Hymenoptera venom immunotherapy. Its use for bullous pemphigoid, contact dermatitis and idiopathic non-clonal mast cell activation syndrome is mainly anecdotal and is not recommended.

FORMULATIONS/PRESENTATION

Xolair® 150 mg solution of omalizumab in a pre-filled syringe is given only by subcutaneous injection. The dose per injection site must not exceed 150 mg.

DOSAGES AND SUGGESTED REGIMENS

The licensed dosing regimen for CSU in the UK is 300 mg omalizumab every 4 weeks. Patients' response to treatment varies. If there is no response to treatment before/at injection 4, treatment should be stopped. If patients are in remission after injection 6, treatment should be stopped to assess if continued treatment is needed. If patients relapse after cessation of treatment, it can be restarted. Prescribers should periodically reassess the need for continued therapy.

If omalizumab is used nonstop for more than 6 months, it can be stopped abruptly (the patient can be retreated if CSU relapses), or injection intervals can be increased by 1 week until an 8-week interval is reached and then stopped.

Previous data suggests that there is no need for dose adjustment in patients with CSU for age (≥12), gender, race, body mass index (BMI), baseline IgE and anti-FcεRI autoantibodies. However, more recent data supports off-license dosing protocols. In chronic inducible urticaria, treatment can start at 150 mg every 4 weeks and increased to 300 mg every 4 weeks if needed. In some patients with CSU, the dosing interval might need to be shortened to every 2 weeks and/or the dose might need to be increased to 450 or even 600 mg per dose to achieve symptom control. This is not endorsed by UK NICE. In some well-controlled patients, the dose can be reduced to 150 mg every 4 weeks and/or the interval extended to 5–8 weeks, instead of the standard 4 weeks. In recent studies patients who required a higher dose of omalizumab had a higher BMI, lower total IgE level and lower pre-omalizumab urticaria control test (UCT) scores. (The UTC is a patient-reported outcome measure ranging from 0 to 16, and lower scores (≤ 11) indicate poorer disease control.)

In December 2018, the European Medicine Agency approved omalizumab for self-administration in patients with no history of anaphylaxis who may self-inject or be injected by a caregiver from the 4th dose onwards. The patient or the caregiver must be trained in the correct injection technique and the recognition of anaphylaxis. Virtual and face-to-face training methods can be used. Standard antihistamine therapy should be continued throughout omalizumab treatment.

In recalcitrant severe CSU that has only partially responded to omalizumab, disease control may be achieved by combining omalizumab with methotrexate or ciclosporin under specialist guidance.

BASELINE INVESTIGATIONS AND CONSIDERATIONS

No specific laboratory investigations are required before and during treatment. However, pre-treatment total serum IgE <40 kU/L might be linked to a lower response rate. Moreover, a negative basophil histamine release assay (BHRA) can predict a fast response to omalizumab; a positive test might suggest the opposite. In the UK, all patients need to document at least 2 weeks of the UAS7/Angioedema Activity Score (AAS7) before treatment and have to document a UAS7 score ≥28 or AAS7 ≥28 to be eligible for treatment according to the NICE recommendations. Other validated patient-reported outcome measures (PROM) such as the UCT, angioedema control test (ACT), chronic urticaria life quality questionnaire (CU-QoL), angioedema life quality questionnaire (AE-QoL) and dermatology life quality index (DLQI) can also be used, although decision point thresholds have not been published except for UAS7.

MONITORING

The first 3 doses must be administered in a healthcare setting, and the patient must be monitored for an appropriate period (usually 1–2 hours) to ensure no adverse reaction (anaphylaxis) occurs. Routine provision of adrenaline autoinjectors is not required but can be considered in home therapy patients with a history of unexplained (idiopathic) anaphylaxis or anaphylaxis to other injectable drugs.

CONTRAINDICATIONS

Hypersensitivity to omalizumab or the excipient, polysorbate (Tween), found in Xolair are the main contraindications. The needle cap of the pre-filled syringe contains a derivative of natural rubber latex but not natural rubber latex itself.

IMPORTANT DRUG INTERACTIONS

No formal studies have been conducted, but interactions are not likely. Drug-drug interactions are unlikely as cytochrome P450, efflux pumps and protein-binding mechanisms are not involved in the clearance of omalizumab. Therefore, there is no reason to expect that drugs commonly used in the treatment of CSU will interact with omalizumab. Information on the use of omalizumab in combination with immunosuppressive (ciclosporin, methotrexate and mycophenolate) and anti-inflammatory (dapsone) therapies in patients with CSU available so far is reassuring but not sufficient to allow a formal assessment. As IgE is involved in the immunological response to some helminth infections, omalizumab may reduce the body's natural response to gut parasites and pharmacological treatments. If patients do not respond to anti-helminth treatment, omalizumab might need to be discontinued.

ADVERSE EFFECTS AND THEIR MANAGEMENT

Omalizumab used for CSU is generally well-tolerated.

- The most common adverse reactions reported in patients with CSU include nasopharyngitis, sinusitis, upper respiratory tract infections, nausea, arthralgia, headache and cough. These reactions are generally mild and do not lead to cessation of treatment.
- Injection site reactions have been reported but are usually tolerated by patients. Paracetamol is preferred for analgesia, as NSAIDs may aggravate CSU.
- Type I hypersensitivity reactions (anaphylaxis) to omalizumab have been reported, but they are very rare (0.2%). Most occurred within 2 hours after the injection and within the first 3 doses of Xolair. It is possible that some reactions were actually to the excipient, polysorbate 20 (Tween 20), rather than omalizumab; others might have simply represented a flare-up of the underlying CSU, which was confused with an allergic reaction.
- Type III hypersensitivity reactions (serum sickness) occur 1–5 days after administration and may start after the first or subsequent injections or after prolonged treatment. Symptoms include fever, arthralgia, rash and lymphadenopathy.
- Infections: Omalizumab may increase the risk of some helminth infections in patients who are at high risk. Such individuals might benefit from screening for such infections before treatment.

- Malignancies have been observed anecdotally, but subsequent data do not suggest an association between omalizumab and solid tumors.
- Arterial thromboembolic events (ATE) in controlled clinical trials and an observational study, a numerical imbalance of ATE was observed that was not found in a separate analysis of pooled clinical trials or observed in clinical practice.

USE IN SPECIAL SITUATIONS

PREGNANCY AND LACTATION

Omalizumab was classified as an FDA Category B drug (animal studies do not demonstrate a risk to the fetus, but there are no adequate studies in pregnant patients). It crosses the placenta, but a prospective study of pregnant patients treated with this drug for asthma did not confirm increased risk of major congenital abnormalities. Case reports have not shown any adverse effect in their children up to 4 years of follow-up. Case reports of patients treated for CSU during pregnancy confirm these findings. The amount of omalizumab in breast milk is minimal, so its use is considered acceptable during breastfeeding in patients with severe CSU. There is no human data, but in non-clinical fertility studies in primates, there was no impairment of male and female fertility and no genotoxic effects.

CHILDREN

Omalizumab is not licensed for treatment of urticaria in children younger than 12 years. However, case series have documented successful and well-tolerated treatment in children as young as 2 years with CIU and CSU.

OLDER PATIENTS

There is limited data available on the use of omalizumab in patients over the age of 65 years, but there is no clinical reason to suspect that this age group requires a different dosing protocol or is at higher risk of side effects.

ESSENTIAL PATIENT INFORMATION

Patients must be aware that omalizumab is approved for CSU as an add-on treatment to H_1 antihistamines. They can consider stopping antihistamines if completely symptom-free but should otherwise continue antihistamines while completing UAS7 between courses of omalizumab to identify those patients who are well-controlled without the need for further omalizumab therapy. Patients taking regular oral steroids before starting omalizumab must not stop them abruptly, due to risk of adrenal crisis secondary to iatrogenic adrenal insufficiency.

Patients or their caregivers who are going to (self)-administer omalizumab must receive training in injection techniques and management of anaphylaxis.

FURTHER READING

Agache I, Rocha C, Pereira A, et al. Efficacy and safety of treatment with omalizumab for chronic spontaneous urticaria: A systematic review for the EAACI biologicals guidelines. Allergy. 2021;76:59–70. https://onlinelibrary.wiley.com/doi/epdf/10.1111/all.14547.

National Institute for Health and Care Excellence (NICE). Omalizumab for previously treated chronic spontaneous urticaria. Technology appraisal guidance 339; published date, 8 June 2015.

Online resources: www.bad.org.uk and www.xolair.com can be useful for the patients and caregivers.

Rutkowski K, Wagner A, Jui-Lin Choo K, et al. 'Omalizumab plus': Combining omalizumab with immunosuppression for treatment of refractory chronic urticaria: A multicenter UK series. J Allergy Clin Immunol Pract. 2021;9:1400–1.e2. https://www.jaci-inpractice.org/article/S2213-2198(20)31212-5/fulltext.

30 Potassium Iodide

Genevieve Osborne

CLASSIFICATION AND MODE OF ACTION

Iodine is an essential dietary mineral used for the biosynthesis of tri-iodothyronine and thyroxine by the thyroid gland. From the 1940s, the practice of fortifying table salt with iodine as potassium iodide (KI) or iodate in some countries has eliminated endemic goitre locally, yet iodine deficiency still remains a serious health problem globally.

KI was first isolated in seaweed in the 19th century and thereafter used to treat thyroid disease and various dermatological and infectious diseases. Its use dwindled until the 1970s, when reports appeared of its benefit in treating the neutrophilic dermatoses erythema nodosum and nodular vasculitis.

KI is well-absorbed orally and is distributed into the thyroid gland, salivary glands, gastric mucosa, breasts and choroid plexus of the eye. It readily crosses the placenta, is distributed into milk and is excreted mainly in the urine and to a lesser extent via the faeces, saliva and sweat.

KI has an immunomodulatory mode of action with specific effects on neutrophil function. In vitro studies demonstrate that KI inhibits neutrophil chemotaxis and suppresses neutrophil generation of toxic oxygen intermediates that cause tissue damage. Its anti-fungal mode of action is uncertain, but it may enhance macrophage activation.

INDICATIONS AND DERMATOLOGICAL USES

KI is a thyroid-blocking drug causing inhibition of thyroxine production and may be used preoperatively before partial thyroidectomy in thyrotoxicosis. It is also used as emergency protection of the thyroid following accidental exposure to radiation. KI solution is also used as an expectorant in cough medicines.

DERMATOLOGICAL USES

Fungal infections
- Cutaneous and lymphocutaneous sporotrichosis: This is the most common global use of KI where itraconazole (first-line treatment) isn't available or there are cost pressures given the low comparative cost of KI. Both agents have level A-II evidence to support use in this infection.
- A benefit has also been reported in treatment of some other subcutaneous mycoses such as phycomycosis, human pythiosis, rhinophycomycosis as well as cutaneous cryptococcus and Nocardia brasiliensis.

Inflammatory dermatoses: The evidence to support use of KI is based on small case series or case reports.
- Panniculitis: Both erythema nodosum and nodular vasculitis.
- Neutrophilic dermatoses: Sweet syndrome, pyoderma gangrenosum (used second-line or when other treatments are contraindicated).
- Palmo-plantar pustulosis.

FORMULATIONS/PRESENTATION

- Aqueous solution in various concentrations, commonly a saturated solution of KI ('SSKI') containing 1000 mg of KI/mL with sodium thiosulphate as a preservative.

DOI: 10.1201/9781003016786-30

- SSKI should be stored in a light-resistant container between 15 and 30°C.
- 65 mg and 130 mg tablets (used as thyroid blockers) are less widely available globally.
- Supplements containing much lower doses of KI (e.g. 150 micrograms) can be obtained from health food shops.

DOSAGES AND SUGGESTED REGIMENS

Tablets have a bitter taste and should be swallowed whole with plenty of water. Aqueous solution of KI may be diluted with water, juice or milk and drunk with a straw to limit dental staining. Improved tolerance to gastrointestinal side effects is achieved by administering in 2–3 divided daily doses and by gradual dose increments over a few weeks to the treatment dose.

- Fungal infections: Higher doses used, typically 1.8–7.2 g total daily (600–2,400 mg Tds) for 3–6 months.
- Erythema nodosum: 300–900 mg daily (100–300 mg Tds) for 1–3 months; response may be rapid (within 48 hours).
- Sweet syndrome, pyoderma gangrenosum: 900 mg total daily (300 mg Tds); used for recalcitrant disease as adjunctive or steroid-sparing treatment.
- Palmoplantar pustulosis: 2.7 g total daily (900 mg Tds) for 3 months.

Children typically take one-third to one-half of the adult dose.

BASELINE INVESTIGATIONS AND CONSIDERATIONS

Baseline tests:

- Urea, electrolytes and creatinine.
- Thyroid function and thyroid autoantibodies.

MONITORING DURING TREATMENT

- Thyroid function every 2 months.
- Electrolytes/K^+ monitoring if given with drugs known to cause hyperkalaemia.

CONTRAINDICATIONS

- Impaired renal function.
- Hyperkalaemia.
- Cardiac disease.
- Iodine hypersensitivity.
- Pregnancy.
- Lactation.
- Addison disease.
- Dermatitis herpetiformis and hypocomplementaemic vasculitis.
- Untreated thyroid disease.

CAUTIONS

- Previous thyroid disease and/or positive thyroid autoantibodies, which increase the risk of hypothyroidism due to impaired thyroid autoregulation.
- Drugs that cause hyperkalaemia.

IMPORTANT DRUG INTERACTIONS

- Drugs that cause hyperkalaemia, including spironolactone, angiotensin-converting enzyme inhibitors, potassium sparing diuretics and ciclosporin.
- Iodine-containing drugs, such as amiodarone and thyroid-inhibiting drugs such as lithium and possibly sulphonamides, as they can cause hypothyroidism.

ADVERSE EFFECTS AND THEIR MANAGEMENT

- Gastrointestinal adverse effects: These are the most common side effects, and they are usually mild to moderate and dose-related. There is rarely small bowel ulceration.
- Thyroid dysfunction: This is more likely with pre-existing thyroid disease and when the treatment duration is longer and is caused by loss of thyroid gland autoregulation. It is usually reversible. Both hypothyroidism (Wolff-Chaikoff effect) and hyperthyroidism (Jod-Basedow effect) may occur.
- Metabolic: Hyperkalaemia and metabolic acidosis may cause confusion, arrhythmias, weakness and paraesthesia.
- Iodism (KI excess): This usually occurs at high doses or after prolonged use and causes metallic taste, oral soreness or ulceration, hyperlacrimation, enlarged salivary and lacrimal glands and blurred vision. It resolves within a few days of discontinuing KI.
- Hypersensitivity: Angioedema, urticaria, bronchospasm, pulmonary oedema, headache, fever, arthralgia and vasculitis.
- Dermatological: Pustular, cystic and acneiform lesions (iododerma). Ulcerating plaques appear more commonly where there is coexisting systemic disease. Immunobullous diseases (dermatitis herpetiformis and bullous pemphigoid) may be exacerbated.

USE IN SPECIAL SITUATIONS

PREGNANCY

KI should not be used in pregnancy, as it crosses the placenta and will cause fetal goitre and hypothyroidism.

LACTATION

KI is contraindicated, as it is excreted in breast milk.

ESSENTIAL PATIENT INFORMATION

Patients should be instructed to discontinue treatment and seek urgent medical attention if they develop symptoms of iodism, hyperkalaemia, angioedema, shortness of breath, severe abdominal pain or dark stool.

FURTHER READING

Anzengruber F, Mergenthaler C, Murer C, et al. Potassium iodide for cutaneous inflammatory disorders: A monocentric retrospective study. Dermatology. 2019;235:137–43.

Costa RO, de Macedo PM, Carvalhal A, et al. Use of potassium iodide in dermatology: Updates on an old drug. Ann Bras Dermatol. 2013;88(3):396–402.

Hayashi S, Shimaoka Y, Hamasaki Y, et al. Palmoplantar pustulosis and pustulotic arthro-osteitis treatment with potassium iodide and tetracycline, a novel remedy with an old drug: A review of 25 patients. Int J Dermatol. 2017;56:889–93.

Macedo PM, Lopes-Bezerra LM, Bernardes-Engemann AR, et al. New posology of potassium iodide for the treatment of cutaneous sporotrichosis: Study of efficacy and safety in 102 patients. J Eur Acad Dermatol Venereol. 2015;29:719–24.

Sterling JB, Heyman WR. Potassium iodide in dermatology: A 19th century drug for 21st century uses: Pharmacology, adverse effects and contraindication. J Am Acad Dermatol. 2000;43:691–7.

31 Propranolol

Susannah Baron

CLASSIFICATION AND MODE OF ACTION

Propranolol was the first successful beta-adrenoceptor antagonist (beta-blocker) to be used medically following its discovery by James Black in 1962. It is a non-selective beta-blocker and has been widely used in cardiovascular medicine to treat hypertension, angina and tachyarrhythmias. Infantile haemangiomas (IH), also known as strawberry naevi, are vascular tumours that appear in the first few weeks of life, undergo a proliferative phase (6–12 months) followed by stabilization and eventual spontaneous involution. They affect about 5% of all infants, predominantly on the head and neck. The first report of successful use of propranolol in IH was in 2008, and since then it has become the treatment of choice for this condition although it is unlicensed for IH. Its therapeutic effectiveness in IH may relate to peripheral vasoconstrictive actions, the reduced expression of pro-angiogenic factors and downregulation of the renin-angiotensin-aldosterone axis.

INDICATIONS AND DERMATOLOGICAL USES

Consider using propranolol for proliferating IH which are at risk of causing functional impairment to vision, feeding, breathing, hearing or those at risk of scarring/disfigurement (e.g. central face/ears), ulcerating IH, in segmental IH (facial, lumbar, sacral) and in liver IH (which can occur with multipe cutaneous IH). Propranolol should be initiated under specialist supervision.

CONTRAINDICATIONS

Relative:

- Frequent wheezing.
- BP +/– heart rate (HR) outside normal range; obtain advice from paediatrician.

Absolute:

- Recent/ongoing hypoglycaemic episodes.
- 2nd- and 3rd-degree heart block.
- Hypersensitivity to propranolol.

FORMULATIONS/PRESENTATION

Oral solutions of propranolol (which are of relevance for infants) are available in several concentrations ranging from 1 mg/mL–10 mg/mL. For simplicity and to reduce the risk of dose error, it is advised to routinely use the 5 mg/5 mL solution.

DOSAGES AND SUGGESTED REGIMENS

Guidelines have been published in the UK, United States, Australia and Europe, and while broadly similar, the following regimen is recommended by the British Society of Paediatric Dermatology consensus guidelines published in 2018.

DOI: 10.1201/9781003016786-31

Treatment with propranolol can be started as an outpatient, without monitoring of HR and BP in infants aged >4 weeks, born at term with no significant comorbidities, normal birth weight, established feeds and appropriate weight gain.

Starting doses of 1 mg/kg/day are given in 3 divided doses, at least 6 hours apart, and can be increased after 24 hours to a maintenance dose of 2 mg/kg/day, given in 2 or 3 divided doses with a maximum dose of 3 mg/kg/day. Propranolol should be administered either immediately before, during or right after a feed to minimize risk of hypoglycaemia.

A lower starting dose of 0.5 mg/kg/day should be used for infants with suspected PHACE(S) syndrome, and ideally, cerebral imaging should be performed before starting and increasing to maintenance dosage. For infants <4 weeks, preterm or with comorbidities likely to lead to hypoglycaemia, the starting, incremental and maintenance dosing schedules should be individualized by the supervising paediatrician/paediatric dermatologist.

A drug-dosing card/monitoring booklet is recommended to aid dose adjustments and avoid dosing errors. Treatment should be stopped temporarily if there is significant reduced oral intake/vomiting.

Treatment is usually continued until the end of the proliferative stage at around 14–18 months of age. Most patients with IH do not need treating beyond 18 months of age. Treatment can be stopped abruptly, but it is best to taper the dose, as relapse may occur in up to 15% of patients and treatment can be reinitiated if needed.

BASELINE INVESTIGATIONS AND CONSIDERATIONS

- See Figure 31.1.
- Clinical history and examination, especially of the cardio-respiratory system with heart rate (HR), blood pressure (BP), peripheral pulses and abdominal examination for liver enlargement and signs of hypothyroidism.
- If multiple cutaneous haemangiomas (>5), screen with an ultrasound for liver IH and check thyroid function for consumptive hypothyroidism.
- Document family history of arrhythmias, sudden death, loss of consciousness and maternal connective tissue disease.
- Clinical photography and patient information leaflet.
- ECG in selected patients (e.g. HR outside range for age, strong family history of sudden death/arrhythmia, loss of consciousness, maternal history of connective tissue disease and heart murmur).
- Echocardiogram is required if HR is outside normal range for age or if heart murmur.
- Cardiology assessment may be required according to examination/investigation findings and in those with segmental IH.
- Baseline glucose in selected patients at risk of hypoglycaemia, eg. preterm/low weight (other routine blood tests are not required).
- ENT assessment for suspected airway haemangioma and ophthalmology for periocular haemangioma.
- All patients with cervicofacial segmental IH (suspected PHACE(S) syndrome; see segmental syndromes below) should have an echocardiogram, ECG and assessment by a paediatrician with cardiac expertise. It is important to obtain brain imaging before initiating propranolol, ideally with a cerebral magnetic resonance angiogram (MRA), and if this shows arterial stenosis or agenesis, obtain expert advice from a paediatric neurologist about the safety and dosage of propranolol. If it is not possible to obtain urgent brain imaging, the starting dose of propranolol should be no more than 0.5 mg/kg/day in 3 divided doses.
  - Initiation and dose increments should be carried out during day case admissions for 2–4 hours on initiation and for dose increments >0.5 mg/kg/day.
  - HR and BP should be measured before the first dose and then every 30 min for 2–4 hours.
  - All patients with segmental IH of the perineum or lower back should have further investigation (MRI, ultrasound), as these may be associated with other congenital anomalies.

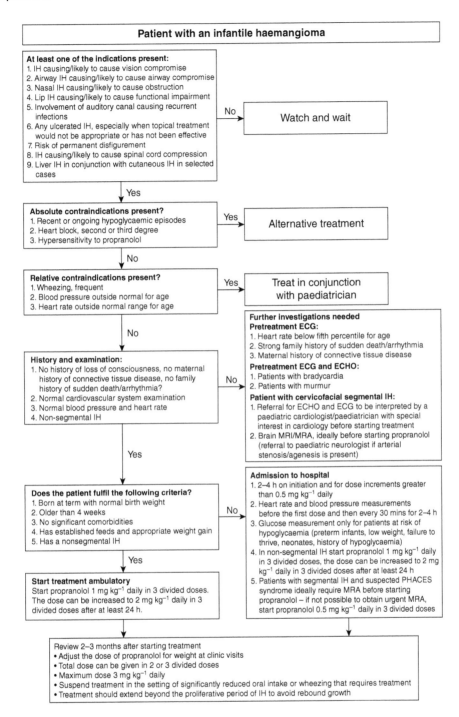

FIGURE 31.1   Propranolol treatment algorithm in IH.

RARE SYNDROMES ASSOCIATED WITH SEGMENTAL HAEMANGIOMAS

- PHACE(S) syndrome: (P)osterior fossa and other brain malformations, large/facial segmental (H)aemangiomas of the head and neck, anatomical abnormalities of the cerebral/cervical (A)rteries, (C)ardiac abnormalities/(C)oarctation of the aorta and (E)ye abnormalities. There may also be clefting of the (S)ternum.

- PELVIS syndrome: Segmental (P)erineal haemangioma, (E)xternal genital malformations, (L)ipomyelomenigocele, (V)esicorenal abnormalities, (I)mperforate anus and (S)kin tag.
- LUMBAR syndrome: Segmental (L)umbosacral haemangioma, (U)rogenital anomalies, (M)yelopathy, (B)ony deformities, (A)norectal malformations/arterial anomalies and (R)enal anomalies.

SUMMARY

Propranolol for IH in healthy, full-term neonates ≥4 weeks:

- Use 5 mg/5 mL propranolol preparation.
- Blood glucose to be checked only in patients at risk of hypoglycaemia (preterm, low weight, faltering growth, neonates or history of hypoglycaemia).
- Obtain baseline photographic record of lesion and serial monitoring photographs at follow-up appointments.
- Starting dose 1 mg/kg/day in 3 divided doses for 24 hours.
- Maintenance dose is 2 mg/kg/day in 2–3 divided doses – Adjust per weight at clinic visits/ by GP or by parents with written instructions.
- Minimum time interval between dose increases is 24 hours.
- Maximum dose for non-responders is 3 mg/kg/day.
- No need for BP or HR monitoring between visits if infant is well.
- Where observations are needed (HR and BP), record at intervals of 30 min for 2–4 hours.
- Routine follow-up should be at 2–3 months.

IMPORTANT DRUG INTERACTIONS

- Avoid lidocaine-containing medications, including teething gels (Bonjela, Dentinox and Calgel), as concurrent use of propranolol increases the risk of lidocaine toxicity.
- Avoid salbutamol or any other selective beta-2-agonists. If bronchodilatation is needed, ipratropium bromide (Atrovent) should be used.
- Cardiac medication may increase the risk of bradycardia and hypotension. Expert advice and closer monitoring are required.
- Corticosteroids may increase the risk of hypoglycaemia due to adrenal suppression.
- Bile acid sequestrants (colestyramine and colestipol) may decrease propranolol levels up to 50%.

ADVERSE EFFECTS AND THEIR MANAGEMENT

- Peripheral vasoconstriction (cold hands and feet) is common. It is usually asymptomatic, but mittens/socks may help and reduce dose if needed.
- Gastrointestinal adverse effects, including nausea, diarrhoea and constipation, are common. Note that propranolol should be stopped if oral intake is reduced due to illness or if the infant has undergone procedures requiring fasting due to the increased risk of hypoglycaemia.
- Sleep disturbance and agitation may occur as propranolol is lipophilic and can passively cross the blood–brain barrier. Use of a hydrophilic beta-blocker such as atenolol may be considered as an alternative. Irritability and agitation may also be features of hypoglycaemia.
- Hypoglycaemia, with symptoms including sweating, shakiness and headache, is uncommon and can usually be avoided by administering propranolol during or immediately after a feed.

- Bronchospasm/wheeze may be induced by viral/respiratory infections. Propranolol should be temporarily discontinued while the child is unwell.
- Cardiovascular adverse effects (bradycardia, hypotension and high-output cardiac failure). Treatment should be stopped and specialist advice should be sought.

If propranolol is not tolerated, treatment with topical Timolol 0.5% gel ×2–3 times per day (ophthalmic formulation) may be considered for small superficial haemangiomas. It is less effective than oral propranolol and rarely can cause skin irritation. Systemic absorption may occur.

The publishers would like to acknowledge the input of Dr. Brid O'Donnell as a contributor to previous versions of this chapter.

FURTHER READING

Hoeger PH, Harper JI, Baselga E, et al. Treatment of infantile haemangiomas: Recommendations of a European expert group. Eur J Pediatr. 2015;174(7):855–65.

Krowchuck DP, Frieden IJ, Mancini AJ, et al. Clinical practice guideline for the management of infantile hemangiomas. Pediatrics. 2019;143(1):e20183475.

Leauge-Labreze C, Harper JI, Hoeger PH. Infantile haemangioma. Lancet. 2017;390:85–94.

Novoa M, Baselga E, Beltran S, et al. Interventions for infantile haemangiomas of the skin. Cochrane Database Syst. Rev. 2018;4:CD006545.

Smithson SK, Rademaker M, Adams S, et al. Consensus statement for the treatment of infantile haemangiomas with propranolol. Australas J Dermatol. 2017;58(2):155–9.

Solman L, Glover M, Beattie P, et al. Oral propranolol in the treatment of proliferating infantile haemangiomas: British Society of Paediatric Dermatology consensus guidelines. Br J Dermatol. 2018;179(3):582–9.

32 Psoralens

Hiva Fassihi

CLASSIFICATION AND MODE OF ACTION

Psoralens are naturally occurring furocoumarins that are found in several plant species. They appear to have a protective role against microbes and inhibit germination of seeds. These aromatic molecules strongly absorb certain ultraviolet (UV) wavelengths and act as photosensitizers when administered orally or topically. Synthetic psoralens have been used therapeutically in dermatology since the 1970s in conjunction with UVA in psoralen-UVA photochemotherapy (PUVA). Three psoralens are in use in dermatology: 8-methoxypsoralen (8-MOP; Methoxsalen), 5-methoxypsoralen (5-MOP; Bergapten) and 4,5,8-trimethylpsoralen (TMP).

Photochemical reactions involve the interaction of light or UV radiation with a specific molecule or chromophore, which absorbs this radiation to induce a photochemical reaction. The precise molecular structure of a chromophore determines the wavelength of radiation absorbed, while the degree of tissue penetration by such radiation regulates the depth at which the photochemical reaction occurs. In PUVA, the chromophore is psoralen, which is distributed throughout the skin by diffusion from dermal blood vessels or trans-dermally following a topical application. Since UVA readily penetrates the skin to the region of the papillary dermis, the therapeutic effects of PUVA are maximal in epidermal and superficial dermal pathologies.

Psoralens intercalate between DNA strands, favouring thymidine-rich portions of the genome. Subsequent absorption of UVA leads to their photoreaction with DNA, binding to both sides of the double-stranded helix (bifunctional adducts) to produce inter-strand cross-links that prevent DNA replication. PUVA also induces reactive oxygen species formation, which leads to cell membrane damage by lipid peroxidation. Skin-infiltrating lymphocytes are suppressed by PUVA, which may explain its therapeutic effects in cutaneous T-cell lymphoma as well as inflammatory skin diseases. PUVA induces pigmentation by enhanced proliferation of melanocytes, increased formation and melanization of melanocytes, and transfer of melanosomes to keratinocytes.

INDICATIONS AND DERMATOLOGICAL USES

Psoralens are unlicensed drugs in the UK and Ireland. 8-methoxypsoralen is approved for dermatological diseases by the FDA in the United States. The main uses of PUVA therapy are as listed below.

PSORIASIS

PUVA is effective in clearing chronic plaque psoriasis, but thick plaques may be slow to respond. Bath and oral PUVA appear to have similar efficacy in the treatment of psoriasis. PUVA should be offered before oral systemic and biological therapy for patients that have not responded adequately to other therapies, including narrowband UVB phototherapy. The overall efficacy is good, with approximately 60–70% of patients achieving a 75% reduction from the baseline Psoriasis Area and Severity Index (PASI 75), and disease remission may last several months. Maintenance PUVA should be avoided in order to minimize cumulative skin damage and carcinogenesis.

DOI: 10.1201/9781003016786-32

VITILIGO

PUVA is usually reserved for patients with deeply pigmented skin (types IV to VI). Widespread small lesions, central body involvement and disease of recent onset respond best, while acral vitiligo and bony areas generally respond poorly. Progress should be documented with clinical photographs (approximately once every 4 months), and treatment should be discontinued once improvement has ceased. In sunny parts of the world, application of topical psoralen creams and use of natural sunlight in low doses is widely practiced. Narrowband UVB phototherapy has now superseded PUVA as the treatment of choice for vitiligo, as it has similar efficacy but induces a better quality of skin repigmentation and has a better safety profile.

CUTANEOUS T-CELL LYMPHOMA (CTCL)

PUVA is an effective treatment for early-stage CTCL. It is used in the treatment of mycosis fungoides (MF), the most common subtype of CTCL, where it is an important treatment modality, particularly in plaque stage disease. PUVA achieves high rates of clearance and prolonged disease-free intervals, although the long-term course of the disease may be unchanged. PUVA can be given in combination with interferon or retinoids if response to monotherapy is slow. Maintenance therapy may be considered in those with quickly recurrent disease. It is also a useful adjunctive therapy for late-stage disease through reducing the tumour burden in the skin and improving quality of life for patients. Extracorporeal photopheresis involves the removal of circulating white blood cells and their irradiation with UVA in conjunction with 8-methoxypsoralen, followed by reinfusion into the patient. It is used in the treatment of advanced CTCL in persons who have not been responsive to other forms of treatment.

ECZEMA

Good-quality randomized control trials on the use of PUVA in the management of atopic eczema (atopic dermatitis) is limited. Eczema is more difficult to treat with PUVA compared to psoriasis, and a higher number of treatments is often required. Narrowband UVB phototherapy should be the first-line phototherapy for atopic eczema, and PUVA should only considered if narrowband UVB has not been adequately effective.

OTHER

Other dermatological conditions that are commonly treated with PUVA include:

- Hand and foot dermatoses: Local PUVA, using oral or topical psoralens, is an effective treatment for hand and foot dermatoses. The three main conditions are hand and foot eczema, psoriasis and palmoplantar pustulosis. In general, oral PUVA is more effective than topical PUVA for these patients. In addition, in palmoplantar pustulosis, there is evidence for increased treatment efficacy when oral PUVA is combined with oral retinoids.
- Photodermatoses (polymorphic light eruption, solar urticaria and chronic actinic dermatitis): The mechanism by which phototherapy induces tolerance to sunlight might involve hyperpigmentation and thickening of stratum corneum, as well as modulation of cutaneous immune response. There is a high risk of provocation, and care must be taken. PUVA for photodermatoses should only be carried out in experienced specialized units. In temperate countries, PUVA is usually administered in early spring and continued natural sunlight exposure is advised to maintain the benefits of phototherapy throughout the spring and summer months.
- Other dermatoses: PUVA is also used with variable effect in other dermatoses such as lichen planus, generalized granuloma annulare, chronic graft-versus-host disease, urticaria pigmentosa and nodular prurigo.

FORMULATIONS/PRESENTATION

Two oral psoralens are currently available:

- 8-MOP (Methoxsalen) is available in two different 10 mg capsule formulations:
  - Oxsoralen-Ultra® soft gelatin capsules taken 1.5–2 hours before UVA exposure for psoriasis treatment.
  - Puvasoralen® hard gelatin capsules taken 2 hours before UVA exposure for psoriasis and 2–4 hours before UVA in vitiligo treatment.
    - If nausea occurs, the dose may be divided and extended to 4 hours before treatment in both diseases.
    - These formulations should not be used interchangeably, as the bioavailability and photosensitization time course is significantly greater and earlier for soft gelatine capsules.
- 5-MOP (Bergapten) is available in 20 mg capsules and is taken 3 hours before UVA.

A variety of other generic and branded topical formulations are available globally:

- 8-MOP 1.2% lotion for dilution to a final concentration of 3.6 mg/L at 37°C for immersion (bath- or hand/foot-PUVA). The patient is immersed for 15 minutes, and UVA exposure is given immediately.
- 8-MOP 0.005% gel for direct application to the diseased area using a gloved hand. UVA exposure is given 30 minutes later.
- Oxsoralen lotion 1%, used topically before UVA for treatment of vitiligo (United States only).
- TMP (tripsoralen/trioxsalen) manufacturing has now been largely discontinued.

DOSAGES AND SUGGESTED REGIMENS

Oral PUVA

8-MOP capsules should be taken at a specified time before UVA exposure (see Formulations/Presentation). The timing of psoralen ingestion should be exact, and the dosage should be based on surface area. The usual dose is 25 mg/m^2 (approximately 0.6 mg/kg). The body surface area is calculated using a nomogram. Basing the dose on body surface area is preferable to basing the dose only on body weight. Ideally, food should be avoided 1 hour before and after dosing, but it is usually necessary to take the dose with a light meal to avoid nausea. In this case, the type and amount of food should be kept constant for the patient to avoid variations in drug bioavailability.

In standard PUVA regimens, the initial UVA exposure should preferably be determined on the basis of prior measurement of the minimal phototoxic dose (MPD) rather than skin type, as this allows more accurate and higher UVA doses during the initial treatment phase. PUVA erythema peaks at 48–96 hours, and as a compromise, MPDs are usually measured at 72 hours. PUVA treatments are usually given twice weekly for psoriasis, and increases in UVA dose are calculated as a percentage of previous exposures, or rarely, by intermittent MPD testing. Treatment regimens vary for other dermatoses; smaller incremental doses of UVA are used in the management of atopic eczema and CTCL, while low doses of UVA are used in the prophylaxis of polymorphic light eruption.

When adding an oral retinoid to patients already receiving PUVA therapy, the UVA dosage needs to be reduced by about 50%. It is best to recheck the MPD to minimize the risk of burning, as the effects of retinoids vary between individuals.

5-MOP is administered at a dose of 50 mg/m^2 (approximately 1.2 mg/kg), and its slower absorption leads to less nausea.

> Retinoid with UVA (RePUVA): RePUVA therapy involves a combination of a systemic retinoid with PUVA. It reduces the number of treatments needed for disease clearance by about one-third, and the total UVA dose often by more than one-half compared with conventional

PUVA. The 'synergistic' action accelerates desquamation of psoriatic plaques and reduces inflammatory infiltrate. Retinoids also provide chemoprevention against non-melanoma skin cancer development. Treatment is initiated with oral retinoid approximately 10–14 days before starting PUVA. The starting dose ranges from 0.1 to 1 mg/kg, as retinoids are variably tolerated by the individual; most people tolerate 0.3–0.5 mg/kg. Acitretin is currently the conventionally used oral retinoid, but isotretinoin can be used instead if prolonged risk of teratogenicity is unacceptable.

Eye and skin protection: Patients should avoid sun exposure for at least 8–12 hours after psoralen ingestion. Eye protection with special protective goggles is mandatory during UVA exposure, and UVA-absorbing wrap-around sunglasses should be worn throughout daylight hours after psoralen ingestion. The sunglasses should be marked UV400 (blocking all wavelengths below 400 nm). In view of the high risk of PUVA-induced genital skin cancer in males, genital protection with a UV opaque garment is strongly recommended. Facial skin, if unaffected, should also be covered during treatment, usually by means of a visor.

TOPICAL PUVA (BATH, IMMERSION OR PAINT)

UVA is administered immediately after immersion for bath PUVA therapy, while an interval of 15–30 minutes should be allowed between application of psoralen paint and UVA exposure. Patients do not need to shower afterwards, but should have sunscreen applied to any areas that will be exposed to sunshine in the next 4 hours.

Topical PUVA is preferable to oral PUVA in patients with hepatic dysfunction, gastrointestinal disease where absorption is impaired (e.g. after ileostomy), cataracts or those unable to comply with eye protection, to permit shorter irradiation times, and where drug interactions are anticipated. However, many patients prefer oral to topical PUVA, as it involves shorter overall hospital attendance times.

SPECIAL POINT

MPD testing should be repeated if patients are changed from oral to bath PUVA, as bath 8-MOP therapy is approximately 5–10 times more photosensitizing than the oral form. Severe burning may therefore result if the UVA dose is not reduced during conversion from oral to bath PUVA.

BASELINE INVESTIGATIONS AND CONSIDERATIONS

- Full blood count (FBC) (complete blood count [CBC]).
- Renal indices.
- Liver function tests (LFTs).
- Antinuclear antibodies if there is a history of photosensitivity.
- Baseline minimal phototoxic dose (MPD).
- Ophthalmological investigation for patients at increased risk of cataracts.
- Careful assessment for skin cancer risk.
- Documentation of concomitant topical and systemic medications.
- Education of patient regarding sun-protective measures with a high factor, broad-spectrum sunscreen and UV protective clothing.

MONITORING

- FBC, renal indices and LFTs should be repeated 6–12 months after initiation of therapy.
- During and particularly after protracted PUVA therapy (more than 150 treatments), patients should undergo regular full skin examination for pre-cancerous and cancerous lesions, as well as receiving advice on self-examination for new or changing skin lesions.

CONTRAINDICATIONS AND CAUTIONS

The absolute and relative contraindications for PUVA are listed below, according to guidelines from the British Photodermatology Group.

ABSOLUTE CONTRAINDICATIONS

There are a number of absolute contraindications to the use of PUVA. These include:

- Photogenodermatoses (xeroderma pigmentosum, Cockayne syndrome, trichothiodystrophy, Bloom syndrome and Rothmund Thomson syndrome).
- Disorders with a genetic predisposition to skin cancers (Gorlin syndrome, hereditary dysplastic naevus syndrome and albinism).
- Lupus erythematosus.
- Previous malignant melanoma.

RELATIVE CONTRAINDICATIONS

Major:

- Age <10 years.
- Previous or current non-melanoma skin cancer.
- Current pre-malignant skin lesions.
- Previous exposure to arsenic or ionizing radiation.
- Concomitant oral immunosuppressive therapy.
- Pregnancy and nursing.
- Porphyria.

Minor:

- Age <16 years.
- Pre-existing cataracts or patients who are aphakic.
- Bullous pemphigoid and pemphigus.
- Significant hepatic impairment.
- Previous internal malignancy.
- Past excessive exposure to natural sunlight, sunbeds or phototherapy.
- Any medical condition causing intolerance of heat or prolonged standing (for example, those with severe cardiovascular or respiratory disease and those with poorly controlled epilepsy).

CAUTIONS

- PUVA should be used with caution in patients with skin type I and II who tend to burn easily.
- PUVA should generally be avoided in patients with a past or current personal history of melanoma or non-melanoma skin cancer; however, cases should be assessed on an individual basis and PUVA could be considered in those where therapeutic options are limited and the benefit of the treatment outweighs the potential risks.
- Concurrent and post-PUVA treatment with ciclosporin or methotrexate must be avoided.
- As oral psoralens are metabolized in the liver, it is sensible to avoid PUVA in severe liver disease, although they may be used in mild impairment. Sporadic reports of hepatitis associated with PUVA treatment have been published. In severe impairment, the use of topical

psoralens is recommended (bath or lotion) because serum levels are low compared with oral therapy.

- Renal excretion is the main route of elimination of psoralen metabolites; thus, oral PUVA can be used in patients with stable renal impairment in a reduced dose, but preferably combined with MPD measurement before treatment, to reduce the risk of burning. Bath PUVA is preferable in such circumstances.

IMPORTANT DRUG INTERACTIONS

- Photosensitizing concurrent drug treatment should be noted, and if started after the onset of PUVA, MPD testing should be undertaken with appropriate UVA dosing to prevent excessive phototoxic reactions. These include retinoids, non-steroidal anti-inflammatory drugs (NSAIDs), fluoroquinolone and tetracycline antibiotics, thiazide diuretics, griseofulvin, phenothiazines and sulphonamides.
- Coumarin anticoagulants may be displaced from binding sites by psoralens.
- Anticonvulsant therapy can result in low serum concentrations of oral psoralens as a result of the induction of hepatic enzymes.
- Hepatic cytochrome 450 (CYP450) 1A2 is inhibited by systemic PUVA and metabolism of theophylline, and other CYP1A2 substrates may be affected (including tricyclic antidepressants and propranolol).

ADVERSE EFFECTS AND THEIR MANAGEMENT

Acute Adverse Effects

- Nausea is a relatively common side effect of oral psoralens occurring in about 3–13% of patients and is usually reduced by taking psoralens with food. A light, low-fat meal is recommended, as high-fat diets can cause a significant decrease in psoralen absorption. Rescheduling UVA treatment for later in the day or taking the dose of psoralen in divided portions over a 30-minute period may help. Severe nausea can be treated with antiemetics, or if intractable, the psoralen dose may be reduced by 10 mg and the UVA dose increased proportionately. Nausea is less frequent with 5-MOP therapy because of slower absorption.
- Erythema and burning may occur due to pronounced sensitivity to psoralen or excessive UVA dosing. Although the erythema is often evident at 24 hours, it will not peak until 96 hours or later. Therefore, early recognition and omission of further treatment is important. Prompt treatment with emollients, topical corticosteroids and oral NSAIDs may be helpful. If the erythema is not too severe, once it has resolved, PUVA might be restarted at a lower UVA dose, using smaller increments.
- Pruritus may be either localized or generalized, and usually occurs in patients receiving oral psoralens. It may rarely be severe and persistent. Treatment with topical and systemic steroids, emollients and antihistamines is often unsatisfactory. The itch has a prickling quality and may persist for weeks to months before eventually resolving. The incidence of pruritus is reported to be lower with 5-MOP than with 8-MOP, and so if PUVA therapy is absolutely necessary thereafter, oral 5-MOP should be used. Generally, however, further PUVA should be avoided.
- Induction of photodermatoses that are associated with UVA photosensitivity can occur with PUVA. There are many reports of polymorphic light eruption and chronic actinic dermatitis being exacerbated by PUVA treatment given for an alternative indication.
- Triggering of herpes simplex virus can occur with PUVA, and the use of a high-factor sunscreen on the lips is recommended. Occasionally, prophylactic acyclovir may need to be prescribed during PUVA treatment.

- Hepatotoxicity is rare. In reported cases, the abnormal liver function tests revert to normal after PUVA treatment is stopped.
- Severe skin pain is very rare and is characterized by persistent burning or dysaesthesia, which can last from hours to weeks or months. An underlying neurogenic mechanism is likely. Analgesics, topical anaesthetics, and topical or systemic steroids are usually ineffective. Capsaicin, gabapentin and phenytoin may be of benefit. PUVA pain is a relative contraindication to further PUVA treatment.
- Allergic and photocontact dermatitis to psoralens is rare but can occur in patients being treated with topical PUVA.
- Anaphylaxis is an extremely rare event.

CHRONIC ADVERSE EFFECTS

- Cutaneous photocarcinogenesis and photoaging are the most significant long-term complications of PUVA. A significant increase in squamous cell carcinoma (SCC) is noted in patients exposed to more than 150 treatments, and there is also an associated increase in basal cell carcinoma (BCC). An increased rate of melanoma has been reported with high cumulative doses of PUVA, but there may be a latent period of many years and the relationship remains to be clarified. Ciclosporin should be avoided in those with a history of PUVA treatment, as this increases the risk of SCC development.
- PUVA lentigines (irregular, stellate, darkly pigmented macules) may develop in fair-skinned individuals, particularly after a high cumulative number of PUVA treatments. Other skin changes related to high exposure include PUVA keratoses, porokeratoses and poikiloderma.
- Induction of cataracts is a theoretical risk but is virtually unheard of in practice. The use of UVA protective goggles in the UVA cabinet and the wearing of UV protective glasses on treatment days prevents this potential side effect, which dissipates after 24 hours. Protective glasses are not needed after bath PUVA.

USE IN SPECIAL SITUATIONS

PREGNANCY

Oral psoralen is associated with reduced birth rate and teratogenicity in animal studies, but this was not found in humans. Small studies did not reveal a higher rate of congenital malformations in humans, although there was an increase in low–birth-weight babies born to females who received PUVA during pregnancy. It was assumed that this finding was the effect of the underlying inflammatory skin disease rather than PUVA. Nevertheless, it is recommended that patients should avoid conception during PUVA therapy.

LACTATION

There is a minor risk of transmission of psoralen in breast milk, with the consequent possibility of induction of photosensitization in infants. PUVA in all forms is therefore contraindicated during lactation.

CHILDREN

Oral psoralens should not be used routinely in children under the age of 10 years, due to long-term risk of carcinogenicity. Treatment can be undertaken in special circumstances with great caution.

ESSENTIAL PATIENT INFORMATION

Before starting PUVA, it is recommended that written patient consent is obtained. This should supplement careful verbal explanation and helps to document that the patient has been informed of potential risks of treatment.

With acknowledgement to Gillian Murphy and Veronika Dvorakova, who contributed this chapter to the previous edition.

FURTHER READING

Elmets CA, Lim HW, Stoff B, et al. Joint American Academy of Dermatology – National Psoriasis Foundation guidelines of care for the management and treatment of psoriasis with phototherapy. J Am Acad Dermatol. 2019;81(3):775–804.

Ling TC, Clayton TH, Crawley J, et al. British Association of Dermatologists and British Photodermatology Group guidelines for the safe and effective use of psoralen-ultraviolet A therapy 2015. Br J Dermatol. 2016;174(1):24–55.

Stern RS. The risk of squamous cell and basal cell cancer associated with psoralen and ultraviolet A therapy: A 30-year prospective study. J Am Acad Dermatol. 2012;66(4):553–62.

UK service guidance and standards for Phototherapy Units and examples of PUVA treatment schedules can be found on the following websites:

British Association of Dermatologists: https://www.bad.org.uk/healthcare-professionals/clinical-services/service-standards/phototherapy

The South-East of England Phototherapy Network: http://www.phototherapysupport.net

33 Rituximab

Richard W. Groves

CLASSIFICATION AND MODE OF ACTION

Rituximab (Rituxan) and biosimilars such as Truxima and Rixathon are chimeric, murine–human monoclonal antibodies of the immunoglobulin (Ig) G1 subclass directed against the B-lymphocyte–specific antigen CD20, expressed by pre-B- and mature B-cells. These include early B-cells in the bone marrow, autoantigen-specific B-cells, memory B-cells and mature B-cells. Haematopoietic stem cells and plasma cells lack the CD20 antigen and are therefore not directly affected by rituximab treatment. CD20 is thought to regulate cell cycle initiation and differentiation of the B-cell lineage and possibly functions as a calcium channel. Interestingly, rituximab seems predominantly to affect autoantigen-specific B-cells in comparison to memory B-cells directed against microbial antigens, which may be protected by their privileged location in the bone marrow and solid organs. The fragment antigen-binding (Fab) domain of rituximab binds to the CD20 antigen on B-lymphocytes, and the Fc domain recruits immune effector cells that mediate B-cell lysis. Three mechanisms of B-cell depletion have been proposed, including complement dependent cytotoxicity, antibody-dependent cell-mediated cytotoxicity and induction of apoptosis. Thus, rituximab results in a rapid and sustained depletion of circulating and tissue-based B-cells, which can be maintained for at least 6–12 months. Recent data suggest that rituximab may also affect T-cell function and might modulate autoreactive T-cells and production of T-cell cytokines.

The half-life of the monoclonal antibody in the peripheral circulation is approximately 22 days. It is thought that non-specific degradation of rituximab occurs in the liver, followed by renal excretion.

INDICATIONS AND DERMATOLOGICAL USES

Rituximab has been widely used in the treatment of B-cell malignancies, with use in over a million patients. The licensed indications in the UK are:

- B-cell haematological malignancies: CD20 positive non-Hodgkin lymphoma (NHL) and chronic lymphocytic leukaemia.
- Rheumatoid arthritis.
- Granulomatosis with polyangiitis and microscopic polyangiitis.
- Pemphigus vulgaris.

Rituximab has also been reported to be of benefit in the treatment of other autoimmune diseases, including idiopathic thrombocytopenic purpura, haemolytic anaemia and connective tissue diseases such as dermatomyositis and Sjögren syndrome. Its main use within dermatology has been in the treatment of immunobullous disorders.

Patients suffering from immunobullous skin diseases who have failed conventional immunosuppressive therapy (systemic corticosteroid with other immunosuppressive agents) or have developed intolerable side effects from these drugs may benefit from rituximab. The most common disease that has been treated is pemphigus vulgaris, and high response rates have been reported, mostly when used in conjunction with concurrent immunosuppressive medication. There have also been several reports and studies indicating effectiveness in pemphigus foliaceus,

DOI: 10.1201/9781003016786-33

paraneoplastic pemphigus, mucous membrane pemphigoid, epidermolysis bullosa acquisita and bullous pemphigoid.

Other dermatoses that have been reported to respond to rituximab include atopic dermatitis, chronic graft-versus-host disease, cutaneous lupus, cryoglobulinaemia and cutaneous B-cell lymphoma.

FORMULATIONS/PRESENTATION

Rituximab for IV infusion is typically available as follows:

- Vials of 10 mL containing 100 mg of rituximab.
- Vials of 50 mL containing 500 mg of rituximab.

DOSAGES AND SUGGESTED REGIMENS

The licensed dosing regimens in the UK for rituximab are as follows:

- Weekly infusions of 375 mg/m^2 for 4–8 consecutive weeks, as a single agent or in combination with chemotherapy (NHL regimen).
- Two infusions of 1000 mg given 2 weeks apart.

In the initial reports of immunobullous disease treatment, the NHL regimen was used. However, the 1000-mg-2-weeks-apart regimen is generally favoured nowadays.

Rituximab should be administered under close supervision in a setting with full resuscitation facilities. Since transient hypotension may occur during infusion, consideration should be given to withholding antihypertensive medications 12 hours before and throughout infusion with rituximab. Treatment with paracetamol (acetaminophen) and H1-antihistamines is recommended before and throughout each infusion to reduce the risk of infusion reactions. Pre-medication with corticosteroids may be considered in order to reduce the frequency and severity of infusion-related reactions. Patients should receive 100 mg IV methylprednisolone to be completed 30 minutes before each infusion.

Patients with pre-existing cardiac conditions such as angina and arrhythmias or patients who develop clinically significant arrhythmias should undergo cardiac monitoring during and after subsequent infusions of rituximab.

For the first infusion, rituximab should be administered at an initial rate of 50 mg/h. If hypersensitivity or infusion-related events do not occur, this can be increased in 50 mg/h increments every 30 minutes, to a maximum of 400 mg/h. If hypersensitivity or an infusion-related event develops, the infusion should be temporarily slowed or interrupted. The infusion can continue at half of the previous rate upon improvement of the patient's symptoms.

Subsequent infusions of rituximab can be administered at an initial rate of 100 mg/h and increased by 100 mg/h increments at 30-minute intervals, to a maximum of 400 mg/h as tolerated. No dose adjustment is required in older patients (aged >65 years).

The onset of therapeutic effects in autoimmune bullous dermatoses is usually 2–3 months after initiation, though responses as late as 12 months have been reported. If disease relapses, further courses of rituximab can be safely administered without an increased risk of adverse effects.

Adjuvant systemic immunosuppressive drugs can be continued with concomitant use of rituximab, but dose reduction should be considered to decrease the risk of infections and other adverse effects related to immunosuppression.

Treatment of cutaneous B-cell lymphoma with intralesional injections of rituximab is also reported to be effective.

BASELINE INVESTIGATIONS AND CONSIDERATIONS

- Full blood count (FBC) (complete blood count [CBC]) and lymphocyte subsets, including B-lymphocyte count.
- Urea, electrolytes and creatinine.
- Liver function tests (LFTs).
- Ig levels.
- Hepatitis B and C serology.
- HIV testing.
- Pregnancy test.

These investigations should be repeated before each subsequent course of rituximab. Immunization status should be assessed before initiation of rituximab and consideration given to vaccination if appropriate.

MONITORING

- FBC (CBC) and lymphocyte subsets (B-cell count).
- Ig levels.
- Urea, electrolytes and creatinine.
- LFTs.

These should be checked 1 month after the last infusion, then every 3 months.

In pemphigus, serum desmoglein 1 and desmoglein 3 antibody levels should be measured by indirect immunofluorescence and/or enzyme-linked immunosorbent assay (ELISA) before first treatment, 1 month after the last infusion, then every following 3 months, as they reflect disease activity and can predict relapse. In the majority of patients with pemphigus vulgaris, the level of these autoantibodies parallels disease activity and decreases 3–10 months after treatment with rituximab. Rarely, clinical improvement occurs in the absence of a significant fall in antibody titer.

Circulating B-lymphocyte levels usually recover before disease activity relapses, but in some patients, relapse may occur despite persisting B-cell depletion.

CONTRAINDICATIONS

- Hypersensitivity to rituximab or to murine proteins.
- Progressive multifocal leukoencephalopathy (PML).
- Live virus vaccines.
- Severe active infection, including active hepatitis B disease.
- Severely immunocompromised patients.

CAUTIONS

- Severe heart failure (New York Heart Association Class IV) or severe uncontrolled cardiac disease.
- Patients with positive hepatitis B serology but no active disease should be referred to a hepatologist for assessment before starting rituximab, for advice on further management and monitoring.
- Patients may be immunized with non-live vaccines during treatment with rituximab. However, because of the B-cell depletion from the drug, the vaccine response is likely to be attenuated. Consequently, it is advised that important vaccines, including influenza, pneumococcus and COVID-19, are administered at least 4 weeks before the initiation

of rituximab. Should prior vaccination not be possible, at least 3 months should elapse from the final rituximab infusion before vaccination commences. Prescribers are advised to consult the latest recommendation on COVID-19 vaccine and booster scheduling (see e.g. https://www.nhs.uk/conditions/coronavirus-covid-19/coronavirus-vaccination/health-conditions/).
- Current COVID-19 guidelines should be consulted for dermatology patients with immune-mediated inflammatory disorders (IMID) who are eligible for treatment with neutralising monoclonal antibodies or antivirals.

IMPORTANT DRUG INTERACTIONS

There are limited data on drug interactions with rituximab. It is unlikely that rituximab affects the pharmacokinetics of drugs that are used in combination with it.

- Concomitant use of other immunosuppressive or immunomodulatory drugs can enhance the degree of immunosuppression and increase the risk of severe infections.

ADVERSE EFFECTS AND THEIR MANAGEMENT

Rituximab is generally well-tolerated.

- Infusion reactions are usually mild to moderate and occur within 30–120 minutes of infusion. They can present with fever, chills, headache, weakness, hypotension, nausea, dizziness, cough, pruritus and urticaria. The majority of reactions occur during the first infusion of rituximab and are less frequent with subsequent infusions. The symptoms are reversible when the infusion is discontinued and can usually be prevented by use of pre-treatment with antihistamines, cortico-steroids and paracetamol. When infusion reactions happen, treatment should be discontinued. If symptoms resolve, the infusion can be restarted at a reduced rate (half of the flow rate). More severe (occasionally fatal) infusion reactions have been reported rarely with acute respiratory distress syndrome, myocardial infarction (MI), ventricular fibrillation, cardiogenic shock and/or anaphylaxis. Stop the infusion immediately and start appropriate supportive management.
- Infections may occur due to immunosuppressive effects. The most common are respiratory tract infections, urinary tract infections and nasopharyngitis. Serious infections and fatal out-comes have been reported in patients treated for autoimmune bullous diseases with rituximab. In other indications, severe opportunistic, bacterial and viral infections such as pneumonias, pyelonephritis, skin infections, sepsis and systemic varicella zoster virus infections have been fatal. Reactivation of hepatitis B may occur (see Cautions), leading to fulminant hepatitis. Skin disease severity and concomitant immunosuppressant therapy affect the risk of severe infections. It is therefore advisable to try to reduce other immunosuppressive drugs to the minimal effective dose. Data from patients with primary cutaneous B-cell lymphoma sug-gest that the risk of infection is less frequent when rituximab is used as a monotherapy.
- PML due to reactivation of latent JC virus has been reported in at least 50 patients treated with rituximab for lymphoproliferative disorders, rheumatoid arthritis or SLE. Most cases were diagnosed within 12 months of treatment. Confusion, disorientation, motor weakness, diplopia, altered speech, dysphagia and ataxia should raise suspicion for PML. Discontinuation of rituximab and urgent neurological evaluation are advised.
- Hypogammaglobulinaemia may be associated with severe infections in patients treated with rituximab.
- Leukopaenia, neutropenia and thrombocytopenia have been reported in about 10% of patients. Closer monitoring of blood counts is indicated in such cases. Late neutropenia may occur up to 6 months after therapy. The mechanism of these reactions is unclear.

- Cardiac adverse effects such as angina, arrhythmia, heart failure and MI have been reported, so close monitoring is required in patients with a history of cardiac disease.
- Other severe adverse effects include tumour lysis syndrome and renal failure in patients with NHL.
- Severe mucocutaneous reactions (lichenoid dermatitis, paraneoplastic pemphigus, Stevens–Johnson syndrome, toxic epidermal necrolysis and vesiculobullous dermatitis) have been reported, though whether these relate to the drug or to the underlying condition being treated is unclear. In cases of doubt, immediate cessation of treatment is required.

It is not clear if there is an increased risk of malignancy relating to the immunosuppressant actions of rituximab.

USE IN SPECIAL SITUATIONS

PREGNANCY

IgG is known to cross the placental barrier, and transient B-cell depletion and lymphocytopenia have been reported in some infants born to mothers exposed to rituximab during pregnancy. For these reasons, the use of rituximab is advised against in pregnancy.

Females of childbearing potential should use effective contraceptive methods during treatment and for 12 months following the last infusion.

LACTATION

Maternal IgG is excreted in human milk, and mothers should not breastfeed while receiving rituximab and for 12 months following the last infusion.

CHILDREN

There are limited safety data for the use of rituximab in children, but uncontrolled studies have shown effectiveness in idiopathic nephrotic syndrome and severe rheumatic diseases. Transient and persistent hypogammaglobulinemia has been reported in rare cases of children with immunobullous diseases.

ESSENTIAL PATIENT INFORMATION

- Patients should be advised to seek prompt medical attention if they develop signs or symptoms of infection following treatment with rituximab.
- Patients should be informed of the potential risk of PML, though the magnitude of risk is unclear for patients with immunobullous disease.

FURTHER READING

Joly P, Horvath B, Patsatsi A, et al. Updated S2K guidelines on the management of pemphigus vulgaris and foliaceus initiated by the European Academy of Dermatology and Venereology (EADV). J Eur Acad Dermatol Venereol. 2020 Sep;34(9):1900–13.
Kushner CJ, Wang S, Tovanabutra N, et al. Factors associated with complete remission after rituximab therapy for pemphigus. JAMA Dermatol. 2019 Oct 23;155(12):1404–9.
Shimanovich I, Baumann T, Schmidt E, et al. Long-term outcomes of rituximab therapy in pemphigus. J Eur Acad Dermatol Venereol. 2020 Dec;34(12):2884–9.

34 Sulfapyridine and Sulfamethoxypyridazine

Ellie Rashidghamat

CLASSIFICATION AND MODE OF ACTION

The sulfonamide (sulphonamide) antibacterial drugs, sulfapyridine (SP) and sulfamethoxypyridazine (SMP) are structurally related to para-aminobenzoic acid (PABA). Their antibacterial effects are related to competitive inhibition of the bacterial enzyme dihydropteroate synthase, which plays a key role in converting PABA to dihydrofolic acid (a precursor of folic acid). Folic acid is required for the biogenesis of nucleic acids in DNA and RNA synthesis in both bacteria and in mammals.

Sulfonamides do not affect human cells by this mechanism, as they require pre-formed folic acid. Enzyme inhibition is reversible, so sulfonamides have bacteriostatic rather than bactericidal activity. They are rarely used as antibiotics nowadays due to adverse effects and bacterial resistance, with resistance to one sulfonamide conferring resistance to all.

SP was introduced in 1938 as M&B (May and Baker) 693 and was one of the first generation of sulfonamide antibiotics before being followed by several other related drugs. Shortly afterwards, their effectiveness in treating non-infective skin disorders was recognized. The current main use of SP and SMP is in inflammatory dermatoses mediated by activated neutrophils. They impair neutrophil cytotoxicity by inhibiting myeloperoxidase activity and preventing the formation of activated oxygen species, leading to anti-inflammatory actions. It is thought that the inhibitory effects on neutrophil function are similar to those of dapsone (see Chapter 17). They may also affect the protein moiety of glycosaminoglycans, leading to a reduction in tissue viscosity, oedema and vesicle formation.

Sulfonamides are slowly and incompletely absorbed from the gastrointestinal (GI) tract and do not undergo first-pass metabolism. They are protein-bound to variable degrees in the circulation, and unbound sulfonamide diffuses throughout the body, especially to sites of inflammation. Sulfonamides are metabolized to inactive compounds by hydroxylation, acetylation and glucuronidation in the liver. The enzyme N-acetyltransferase (NAT2) acetylates sulfapyridine into N-acetylsulfapyridine and, depending on polymorphisms, the rate of acetylation may vary across individuals. Parent drugs and their metabolites undergo renal excretion, and some sulfonamides are actively reabsorbed in the renal tubule. SP has a half-life of about 6–14 hours, depending on acetylator status, and SMP is longer-acting, with a half-life of 22 hours.

INDICATIONS AND DERMATOLOGICAL USES

The produce license for SP and SMP has lapsed, and they are now only available on a named-patient basis. The main use for these drugs is in the treatment of immunobullous diseases:

- Dermatitis herpetiformis.
- Linear IgA disease, chronic bullous dermatosis of childhood.
- Cicatricial (mucous membrane) pemphigoid.

Dapsone is usually the treatment of choice for these conditions; however, in patients that are intolerant of dapsone, or experience adverse effects, including haemolysis, methemoglobinemia and agranulocytosis, SP and SMP may be preferable. The risk for intolerance may increase with advancing age and in those with underlying cardiorespiratory disease (see Chapter 17), and in such patients,

DOI: 10.1201/9781003016786-34

SP or SMP are favoured options. Combination therapy with 2 or 3 (dapsone, SMP and SP) is occasionally used in patients with treatment-resistant disease. It also reduces the risk of renal toxicity from crystalluria (see Adverse Effects and Their Management).

Other, rarer uses of SP and SMP include pustular disorders such as subcorneal pustular dermatosis, pyoderma gangrenosum, pustular psoriasis and cystic or conglobate acne. There have also been reports of benefit in acrodermatitis continua, erythema elevatum diutinum and vasculitides, including leukocytoclastic vasculitis.

The pro-drug sulfasalazine (SSZ), which is licensed for the treatment of inflammatory bowel disease and rheumatoid arthritis, is converted to 5-aminosalicylic acid and SP by colonic bacterial enzymes. SP is almost fully absorbed, while most of the 5-aminosalicylic acid is excreted in the faeces. SSZ has been used off-label for a range of inflammatory dermatoses, but large studies are lacking. It is less expensive and may be a more accessible alternative to SP and SMP. It has fewer gastric side effects than SP, due to a lack of absorption in the upper gastrointestinal tract.

FORMULATIONS/PRESENTATION

- SP is available as 250 mg capsules under the brand name 'Concord 693.' It is manufactured by Kyowa Kirin Limited (acquired by Archimedes Pharma UK Ltd).
- SMP is currently available as 500 mg tablets by HAUPT Pharma. It is manufactured as an unlicensed product in Germany and imported by Clinigen (previously known as IDIS).

Both drugs should be protected from exposure to light.

- SSZ is available as 500 mg tablets and an oral suspension of 250 mg/5 mL.

DOSAGES AND SUGGESTED REGIMENS

SP and SMP are used as second-line agents when treatment with dapsone has failed or is contraindicated. They may be used in combination or with low-dose corticosteroid if monotherapy does not adequately control the disease.

In the treatment of adults with dermatitis herpetiformis (Table 34.1) a typical starting dose of SP is 500 mg twice a day, increased to 3 g daily, in accordance with disease control, tolerability and dose-related side effects. In most patients, the rash is controlled within this dose range. The maximum dose is 4.5 g daily. The clinical response should be assessed within 2 weeks, and dosage should be adjusted as necessary. The maintenance dose should be the lowest dose that prevents disease breakthrough. This may require frequent adjustment because of irregular absorption. With longer-term use, drug requirements should fall as dietary measures become effective. With a strict

---

TABLE 34.1

Dosage Schedule for the Treatment of Dermatitis Herpetiformis

Dose/Day	Sulfapyridine	Sulfamethoxypyridazine
Initial dose	1 g	500 mg
If good disease control, reduce to[a]:	0.5 g	500 mg on alternate days
If disease not controlled, incrementally increase dose to:	3 g	1 g
Maximum dose	4.5 g	1.5 g

[a] If control is maintained, reduce the dose further at 2–3 day intervals until breakthrough occurs. Maintain at the dose required to prevent breakthrough.

gluten-free diet, drug requirements usually diminish after an average of 8 months, but it usually takes 2 years of a strict gluten-free diet before drug discontinuation is possible. A partial gluten-free diet usually requires ongoing drug therapy.

SSZ may be considered as an alternative to SP. Two grams of SSZ is the molar equivalent of 800 mg of SP. The initial dose is 500 mg SSZ per day, increased up to 4 g daily in divided doses.

SMP has a longer half-life, and the usual starting dose in dermatitis herpetiformis is 500 mg once daily, increasing as below according to disease response, up to a maximum daily dose of 1.5 g.

Lower doses are used in the treatment of other pustular and immunobullous diseases.

SP and SPM should be taken with plenty of water, and a high fluid intake is recommended.

BASELINE INVESTIGATIONS AND CONSIDERATIONS

- Full blood count (FBC) (complete blood count [CBC]).
- Reticulocyte count.
- Urea and electrolytes.
- Liver function tests (LFTs).
- Glucose-6-phosphate dehydrogenase (G6PD) level (see Chapter 17).
- Urine microscopy with urinalysis to assess renal function.

MONITORING

- FBC and urinalysis at monthly intervals for the first 3 months and then every 3–6 months.
- Urea and electrolytes and LFTs: In the absence of specific advice, a similar monitoring schedule is reasonable, i.e. monthly for the first 3 months, then every 3–6 months.
- More frequent monitoring is recommended by the manufacturers for SSZ, with FBC and LFTs tested every 2 weeks for the first 3 months, then monthly for 3 months, and thereafter every 3 months if clinically stable.

CONTRAINDICATIONS

- Pregnancy and lactation.
- Hypersensitivity to sulfonamides[*].
- Infants (<1 year).
- Acute porphyrias.
- G6PD deficiency.
- Pre-existing significant anaemia or history of haemolytic anaemia.
- Interstitial lung disease (SMP).

SSZ is contraindicated in patients with salicylate hypersensitivity, e.g. aspirin.

CAUTIONS

Extra caution should be taken when SP/SMP is prescribed in the following:

- Liver dysfunction: Use the lower dose.
- Renal impairment: Use the lower dose.

---

[*] The sulfonamide chemical moiety is present in a range of other non-antimicrobial drugs, including certain diuretics, sulfonylureas and cyclo-oxygenase 2 inhibitors. However, the reactive arylamine group present in sulfonamide antibiotics that is a cause of drug hypersensitivity is absent in other non-antimicrobial sulfonamides, and the latter do not routinely need to be avoided in patients with a history of hypersensitivity to sulfonamide antimicrobials.

- Blood dyscrasias: Requires closer blood test monitoring.
- SSZ should be avoided in the above unless benefits outweigh risks. It should be given with caution in patients with asthma.

IMPORTANT DRUG INTERACTIONS

SP and SMP bind to plasma proteins and may displace other protein-bound drugs, resulting in increased free levels of the displaced drug with potential toxicity. Drugs affected include:

- Ciclosporin (cyclosporine).
- Clozapine: Increased risk of agranulocytosis.
- Coumarin anticoagulants (warfarin).
- Methotrexate.
- Phenytoin.
- Procaine (amino ester) local anaesthetics.
- Sulfonylurea oral hypoglycaemic agents.
- Non-steroidal anti-inflammatory drugs (NSAIDs): Sulfonamides may be displaced from the binding sites by highly acidic drugs such as NSAIDs, increasing the risk of toxicity.
- Zidovudine: Hepatic metabolism and clearance may be inhibited by SP.
- Live typhoid vaccine: Sulfonamides possess bacterial activity against Salmonella typhi and may thus interfere with the immunological response to the live typhoid vaccine. Allow 24 hours or more to elapse between the last dose of the antibiotic and the live typhoid vaccine. SP is also an inhibitor of cytochrome P450 2C9, and this may also contribute to interactions.

SSZ inhibits thiopurine methyl transferase enzyme activity and may potentiate azathioprine toxicity.

ADVERSE EFFECTS AND THEIR MANAGEMENT

Adverse effects are uncommon with the low doses used in dermatology. Sulfonamides undergo hepatic metabolism to inactive compounds, and slow acetylators appear to be at greater risk of severe adverse drug reactions. The adverse effect profile of SP and SMP is similar.

- Haematological: Adverse effects include blood dyscrasias (leukopenia, agranulocytosis and aplastic anaemia), methemoglobinemia and sulphaemaglobinemia. These can usually be prevented by careful FBC monitoring and early drug withdrawal. Haemolysis particularly affects those with G6PD deficiency but can occur with normal G6PD levels. Macrocytosis may also occur with or without folate deficiency.
- Dermatological: Urticarial/immediate-type hypersensitivity reactions and delayed-type hypersensitivity reactions may occur. The latter include severe cutaneous adverse drug reactions (Stevens–Johnson syndrome/toxic epidermal necrolysis and hypersensitivity vasculitis). The appearance of any of these necessitates immediate drug withdrawal. Milder adverse effects include uncomplicated exanthems and fixed drug eruptions. Desensitisation may be considered in special situations in patients with milder rashes. It has been successfully reported in patients with cystic fibrosis and human immunodeficiency virus (HIV) who require antimicrobial sulfonamide therapy. Photosensitivity has been reported with various sulfonamides but is rarely a clinical problem with SP and SMP.
- Gastrointestinal: Nausea and vomiting, stomatitis (SP > SMP) and abdominal pain are usually mild and may be helped by dose reduction. Nausea and vomiting often settle as

treatment continues, so immediate dose reduction may not be needed. Enteric-coated formulations may help if available.

- Hepatotoxicity: This ranges from mildly abnormal LFTs to severe hypersensitivity hepatitis with jaundice, fever and rash. Abnormalities usually occur within the first month of treatment, but later reactions have been described, so continued monitoring is important. Pancreatitis has also been reported as an idiosyncratic reaction with SP.
- Renal and urinary: Crystalluria and nephrolithiasis are more common with rapidly excreted sulfonamides (SP > SMP) and relate to a reduction in drug solubility in the acidic pH of the urinary tract. They may be asymptomatic or cause renal colic, haematuria, or chronic or even acute renal failure. A daily fluid intake of 2.5–3.5 L is recommended to maintain a urinary output of 1.2–1.5 L. Other measures that reduce crystal precipitation include alkalinisation of the urine and using triple sulfonamide combinations. Nephritis and albuminuria have also been rarely reported.
- Endocrine: Goitre and thyroid dysfunction have been reported with SP.
- Neurological: Fever, headaches, dizziness and drowsiness may respond to dose reduction. Paraesthesia and motor neuropathy have rarely been reported.
- Respiratory adverse effects that have been reported specifically with SMP include pneumonitis, alveolitis and obliterative bronchiolitis. These are potentially serious complications and usually present with progressive breathlessness and cough. Chest radiographs show diffuse interstitial shadowing, and a restrictive pattern is seen on lung function tests (reduced FEV1 and FVC). A peripheral eosinophilia has been found in a minority of cases, and an underlying vasculitis has been implicated. Most cases have occurred during prolonged drug administration. The condition generally responds to drug withdrawal and oral corticosteroid therapy, but rare fatalities have occurred.
- Hypersensitivity myocarditis is one of the most serious adverse effects, and it presents with cardiac failure.

USE IN SPECIAL SITUATIONS

PREGNANCY AND PRE-CONCEPTION

SP has been shown to cause oligospermia and infertility in males. This is reversible upon discontinuation of SP. Sulfonamides can cross the placenta and are relatively contraindicated in pregnancy, especially in the last trimester, due to potential neonatal toxicity.

LACTATION

SMP is contraindicated. The use of SP is controversial; it is excreted into breast milk at a concentration of 30–60% of that in maternal serum. Infants with G6PD deficiency may develop haemolytic anaemia. Kernicterus is theoretically possible due to bilirubin displacement from albumin binding sites by SP, but breastfeeding, according to the manufacturers, does not pose a significant risk for the healthy, full-term neonate. However, its use should be avoided in pre-term, stressed or ill infants.

CHILDREN

Both drugs have been used safely in a limited number of children, especially for chronic bullous disease of childhood (childhood linear IgA disease) (Table 34.2). The usual recommendation is to use half the adult dose for SP or 15–60 mg/kg/d. For SMP, dosing is weight-dependent as below (based on the manufacturer's advice for Lederkyn®, the previously available formulation of SMP).

TABLE 34.2

Sulfamethoxypyridazine Dosing in Children

Age in Years (Approx. Weight)	Initial SMP Dose/Day	Maintenance SMP Dose/Day
1–3 (9 kg)	250 mg	125 mg
4–6 (18 kg)	500 mg	250 mg
6–10 (27 kg)	750 mg	375 mg

ESSENTIAL PATIENT INFORMATION

- Patients should be advised to maintain a high fluid intake during treatment to reduce the risk of crystalluria.
- Patients should report any signs of bone marrow suppression (bleeding, bruising, etc.) or new rashes immediately.
- Due to the possible risk of photosensitivity, patients taking sulfonamide drugs should be advised to avoid excessive sun exposure.

With acknowledgements to Jonathan Leonard, Eirini Merika and Catherine Hardman, authors of this chapter in previous editions.

FURTHER READING

Caproni M, Antiga E, Melani L, et al. Guidelines for the diagnosis and treatment of dermatitis herpetiformis. J Eur Acad Dermatol Venereol. 2009;23(6):633–8.

Fortuna G, Marinkovich MP. Linear immunoglobulin A bullous dermatosis. Clin Dermatol. 2012;30(1):38.

Ingen-Housz-Oro S. Linear IgA bullous dermatosis: A review. Ann Dermatol Venereol. 2011;138(3):214–20.

Ingen-Housz-Oro S, Bernard P, Bedane C, et al. Linear IgA dermatosis. Guidelines for the diagnosis and treatment. [Centres de référence des maladies bulleuses auto-immunes. Société française de dermatologie]. Ann Dermatol Venereol. 2011;138(3):267–70.

Lings K, Bygum A. Linear IgA bullous dermatosis: A retrospective study of 23 patients in Denmark. Acta Derm Venereol. 2015;95(4):466–71.

Paniker U, Levine N. Dapsone and sulfapyridine. Dermatol Clin. 2001;19(1):79–86.

Pfeiffer C, Wozel G. Dapsone and sulfones in dermatology: Overview and update. J Am Acad Dermatol. 2003;48(2):308–9.

35 Thalidomide

Elaine Agius and Robert P.E. Sarkany

CLASSIFICATION AND MODE OF ACTION

Thalidomide (alphapthalimido-glutaramide) is a derivative of glutamic acid and was first introduced in 1957 as a non-barbiturate sedative hypnotic. However, it was withdrawn several years later when an association with severe congenital abnormalities became clear. Thalidomide is a potent teratogen, and up to 12,000 newborn infants were affected, particularly with phocomelias (congenital limb foreshortening). Interest in thalidomide and its analogues has re-emerged in recent years, as it has significant anti-inflammatory, immunomodulatory and anti-cancer effects. Thalidomide was approved by the FDA in the United States for the treatment of erythema nodosum leprosum in 1998, and then later by the FDA and European Medicines Agency for the treatment of multiple myeloma. Thalidomide has orphan drug status. This provides the financial structure for a company to produce a drug for a rare medical condition that might otherwise be uneconomic. In the United States, thalidomide is prescribed in accordance with the mandatory THALOMID REMS® (Risk Evaluation and Mitigation Strategy) program (www.thalomidrems.com). In Europe, it is dispensed according to the Thalidomide Celgene Pregnancy Prevention Programme.

Thalidomide has complex immunomodulatory effects which are not fully understood. It has a direct suppressive effect on tumour necrosis factor (TNF)-α synthesis and reduces production of other cytokines such as interleukin (IL)-6 and Il-12 and free radicals that may cause oxidative DNA damage. It also activates apoptotic pathways and inhibits angiogenesis. New analogues of thalidomide, lenolidamide and pomalidomide, with greater anti-TNF activity and reduced toxicity, have been licensed for use in oncology.

INDICATIONS AND DERMATOLOGICAL USES

Thalidomide is only licensed in Europe for the treatment of multiple myeloma. It is widely used to treat leprosy reactions (erythema nodosum leprosum) and licensed for this indication in the United States. It has also been reported to be of benefit in a range of inflammatory skin diseases, including:

- Actinic prurigo.
- Cutaneous lupus erythematosus.
- Erythema nodosum leprosum.
- Nodular prurigo.
- Pyoderma gangrenosum.
- Severe aphthous stomatitis and Behçet's syndrome.
- Chronic graft-versus-host disease.
- Cutaneous sarcoidosis.
- Erythema multiforme.
- Kaposi sarcoma.
- Lichen planus.
- Uraemic pruritus.
- Scleromyxoedema.
- Systemic mastocytosis.

DOI: 10.1201/9781003016786-35

FORMULATIONS/PRESENTATION

Thalidomide is available in 25 mg tablets and 50 mg hard capsules in the UK and in 50 mg, 100 mg, 150 mg and 200 mg capsules in the United States.

DOSAGES AND SUGGESTED REGIMENS

The onset of action is slow, and therapeutic effects may be delayed for several months except in cases of resistant oral ulceration, where a more rapid response is typical. Dosing for chronic dermatological conditions such as actinic prurigo, cutaneous lupus erythematosus or nodular prurigo is usually in the range of 25–150 mg per day taken at bedtime more than 1 hour after the evening meal. It is best to initiate treatment at a low dose for the first 3 months and titrate the dose upwards if tolerated. At body weights of <50 kg and in adults over the age of 75, we recommend starting at the lower end of the dosing range. Shorter courses at higher doses are used to treat erythema nodosum leprosum: A starting dose of 100–400 mg nocte, continued until symptoms and signs subside (usually about 2 weeks) and then slowly stopped using a 50 mg reduction in dose every 2–4 weeks. For all other dermatological conditions treated with thalidomide, an attempt should be made to reduce the dose to the lowest dose necessary every 3–6 months.

BASELINE INVESTIGATIONS AND CONSIDERATIONS

Disease severity should be quantified with a clinical score, if available, and Dermatology Life Quality Index (DLQI). A full medical history is necessary to assess risk factors for cardiac disease, thromboses and neuropathy. The following baseline investigations are required before starting treatment:

- Full blood count (FBC) (complete blood count [CBC]) and differential white cell count (WCC).
- Urea, electrolytes and creatinine.
- Liver function tests (LFTs).
- Thyroid function tests (TFTs).
- Simple coagulation screen (INR, activated partial thromboplastin time [APTT] and derived fibrinogen).
- In HIV patients: Viral load.
- Nerve conduction studies.
- Pulse rate, blood pressure and weight.
- Contraception and pregnancy prevention programme (PPP; including a pregnancy test) (Table 35.1).

Before starting the treatment:

- In Europe, complete the Prescription Authorisation Form (Thalidomide Celgene Pregnancy Prevention Programme).
- In the United States, patients must be enrolled in the THALOMID REMS® program. Physicians enroll their patients, fill out a prescription form and complete mandatory confidential surveys using CelgeneRiskManagement.com. Patients also complete a mandatory confidential survey at the same website.
- Any immunizations should be carried out before starting treatment: For live vaccines, at least 4 weeks before starting treatment, for inactivated vaccines at least 2 weeks before starting treatment. An exception is the influenza vaccine which can be given while taking thalidomide.

TABLE 35.1

Contraception and Pregnancy Prevention Programme for Thalidomide

Female Patients of Childbearing Potential

Counselling:

- Ensure the patient understands the teratogenic risk and the absolute requirement for a reliable form of contraception without interruption for 4 weeks before starting, throughout the entire duration of treatment and for 4 weeks after stopping
- Assess capability to comply with effective contraceptive measures and explain the need to consult rapidly if there is a risk of pregnancy. Explain the need to commence the treatment as soon as thalidomide is dispensed following a negative pregnancy test
- Explain the need and check that the patient agrees to undergo pregnancy testing every 4 weeks

Contraception: The patient must have been using 1 highly effective method of contraception for at least 4 weeks before therapy: Implant, levonorgestrel-releasing intrauterine system (IUS), medroxyprogesterone acetate depot, previous tubal ligation, partner's vasectomy or an ovulation inhibitory progesterone-only pill, e.g. desogestrel (NOT a combined oral contraceptive, since the oestrogen component increases the risk of thromboembolism). In the United States, an additional effective method of contraception – diaphragm, cervical cap or male latex/synthetic condom – is mandatory

Pregnancy testing: Should be carried out once the patient has been on effective contraception for at least 4 weeks, and on the same day that the prescription is issued

Prescribing and dispensing:

- Prescriptions must be limited to 4 weeks of treatment
- Pregnancy test, writing of prescription and dispensing of thalidomide should be carried out all on the same day
- The prescription should only be valid for 7 days from the date that it is written, as a safety measure

Treatment initiation form

To be signed by both patient and physician:

- Thalidomide Celgene Pregnancy Prevention Programme Females of Childbearing Potential Treatment Initiation form in Europe
- THALOMID REMS program Patient-Physician agreement form in the United States

Female Patients of Non-Childbearing Potential

Check that patient is either post-hysterectomy and/or bilateral oophorectomy or 1 year post-menopause (2 years in the United States) or a female child who has not started menstruating

In Europe: Thalidomide Celgene Pregnancy Prevention Programme Females of Non-Childbearing Potential Treatment Initiation form signed by the patient

In the United States: Initial mandatory confidential survey completed by the patient by visiting www. CelgeneRiskManagement.com and patient surveys completed every 6 months throughout treatment

Male Patients

Check that the patient understands the need for the use of a condom if engaged in sexual activity with either a pregnant female or a female of childbearing potential who is not using effective contraception

This applies during the treatment period and for 1 week after stopping treatment (4 weeks in the United States)

Treatment initiation form (Thalidomide Celgene Pregnancy Prevention Programme Male Potential Treatment Initiation form) signed by patient

MONITORING

- General blood tests: FBC, urea, electrolytes, creatinine and liver function tests monthly for first 3 months and every 3 months after that.
- Thyroid function tests: Every 3 months.
- Nerve conduction studies: Monitor for clinical features of neuropathy monthly for the first 3 months and every 3–6 months after that. Nerve conduction studies must be carried out every 6 months to detect asymptomatic neuropathy, and more frequently if there is any clinical reason that arises.

- Pulse rate and blood pressure: Repeat every 3 months.
- Pregnancy test: In female patients of childbearing potential, repeat every 4 weeks during treatment and once more 4 weeks after stopping treatment. In the United States, weekly pregnancy testing is required for the first 4 weeks of treatment.

CONTRAINDICATIONS

- Known hypersensitivity to thalidomide.
- Pregnancy.
- Females of childbearing potential, unless all the conditions of the Pregnancy Prevention Programme (Thalidomide Celgene in Europe and THALOMID REMS in the United States) are met.
- Patients unable to fully adhere to the required contraceptive measures.

CAUTIONS

- Presence of risk factors for myocardial infarction (MI), bradycardia, atrioventricular (AV) block or cardiac failure.
- Existing peripheral neuropathy (which may be made more severe).
- A history of or risk factors for thromboembolism, including smoking, hypertension and hyperlipidaemia.
- Older people (age over 65 years) are more susceptible to the adverse effects of thalidomide, and as a result lower dosages should be considered.
- Presence of renal or hepatic impairment.
- Presence of anaemia, thrombocytopenia or leukopenia.

IMPORTANT DRUG INTERACTIONS

There is evidence that thalidomide requires cytochrome P450-catalysed biotransformation to exert its pharmacological activity and that the CYP2C subfamily may be primarily involved. The potential for clinically relevant interactions with medicinal products appears to be low. Special precautions should be taken with:

- Beta-blockers or anticholinesterase agents (e.g. neostigmine), due to increased risk of bradycardia.
- Sedatives such as anxiolytics, hypnotics, antipsychotics, antihistamines, opiate derivatives, barbiturates and alcohol, due to thalidomide's sedative effect.
- Drugs known to be associated with peripheral neuropathy (e.g. vincristine and bortezomib).
- Combined hormonal contraceptive pills and hormone replacement therapy, due to the increased risk of venous thromboembolic disease.
- Erythropoiesis-stimulating agents, due to the increased risk of thromboembolism while taking thalidomide.
- Live vaccines, since thalidomide is an immunosuppressant.
- Myelosuppressant drugs, since thalidomide is a myelosuppressant.

ADVERSE EFFECTS AND THEIR MANAGEMENT

- Teratogenicity: The risk of intrauterine death or severe birth defects, particularly phocomelia, is extremely high. Thalidomide must not be used at any time during pregnancy.
- Venous and arterial thromboembolic events: An increased risk of venous thromboembolism (such as deep vein thrombosis and pulmonary embolism) and arterial thromboembolism (MI

and cerebrovascular events) has been reported in patients treated with thalidomide, especially during the first 5 months of therapy. Although the majority of data are associated with its use in patients with malignant disease (multiple myeloma), there have been isolated cases reported in a non-cancer setting: In a recent meta-analysis, 2% of 548 patients treated with thalidomide for cutaneous lupus erythematosus had a thromboembolic event during treatment. Patients should be advised to seek urgent attention if they develop shortness of breath, limb pain or limb swelling.

- Cardiac: Thalidomide can induce bradycardia and AV block. This complication may present with orthostatic hypotension, syncope and signs of cardiac failure. Blood pressure and the pulse rate must be monitored regularly.
- Neurological: Peripheral neuropathy is a very common and potentially severe effect, as it may be irreversible. Sensory neuropathy typically precedes motor neuropathy. The incidence of this side effect is linked to higher daily doses and higher cumulative doses, and therefore it generally occurs following long-term use. However, it can less commonly occur following relatively short-term use, and symptoms may also develop after treatment has stopped. There is no evidence that the prevalence of thalidomide neuropathy differs between groups of patients being treated for different diseases. The typical presentation is symmetrical painful distal limb paraesthesia. In a recent meta-analysis, 16% of 548 patients with cutaneous lupus erythematosus experienced this complication. The prevalence of peripheral neuropathy in patients with inflammatory bowel disease who were treated with thalidomide has been estimated with a range from 20–56%. All patients require careful monitoring for symptoms of neuropathy, including pain, tingling, numbness, abnormal coordination or weakness. Expert neurological assessment should be sought if these symptoms develop. Six monthly nerve conduction studies are important for detecting asymptomatic neuropathy (about a quarter of patients with this complication are asymptomatic) before it becomes more severe. Clearly, thalidomide must be stopped if neuropathy is found to be developing.
- Sedative: Somnolence/drowsiness is an expected effect, so thalidomide should be taken before bed. Patients should be advised about possible impairment of mental or physical abilities for hazardous tasks such as driving or operating machinery.
- Haematological: Neutropenia, lymphopenia, thrombocytopenia and anaemia may occur. If the white blood cell count (WBC) is $<3.5 \times 109/L$, neutrophils $<2.0 \times 109/L$, lymphocytes $<0.5\ 0 \times 109/L$ or platelets $<150 \times 109/L$, the thalidomide should be stopped until a haematologist has assessed the situation.
- Hepatitis: Biochemical evidence of hepatocellular, cholestatic and mixed abnormalities may occur, usually within the first 2 months of therapy. Most of these hepatic adverse reactions resolve with dose reduction or drug discontinuation. Closer monitoring for liver disease is required in patients with pre-existing liver disease or with concomitant use of hepatotoxic medication.
- Cutaneous: Severe adverse effects include angioedema, Stevens–Johnson syndrome and toxic epidermal necrolysis. Immediate discontinuation of the thalidomide is required.
- Gastrointestinal: These include dry mouth and constipation.
- Endocrine: Thyroid abnormalities have been reported rarely. Common side effects of thalidomide (bradycardia, oedema and weight gain) may be indistinguishable from the symptoms of hypothyroidism, so biochemical monitoring of thyroid function is necessary.

USE IN SPECIAL SITUATIONS

PREGNANCY AND PRE-CONCEPTION

- Thalidomide is absolutely contraindicated, due to the high risk of teratogenicity.
- Thalidomide is excreted in semen; males are advised not to father children during treatment or for 1 week after the last dose (1 month in the United States).

LACTATION

The safety of thalidomide in lactation is not established. Mothers taking thalidomide should not breastfeed.

CHILDREN

Thalidomide has been used successfully in children, particularly in actinic prurigo. It should only be considered if clinically necessary and after alternative treatments have failed.

ESSENTIAL PATIENT INFORMATION

- Patients should be informed whether the drug is being used for a licensed indication or not.
- It should be explained that the onset of action is slow and that benefit may not appear until after 2–3 months of treatment.
- All patients must be aware of the extremely high risk of teratogenicity with thalidomide used during pregnancy or around conception by both males and females.
- Patients must clearly understand the need for regular monitoring in order to minimize the risk of adverse effects, and they must be able to comply with this.
- Patients should be advised that they are at increased risk of thromboembolic events and should seek urgent medical attention if they develop the following symptoms and signs: Calf pain, chest pain, shortness of breath or haemoptysis.
- Patients should be told about common adverse effects, including sedation and peripheral neuropathy.
- It must be explained that medication must not be shared with anyone and that the patient should not donate blood/semen.

FURTHER READING

Bastuji-Garin S, Ochonisky S, Bouche P. Incidence and risk factors for thalidomide neuropathy: A prospective study of 135 dermatologic patients. J Invest Dermatol. 2002;119:1020.

Chasset F, Tounsi T, Cesbron E, et al. Efficacy and tolerance profile of thalidomide in cutaneous lupus erythematosus: A systematic review and meta-analysis. J Am Acad Dermatol. 2018;78:342–50. E4.

Sardana K, Gupta A, Sinha S. An observational analysis of low-dose thalidomide in recalcitrant prurigo nodularis. Clin Exp Dermatol. 2020;45:92–6.

Wu JJ, Huang DB, Pang KR, Hsu S, Tyring SK. Thalidomide: Dermatological indications, mechanisms of action and side-effects. Br J Dermatol. 2005;153:254–73.

Yuki EFN, Silva CA, Aikawa NE, et al. Thalidomide and lenalidomide for refractory systemic/cutaneous lupus erythematosus treatment: A narrative review of literature for clinical practice. J Clin Rheumatol. 2021 Oct 29;27:248–59.

36 Tumour Necrosis Factor Antagonists

Leena Chularojanamontri and Christopher E.M. Griffiths

CLASSIFICATION AND MODE OF ACTION

The tumour necrosis factor (TNF) family is a group of 19 cytokines that produce inflammation, apoptosis, proliferation and angiogenesis. The best-known members of the family are TNF-α and TNF-β.

TNF-α is often simply referred to as 'tumour necrosis factor.' At a low concentration in tissues, TNF-α has beneficial effects, such as prevention of infections, although it can lead to excess inflammation and organ injury at high concentrations. As the name implies, TNF-α has anti-tumour properties and plays a key role in the induction of apoptosis as well as transduction of cell survival signals. Pro-caspase-8 is a key regulator of TNF-α–induced apoptosis, while nuclear factor kappa B (NF-κB) is the major factor in TNF-α–induced survival signals. The role of TNF-α in the regulation of the apoptosis and proliferation cascade indicates its potential for the treatment of malignancy.

TNF-β or lymphotoxin is derived from T-lymphocytes and has a 50% amino acid sequence homology with and binds to the same receptor as TNF-α. Its biological significance is unclear. Much more is known about TNF-α, which is a key pro-inflammatory cytokine that plays a central role in the pathogenesis of psoriasis, psoriatic arthritis and many inflammatory skin diseases. It is released as soluble (sTNF) and membrane-bound forms (transmembrane TNF [tmTNF]). sTNF and tmTNF bind to distinct receptors: TNF receptor 1 (TNFR1, p55) and TNF receptor 2 (TNFR2, p75) leading to activation of NF-κB, inflammation and cell apoptosis, respectively. TNF may also drive keratinocyte proliferation in psoriasis.

- The anti-TNF agents/TNF antagonists commonly used in dermatology can be divided into two groups: Soluble TNF receptors (etanercept) and monoclonal antibodies (infliximab, adalimumab, golimumab and certolizumab pegol). Although all drugs inhibit TNF-α, their structures and pharmacodynamic and pharmacokinetic profiles are different. Etanercept binds primarily to sTNF and TNF-β, whereas all 4 monoclonal antibodies bind primarily to TNF-α, but not TNF-β.
- Etanercept is a soluble TNF receptor protein consisting of the extracellular portions of human TNFR2 (p75) linked to the Fc domain of human immunoglobulin (Ig) G1.
- Infliximab is a chimeric IgG1 human–murine monoclonal antibody (~25% mouse-derived protein).
- Adalimumab and golimumab are fully human monoclonal IgG1 antibodies.
- Certolizumab pegol is a humanized anti-TNF Fab' fragment conjugated to polyethylene glycol to prolong serum half-life, which facilitates once-monthly dosing.

Notably, all drugs can bind to both sTNF and tmTNF and block their abilities to activate TNF receptors, but only infliximab, adalimumab and golimumab can activate complement-dependent cytotoxicity and induce apoptosis in T-cells and monocytes. Golimumab induces a weaker apoptotic effect than either infliximab or adalimumab. This may explain the greater efficacy of infliximab and adalimumab compared to etanercept, as well as the potentially higher risk of infections associated with their uses, especially with infliximab. Data from the British Association of Dermatologists Biologics and Immunomodulators Register (BADBIR) has shown that infliximab is associated with

DOI: 10.1201/9781003016786-36

an overall increase in the risk of serious infection compared with non-biologics (methotrexate, ciclosporin, acitretin, fumaric acid esters, psoralen ultraviolet A and hydroxycarbamide).

INDICATIONS AND DERMATOLOGICAL USES

TNF antagonists are approved for management of psoriasis, psoriatic arthritis (PsA) and other inflammatory diseases, such as ankylosing spondylitis (AS), inflammatory bowel disease (IBD), juvenile idiopathic arthritis (JIA) and rheumatoid arthritis (RA). Off-label prescribing is also used in several dermatological conditions (Table 36.1).

The Psoriasis Area and Severity Index (PASI) is a widely used measure of the clinical severity of psoriasis, whereas the Dermatology Life Quality Index (DLQI) is a validated tool used to evaluate the impact of skin disease on quality of life. In the UK, patient eligibility for treatment with TNF antagonists is dictated by eligibility criteria mandated by the National Institute for Health and Care Excellence (NICE), which include:

- Chronic plaque psoriasis of at least 6 months' duration.
- Documented failure to respond to and/or unsuitability for conventional systemic treatments.
- A PASI of ≥10, and a DLQI of >10 for etanercept, adalimumab and certolizumab pegol; and a PASI of ≥20 and a DLQI of >18 for infliximab.
- PASI and DLQI, both of which are calculated before and during treatment.

The definition of treatment response is either:

- PASI 50: A 50% or greater reduction from baseline PASI or % of body surface area where PASI is not applicable, and at least a 5-point reduction in DLQI.
- PASI 75: A 75% reduction from baseline PASI.

TNF antagonists should be discontinued if patients do not achieve these response criteria. According to NICE guidelines, the time point for reviewing whether to continue therapy is at 16 weeks for adalimumab and certolizumab pegol, and 12 weeks and 10 weeks for etanercept and infliximab, respectively.

TABLE 36.1
Approved Indications and Off-Label Dermatological Uses of Tumour Necrosis Factor Antagonists

TNF Antagonists	Approved Indications	Off-Label Dermatological Uses
Etanercept	Moderate-to-severe adult and paediatric (in patients aged ≥4 years) psoriasis, PsA, AS, JIA and RA	Autoimmune blistering diseases, acute and chronic graft-versus-host disease, Behçet's disease, Granuloma annulare, pyoderma gangrenosum, sarcoidosis, etc.
Infliximab	Moderate-to-severe adult psoriasis, PsA, AS, IBD and RA	
Adalimumab	Moderate-to-severe adult psoriasis, PsA, AS, IBD, JIA, RA, hidradenitis suppurativa and uveitis	Behçet's disease, dermatomyositis, pyoderma gangrenosum, sarcoidosis, Sweet's syndrome, SAPHO syndrome, etc.
Golimumab	PsA, AS, JIA, RA and ulcerative colitis	Psoriasis
Certolizumab pegol	Moderate-to-severe adult psoriasis, PsA, AS, RA and Crohn disease	Limited data

Abbreviations: AS, ankylosing spondylitis; IBD, inflammatory bowel disease; JIA, juvenile idiopathic arthritis; PsA, psoriatic arthritis; RA, rheumatoid arthritis; SAPHO, synovitis, osteitis, hyperostosis and enthesitis.

SPECIAL POINT: TUBERCULOSIS (TB)

The risk associated with TNF antagonists and TB is widely accepted. However, the magnitude of the risk varies between the different available agents. Data from prospective national registries, open-labelled extension studies and retrospective cohorts show that the incidence of TB is highly dependent on its regional prevalence; the monoclonal antibodies (infliximab and adalimumab) carry a higher risk of TB than the soluble receptor (etanercept).

There are less data available regarding the incidence of TB with golimumab and certolizumab pegol due to their more recent approval (2009 and 2010, respectively). In one registry series for golimumab, the incidence of TB was similar to adalimumab, as would be expected because they are both fully humanized monoclonal antibodies. Similarly, national registry data from the UK also showed that the incidence of TB with certolizumab pegol was equal to that of infliximab and adalimumab.

There is a high rate of atypical clinical presentations of TB with these agents. Extrapulmonary disease or disseminated/miliary TB occur in two-thirds and one-third of cases, respectively. The median time to onset of TB was shorter in monoclonal antibody forms of TNF antagonists (3–6 months) compared to etanercept (>1 year). Careful screening for TB before starting therapy and ongoing vigilance for newly acquired disease are therefore essential.

FORMULATIONS/PRESENTATION

- Infliximab: A freeze-dried powder in 100 mg vials for reconstitution with sterile water for intravenous infusion over a period of 2 hours; the drug should be infused within 3 hours after reconstitution or within 24 hours if refrigerated. Among TNF antagonists, infliximab is the only drug that is administered intravenously while the others are administered subcutaneously.
- Etanercept: Preservative-free, lyophilized powder in 25 mg vials for reconstitution with 1 mL of sterile water for subcutaneous administration, pre-filled syringe with 25 mg or 50 mg etanercept and 50 mg pre-filled autoinjector pen.
- Adalimumab: A single-use, sterile, preservative-free solution of 40 mg adalimumab in a pre-filled autoinjector pen device or a pre-filled glass syringe for subcutaneous administration.
- Golimumab: 50 mg/0.5 mL and 100 mg/mL in a single-dose pre-filled autoinjector, 50 mg/0.5 mL and 100 mg/mL in a single dose pre-filled syringe.
- Certolizumab pegol: A 5 mL vial with 200 mg of lyophilized powder; 200 mg/1 mL in a pre-filled syringe.

All the drugs should be stored at 2–8°C and reconstituted before injection.

DOSAGES AND SUGGESTED REGIMENS

TNF Antagonists	Dosages and Suggested Regimens	Achieved a PASI 75 Response
Etanercept	50 mg subcutaneous twice weekly for the first 12 weeks, followed by 50 mg once weekly thereafter	At week 12, 49% of patients
Infliximab	5 mg/kg intravenous at weeks 0, 2 and 6, and thereafter every 8 weeks	At week 10, 75.5% of patients
Adalimumab	80 mg subcutaneous initially, followed by 40 mg the next week and at 2-week intervals thereafter; it can be increased to weekly	At week 16, 71% of patients
Golimumab	50 mg subcutaneous once a month	Limited data for psoriasis
Certolizumab pegol	400 mg subcutaneous every other week – Patient's weight ≤90 kg: 400 mg SC initially and at week 2 and week 4, followed by 200 mg every 2 weeks or 400 mg monthly	At week 12, 83% of patients

Continuous treatment with anti-TNF agents provides better disease control than interrupted therapy, and there may be some loss of efficacy if treatment is reintroduced after a 'drug holiday.' However, intermittent treatment may provide an alternative approach in patients who are unwilling or unable to maintain a continuous regimen. Current evidence suggested that 38% of patients were able to achieve a PASI 75 response at week 50 with as-needed therapy of 5 mg/kg of infliximab, while a PASI 75 response was achieved in ≥60% of patients receiving intermittent regimens of other TNF antagonists (adalimumab, etanercept and certolizumab pegol). A higher incidence of adverse infusion reactions was also found in patients with as-needed therapy of infliximab comparing to continuous dosing.

Loss of efficacy correlates with development of antibodies to TNF antagonists. Co-administration of low-dose methotrexate (5–7.5 mg once weekly) can reduce the incidence of formation of antibodies to infliximab and thereby sustain efficacy. There may be less anti-drug antibody formation, lower rates of immunogenicity and loss of efficacy for certolizumab pegol than with the other TNF antagonists due to its pegylation. Withdrawal of anti-TNF therapy usually leads to a slow relapse of disease, with no evidence of rebound. Switching between biologics may be considered in patients who have experienced poor outcomes and/or adverse effects. Many patients have demonstrated a good response to a second anti-TNF agent, but no firm conclusions on sequential use are currently available.

BASELINE INVESTIGATIONS AND CONSIDERATIONS

- Full blood count (FBC) (complete blood count [CBC]), liver function tests (LFTs) and blood urea nitrogen and creatinine.
- Urinalysis.
- Pregnancy test.
- Hepatitis B virus, hepatitis C virus and human immunodeficiency virus (HIV).
- Chest x-ray.
- TB evaluation, which should be carried out on all patients; this includes a detailed medical assessment of past history of TB and possible exposure to those with active infection.

The tuberculin skin test (TST) or Mantoux test is routinely used as a screening test for latent TB infection in asymptomatic individuals. However, it has several limitations, including the need for follow-up clinic visits at 48 and 72 hours post-test, a lack of specificity for Mycobacterium tuberculosis in those who have received TB immunization (false positive) and attenuated responses in patients receiving immunosuppressant therapy (false negative). Interferon-gamma release assays (IGRA) are a new generation of enzyme-linked immunosorbent (ELISA) laboratory testing based on the measurement of interferon-gamma (IFN-γ) release from sensitized T-cells in response to M. tuberculosis–specific antigens. Since 2016, NICE guidance recommends IGRA to screen for latent TB, if available.

Currently, the British Association of Dermatologists strongly recommends that a plain chest radiograph with an IGRA should be performed to rule out pulmonary pathology at baseline, including granulomas indicative of prior infection and other confounding lung diseases. If positive, assess for active TB and/or management of latent TB in consultation with a TB specialist. In people who require treatment for latent TB (3 months of isoniazid and rifampicin or 6 months of isoniazid), this should be given for at least 2 months before initiation of a biologic.

MONITORING

- Specific assessment for infections, especially in those using TNF-antagonists plus methotrexate, is recommended.
- Screening for skin cancers should be performed.
- In patients who have no other concomitant diseases, there is no evidence to support routine laboratory investigations for monitoring during treatment with TNF antagonists, with the exception of infliximab. Infliximab has been associated with hepatitis; therefore, interval monitoring of LFTs in patients being treated with this biologic is recommended (every 3–6 months).

More frequent monitoring may be needed if patients on infliximab therapy have risk factors for hepatitis or elevated LFTs at baseline.

- Further TB testing may be required according to clinical signs and risks.
- A repeat IGRA should be performed annually on all patients on TNF antagonists, especially in high-risk patients such as health-care workers or following travel to an endemic area.

NB: The response to IGRA may be reduced in patients taking anti-TNF therapy, so their usefulness might be limited once patients have commenced therapy.

CONTRAINDICATIONS

Absolute contraindication:

- Hypersensitivity to any component of the formulation, and infliximab is contraindicated in those with an allergy to murine proteins.

Relative contraindications:

- Severe active infection such as active TB, sepsis, etc.
- Congestive heart failure (NYHA grade III or IV), due to a risk of exacerbation.
- Personal or family history of demyelinating disease/multiple sclerosis.
- History of lymphoreticular malignancy.

CAUTIONS

In addition, the following should be noted.

ASYMPTOMATIC LATENT TB

Patients should be instructed to seek medical advice if signs/symptoms suggestive of a TB infection (e.g. persistent cough, wasting/weight loss, low grade fever or listlessness) occur during or after therapy with anti-TNF agents.

HEPATITIS B VIRUS

Triple serology, including hepatitis B surface antigen (HBsAg), antibodies to HBsAg (anti-HBs) and antibodies to hepatitis B core antigen (anti-HBc) is recommended before TNF-antagonist initiation.

- For anti-HBc+/HBsAg+ patients treated with TNF antagonists, the risk of HBV reactivation is high (≥10%). Therefore, concomitant pre-emptive anti-HBV therapy should be considered. Once therapy is commenced, it is important to check HBV DNA levels and LFTs every 3 months. HBV reactivation typically occurs with immune reconstitution, and therefore antiviral therapy should continue for 6–12 months after stopping a TNF antagonist.
- For anti-HBc+/HBsAg– patients treated with TNF antagonists, risk of HBV reactivation is moderate (1–10%), depending upon their comorbid conditions and the resources made available by the health care system. Monitoring HBV DNA or HBsAg and LFTs is recommended, rather than routine pre-emptive HBV treatment.

HEPATITIS C VIRUS

Unlike HBV reactivation, HCV reactivation is uncommon. TNF antagonists can be used with appropriate evaluation and monitoring during therapy.

HUMAN IMMUNODEFICIENCY VIRUS (HIV)

Patients with HIV may receive a TNF antagonist if they are also receiving highly active antiretroviral therapy and have a stable disease (e.g. low viral load, acceptable CD4 counts and no evidence of active opportunistic infection).

MALIGNANCIES

Patients with prior psoralen plus ultraviolet A (PUVA) therapy and intensive use of immunosuppressive drugs should be evaluated for skin cancer before and during TNF antagonist therapy. It should be noted that TNF antagonists used as monotherapy in patients with psoriasis are not associated with a risk of solid tumour or lymphoreticular malignancy. However, the concomitant use with other immunosuppressive agents can alter the safety profile of TNF antagonists.

Pneumococcal vaccine and annual influenza vaccine are recommended while patients are on therapy; ideally, these inactive vaccines should be administered at least 2 weeks before therapy is started. Prescribers are advised to consult the latest recommendation on COVID-19 vaccine and booster scheduling (see e.g. https://www.nhs.uk/conditions/coronavirus-covid-19/coronavirus-vaccination/health-conditions/).

Current COVID-19 guidelines should be consulted for dermatology patients with immune-mediated inflammatory disorders (IMID) who are eligible for treatment with neutralizing monoclonal antibodies or antivirals.

IMPORTANT DRUG INTERACTIONS

TNF antagonists rarely cause drug interactions. They can be used with acitretin, methotrexate, apremilast and ciclosporin. Glucocorticoids, salicylates (excluding sulfasalazine), nonsteroidal anti-inflammatory drugs (NSAIDs) and analgesics have been used concomitantly with no reports of drug interactions. However, concomitant use of other immunosuppressives or immunomodulatory drugs can enhance the degree of immunosuppression and increase the risk of infection.

ADVERSE EFFECTS AND THEIR MANAGEMENT

Acute problems, including injection site reactions and infusion reactions, are common side effects of TNF antagonists.

- Injection site reactions: Erythema, itching, pain, swelling and cutaneous haemorrhage generally do not result in discontinuation of therapy.
- Infusion reactions: They occur in infliximab treatment, as it is administered intravenously. Infusion reactions are defined as any adverse effects occurring during or within 1 hour after completion of the infusion. Mild-to-moderate symptoms such as flushing, pruritus, chills, headache and urticaria can occur, but severe infusion reactions, include anaphylactic reactions and serum sickness-like reactions, are rare. If mild-to-moderate infusion reactions occur, treatment can usually be continued by decreasing the infusion rate or temporarily stopping the infusion. Pre-treatment with oral antihistamines, paracetamol (acetaminophen) and/or corticosteroids should be considered for future infusions. Serious infusion reactions seem to occur more frequently with intermittent rather than continuous therapy.

Other rare but important adverse effects of TNF antagonists include:

- Demyelinating disorders: They have been reported with TNF antagonists; the risk appears small, and partial or full recovery usually occurs on discontinuation.
- Malignancy: Patients with a history of malignancy who have failed other therapies for psoriasis may in certain circumstances receive TNF antagonists without expectation of an increased risk of tumour recurrence.

- Congestive heart failure: It is a contraindication to anti-TNF therapy, but reports of it occurring de novo with TNF antagonists are rare.
- Drug-induced lupus erythematosus: It has been reported in association with anti-TNF therapy; treatment should be discontinued if symptoms develop, but it can be continued in asymptomatic patients who develop positive antinuclear antibodies.
- Paradoxical side effects: An unexpected onset or exacerbation of an autoimmune disease for which TNF antagonists are indicated other than the one the patient is receiving treatment for. These disorders are mainly reported in patients with rheumatic diseases and inflammatory bowel disease. For paradoxical cutaneous side effects, psoriasiform dermatitis such as eczema, dry skin and psoriasis are the most frequently observed. Palmoplantar pustulosis has been reported. As paradoxical side effects are considered as a class effect seen with all TNF antagonists, switching to another TNF antagonist is mostly not helpful.
- Liver toxicity: Transient and self-limiting transaminitis, cholestatic disease and hepatitis can develop during treatment with anti-TNF treatment and, in some cases, they could be severe and life-threatening. Liver toxicity has been reported to be more associated with infliximab than any other TNF antagonists. The following guidelines can be used with respect to the elevation of alanine aminotransferase (ALT):
  - Isolated increase of ALT <3 times of normal upper limit: Treatment is possible with monitoring ALT up to resolution.
  - Treatment with caution if ALT values are 3–5 times of normal upper limit: Exclusion of other possible causes, consulting a hepatologist, and evaluation of anti-TNF discontinuation.
  - Stop treatment if ALT values are >5 times of normal upper limit.

USE IN SPECIAL SITUATIONS

PREGNANCY AND PRE-CONCEPTION

Meta-analyses found that there was no increased risk of complications during pregnancy or in the neonate in anti-TNF–treated patients compared to those with the same disease state not receiving TNF antagonists. Generally, this offers patients who are afraid of disease flare during pregnancy information to make an informed decision about stopping their biologic in pregnancy. The recommendation is that all anti-TNF biologics can be administered up until the end of the second trimester. If used throughout pregnancy, live vaccines should not be administered to infants until they have reached 6 months of age. The exception is certolizumab pegol which is approved for use throughout the entirety of pregnancy. Certolizumab pegol differs structurally, as it lacks the IgG1 Fc portion. Therefore, it should, in theory, not be transported actively across placenta by the neonatal Fc receptor, leaving passive diffusion as the only explanatory option for any detectable concentrations in exposed infants. This theory was supported by previous case series in which levels of certolizumab pegol at delivery in neonates ranged from undetectable to minimal levels.

LACTATION

The European League Against Rheumatism guideline recommendations state that TNF antagonists are compatible with breastfeeding. This is based on expert opinion and that data that show minimal TNF antagonist levels in breast milk.

CHILDREN

There is limited evidence for the treatment of pediatric patients with TNF antagonists. However, etanercept is FDA approved for the treatment of severe chronic plaque psoriasis in children aged 4 years and older. In Europe, etanercept and adalimumab are approved for children with chronic plaque type psoriasis aged 4 years and older. The dosing schedule is 0.8 mg/kg up to a maximum dose of 50 mg once weekly and 40 mg for etanercept and adalimumab, respectively, by subcutaneous injection.

The British Association of Dermatologists (BAD) has established BADBIR to assess the long-term safety of biologics prescribed for patients with severe psoriasis since September 2007. Following baseline data acquisition, clinicians record changes in therapy, disease activity and adverse events for 5 years (at 6-month intervals for 3 years, then annually thereafter). Collection of long-term effectiveness data is a subsidiary aim. The pharmacovigilance component of BADBIR provides invaluable information for the safe use of biologics in the real-world situation and allows relevant pharmaceutical companies to comply with their regulatory obligations.

ESSENTIAL PATIENT INFORMATION

- Patients should be monitored for early signs and symptoms of infection throughout treatment.
- All patients should be fully assessed for active and latent TB before starting therapy.
- All patients should be assessed for current and past history of malignancy and/or any future risk of malignancy before starting and throughout treatment.
- Patients at risk for hepatitis B infection should be screened for hepatitis B before starting TNF antagonist therapy.
- Patients should not receive live or live-attenuated vaccination within 2 weeks before, during and for 6 months after discontinuation. In the case of shingles (herpes zoster) vaccine, vaccination after discontinuation for 12 months is recommended.
- The pneumococcal and annual influenza vaccines are recommended while patients are on therapy; ideally these inactive vaccines should be administered at least 2 weeks before therapy is started. Prescribers are advised to consult the latest recommendation on COVID-19 vaccine and booster scheduling (see e.g. https://www.nhs.uk/conditions/coronavirus-covid-19/coronavirus-vaccination/health-conditions/).
- Agents should be discontinued at least 4 half-lives before major surgery (2 weeks for etanercept, 4–6 weeks for infliximab, 6–8 weeks for adalimumab, golimumab and certolizumab pegol).
- Where a TNF antagonist therapy is used outside its indication, written consent should be obtained from the patient.

FURTHER READING

Al-Hammadi A, Ruszczak Z, Magariños G, et al. Intermittent use of biologic agents for the treatment of psoriasis in adults. J Eur Acad Dermatol Venereol. 2020;8:doi: 10.1111/jdv.16803.

Godfrey MS, Friedman LN. Tuberculosis and biologic therapies: Anti-tumor necrosis factor-α and beyond. Clin Chest Med. 2019;40:721–39.

Menter A, Strober BE, Kaplan DH, et al. Joint AAD-NPF guidelines of care for the management and treatment of psoriasis with biologics. J Am Acad Dermatol. 2019;80:1029–72.

Smith CH, Yiu ZZN, Bale T, et al. British Association of Dermatologists guidelines for biologic therapy for psoriasis 2020: A rapid update. Br J Dermatol. 2020;18:doi:10.1111/bjd.19039.

Yiu ZZN, Ashcroft DM, Evans I, et al. Infliximab is associated with an increased risk of serious infection in patients with psoriasis in the U.K. and Republic of Ireland: Results from the british association of dermatologists biologic interventions register (BADBIR). Br J Dermatol. 2019;180:329–37.

37 Vismodegib

Faisal R. Ali and John T. Lear

CLASSIFICATION AND MODE OF ACTION

Vismodegib is the first in a new class of orally active anti-cancer drugs that inhibit the hedgehog (Hh) signalling pathway by binding to the smoothened transmembrane protein (Smo) and blocking induction of Hh target genes. Many of these genes are involved in cell proliferation, survival and differentiation. Recent development of Smo inhibitors has led to the current investigation of several drugs as therapy for a range of tumours.

The Hh signaling pathway plays a key role in the morphogenesis of the epidermis and its appendages during embryogenesis and for self-renewal of the skin and hair follicles through-out life. Mutations in PTCH1, the human homolog of the Drosophila gene 'patched,' which is a negative regulator of the Hh pathway, have been found in both hereditary basal cell naevus syndrome (Gorlin syndrome) and the majority of sporadic basal cell carcinomas (BCCs). These result in an unregulated proliferation of basal keratinocytes and the formation of tumours.

Vismodegib is absorbed after oral administration and slowly eliminated by a combination of metabolism by cytochrome P450 (CYP450) 2C9 and CYP3A4/5 and hepatic excretion of the parent drug. Only a small fraction is excreted renally. Its terminal half-life after administration of a single dose is approximately 12 days.

INDICATIONS AND DERMATOLOGICAL USES

Vismodegib was approved in the United States by the FDA in 2012 and in the United Kingdom by the MHRA in 2013. It is licensed for the treatment of adults with advanced BCC in the following contexts:

- Symptomatic metastatic BCC.
- Locally advanced BCC inappropriate for surgery or radiotherapy.

In 2017, NICE (UK) did not recommend that vismodegib be used in patients newly falling into the above two categories, due to lack of cost-effectiveness and studies comparing effectiveness of vismodegib to best supportive treatment. These NICE guidelines did not affect patients who had already commenced treatment with vismodegib.

Short-term studies (median duration of 6 months) have found that approximately 40% of patients with locally advanced BCC had a clinical response (reduction in tumour diameter of >30%) and that there was clearance of the tumour in 20% of patients. The median duration of response was 26.2 months.

In patients with metastatic BCC, approximately one-third showed evidence of a clinical response. The median duration of response was 16.2 months, and median overall survival was 33.4 months.

FORMULATIONS/PRESENTATION

- Hard capsules containing 150 mg vismodegib (Erivedge®).

DOI: 10.1201/9781003016786-37

DOSAGES AND SUGGESTED REGIMENS

One capsule (150 mg) once daily. Capsules should be swallowed whole and taken with water +/– food.

Tumour response should be gauged through serial measurements of tumour diameter and the documentation of the presence of ulceration. Therapy should be continued until disease progression or unacceptable side effect profile. The benefit gained and side effect profile associated with continued treatment should be regularly evaluated in each individual patient.

Adverse effects are common (see Adverse Effects and Their Management), and given its long half-life, interval dosing is being investigated as a means to improve tolerability, though there are no formal guidelines for this. The manufacturers advise that treatment may be interrupted for up to 4 weeks if adverse effects are not tolerated.

Some BCCs continue to grow despite treatment (primary resistance) with vismodegib, and in other cases, there may be regrowth of the BCC after an initial clinical response (acquired resistance). These may reflect mutations in Smo which confer drug resistance, for example, by decreased drug binding.

Vismodegib is curative, and in patients who respond, BCCs have been found to recur within 3 months of stopping treatment. There is interest in using this drug as neoadjuvant therapy, shrinking large primary tumours before complex reconstructive surgery, but further studies are needed to investigate this role.

BASELINE INVESTIGATIONS AND CONSIDERATIONS

For females of childbearing potential, pregnancy testing within 7 days before starting vismodegib and commencement of the manufacturer's pregnancy prevention programme (PPP) are imperative. The plan includes using two forms of contraception before starting treatment, throughout treatment and for 24 months after the last dose, including one highly effective method and a barrier contraceptive. Prescriptions should be limited to 1 month's duration with monthly pregnancy testing during treatment.

For males (including those who have had a vasectomy) having sexual intercourse with females of childbearing potential, counselling should be given of the need for barrier contraception with spermicide throughout treatment and for at least 2 months after the last dose.

Full blood count (FBC), renal indices and liver function tests (LFTs) should be checked.

MONITORING

No specific recommendations currently exist. Intermittent monitoring of routine blood parameters (FBC, LFTs and urea and electrolytes) may be advisable. Females of childbearing potential should follow the PPP, including monthly pregnancy testing.

CONTRAINDICATIONS

- Hypersensitivity to the active substance/excipients.
- Pregnancy or breastfeeding.
- Females of childbearing potential who do not comply with the PPP.

CAUTIONS

Hepatic and renal impairment safety is not established. The manufacturers advise close monitoring in patients with severe renal impairment and moderate-to-severe hepatic impairment.

IMPORTANT DRUG INTERACTIONS

- Antacids, proton pump inhibitors and H2-receptor antagonists may reduce the solubility and bioavailability of vismodegib.
- CYP450 inducers (rifampicin, carbamazepine, phenytoin and St John's wort [Hypericum perforatum]) may reduce the effectiveness of vismodegib.
- Vismodegib is a substrate for the efflux transporter P-glycoprotein and the metabolizing enzymes CYP2C9 and CYP3A4.
- P-glycoprotein inhibitors (e.g. macrolide antibiotics, verapamil and ciclosporin [cyclosporine]), CYP2C9 inhibitors (amiodarone, fluconazole or miconazole) and CYP3A4 inhibitors (including antiretroviral drugs, clarithromycin and azole antifungal drugs) may increase systemic exposure to vismodegib and the risk of adverse effects.

ADVERSE EFFECTS AND THEIR MANAGEMENT

Adverse effects are frequent and may be severe, leading to treatment withdrawal.

- The most common side effects of vismodegib are muscle cramps (72%), alopecia (64%) and taste disturbance (55%), including both abnormal taste and loss of taste.
- Other frequent side effects include weight loss, fatigue, nausea, diarrhoea, decreased appetite, constipation, arthralgia and vomiting.
- Hepatitis with elevated transaminase and/or alkaline phosphatase levels has been noted.
- Rebound of BCCs in hereditary basal cell naevus syndrome has been described on discontinuing therapy.
- Squamous neoplasms have been reported to develop during treatment with vismodegib, including keratoacanthomas and moderate-to-highly-differentiated squamous cell carcinomas.

USE IN SPECIAL SITUATIONS

Pregnancy and Pre-Conception

Animal studies have shown irreversible loss of fertility after treatment with vismodegib. Females taking vismodegib may become amenorrhoeic. Fertility preservation strategies should be discussed with individuals who may wish to have children after completing therapy.

Vismodegib is excreted in semen, and male patients must use a condom when having sex with a female of childbearing potential during treatment and for 2 months after the last dose.

Smo inhibitors, including vismodegib, are potent teratogens, causing severe birth defects and embryo-fetal death. They are absolutely contraindicated during pregnancy. In reality, the majority of female recipients will be beyond an age of childbearing potential. However, for females with childbearing potential, stringent precautions apply, including a strict PPP. The manufacturers advise that pregnancy must be avoided for 24 months after the final dose.

Lactation

Mothers must not breastfeed while taking vismodegib and for 24 months after the final dose.

Children

Animal studies indicate a potential risk of short stature and tooth deformities in infants and children, and vismodegib should not be given to those under the age of 18 years. This may be of relevance in hereditary basal cell naevus syndrome, where BCCs may first appear in early childhood.

OLDER PEOPLE

In clinical trials of vismodegib, approximately 40% of patients are over the age of 65, and vismodegib did not differ in terms of safety or efficacy in this age group compared with younger patients.

ESSENTIAL PATIENT INFORMATION

- Patients and their carers should be advised that this treatment is for symptomatic relief rather than curative; BCCs will likely recur if treatment is discontinued.
- Patients and their carers should be advised of common adverse effects as detailed above.
- Females of childbearing potential must comply with the manufacturer's PPP during treatment and at least 24 months following the final dose.
- Males (including those post-vasectomy) should use barrier contraception with spermicide and must not donate semen while taking treatment and for 2 months after the final dose.
- Patients should not donate blood or blood products while taking vismodegib and for at least 24 months after the final dose.
- Patients must inform their healthcare team should they or their partner become pregnant while taking vismodegib, plan to become pregnant or plan to breastfeed.

FURTHER READING

Ali FR, Lear JT. Systemic treatments for basal cell carcinoma (BCC): The advent of dermato-oncology. Br J Dermatol. 2013;169:53–7.

Chang A, Solomon JA, Hainsworth JD, et al. Expanded access study of patients with advanced basal cell carcinoma treated with the hedgehog pathway inhibitor, vismodegib. J Am Acad Dermatol. 2014;70:60–9.

European Medicines Agency: European Public Assessment Report for Erivedge. https://www.ema.europa.eu/en/medicines/human/EPAR/erivedge.

National Institute for Health and Care Excellence (NICE): Vismodegib for treating basal cell carcinoma. Technology Appraisal Guidance [TA489]. https://www.nice.org.uk/guidance/ta489 (Accessed on 16 January 2021).

Sekulic A, Migden MR, Basset-Seguin N, et al. ERIVANCE BCC investigators. Long-term safety and efficacy of vismodegib in patients with advanced basal cell carcinoma: Final update of the pivotal ERIVANCE BCC study. BMC Cancer. 2017;17(1):332.

Sekulic A, Migden MR, Oro AE, et al. Efficacy and safety of vismodegib in advanced basal-cell carcinoma. N Engl J Med. 2012;360:2171–9.

38 Systemic Therapy in Children and Young People

Susannah Baron

PRINCIPLES OF TREATMENT

Prescribing systemic therapies in children poses several challenges, not least because many drugs are not licensed for use in the paediatric population. While most children tolerate systemic medication well, neonates are at special risk of adverse drug reactions due to their immature liver and renal function. Reliable information on prescribing for children can be found in the British National Formulary for Children (BNFC).

USE OF UNLICENSED AND OFF-LABEL MEDICINES

When a pharmaceutical produce is granted market authorisation ('product license'), the terms of its use are clearly specified in the Summary of Product Characteristics: Dose, regimen, route of administration, patient population, etc. Use of the product outside these terms is said to be 'off-label.' Much prescribing in children is off-label, as the pharmaceutical companies do not usually have sufficient data at the time marketing authorisation is granted. There is little incentive to do so unless the drug is principally for use in children.

Off-label prescribing in children should as far as possible be supported by evidence of safety and efficacy. The use of the product outside the terms of its license should be discussed with the child and their parents. Examples include the use of ciclosporin in childhood psoriasis and azathioprine in atopic dermatitis (atopic eczema). The term 'unlicensed' refers to a product that does not have a license at all and is a less common scenario. Such treatment will usually be initiated and maintained in secondary or tertiary care. Secondary formulations of a product (e.g. dilution or re-formulation) are also considered unlicensed.

PRESCRIPTION, FORMULATION AND ADMINISTRATION OF DRUGS IN CHILDREN

When choosing the best preparation for children, use one that is acceptable to them and that fits in with their daily routine. Some flexibility should be allowed in children to avoid waking them during the night, so their nighttime dose may be given at their bedtime.

For young children, liquid preparations are frequently prescribed. Branded oral liquid preparations that do not contain fructose, glucose or sucrose are described as 'sugar free' and should be prescribed whenever possible to prevent dental caries.

Some drugs are only available in solid dosage. This can pose administration problems for parents. It is important for parents to obtain the correct advice from the dispensing pharmacist on crushing the tablets or emptying the capsules into a suitable vehicle for administration.

Liquid preparations can be available in different strengths, so it is imperative when writing prescriptions to write clearly the drug dosage rather than the amount to be given. Confusion can occur with oral solutions, e.g. methotrexate and propranolol, that are formulated in different strengths. This should be discussed with the pharmacist and the parents and the same strength formulation should be dispensed each time to avoid over- or under-dosage.

Children often tolerate subcutaneous injections very well, and switching to subcutaneous methotrexate can reduce side effects, e.g. nausea, and improve medication efficacy.

DOI: 10.1201/9781003016786-38

SPECIFIC DRUGS

It is recommended that all drugs and dosages are checked in the BNFC or other pharmaceutical database.

ACITRETIN (SEE CHAPTER 1)

- Indications: Licensed for use in children in exceptional circumstances, e.g. severe ichthyosis.
- Children 1 month–12 years: 0.5 mg/kg once daily with food or milk (occasionally up to 1 mg/kg daily) to maximum of 35 mg daily.
- Children 12–18 years: For Darier disease, 10 mg daily for 2–4 weeks then adjusted according to response to 25–50 mg daily; for other conditions, up to 25–30 mg daily for 2–4 weeks, then adjusted for response. Dose may be increased up to 75 mg for short periods.
- Cautions
  - Growth should be monitored to detect premature epiphyseal closure.
  - Concomitant use of keratolytics should be avoided.
  - Discontinue if severe headaches, nausea, vomiting or visual disturbances occur as they could be signs of benign intracranial hypertension.
  - Be aware of teratogenic effect as pregnancy must be avoided for 3 years after stopping treatment.

Acitretin is insoluble in water and light-sensitive. A suspension may be formulated from capsule contents for neonates and infants, but care must be taken that the suspension is dispensed in a dark bottle and not exposed to light.

ACNE ANTIBIOTICS (SEE CHAPTER 2)

- Indications: Infantile and childhood acne.
- In children <12 years: Oral erythromycin is the first-line treatment with oral trimethoprim for resistant acne.
- In children >12 years: Oral tetracyclines are the first-line systemic treatment. Use of a once daily preparation, not taken pre-food, will improve compliance.

ALITRETINOIN (SEE CHAPTER 3)

Not recommended for use in children and adolescents under the age of 18 years.

ANTIBIOTICS COMMONLY USED FOR SKIN INFECTIONS (SEE CHAPTER 5)

Indications: Impetigo/infected atopic eczema.

Impetigo is common in young children and can be caused by Staphylococcus aureus and beta-haemolytic streptococci. These bacteria may also be implicated in infected flares of atopic eczema. Flucloxacillin is the treatment of choice for staphylococcal infections, with erythromycin an alternative for penicillin-allergic children. Virulent and resistant community-onset staphylococcal disease has emerged worldwide, associated with Panton–Valentine leukocidin (PVL) cytotoxin. In the UK, it is present in the majority of community-associated methicillin-resistant S. aureus (MRSA). Clindamycin alone or in combination with rifampicin may be used for PVL-positive S. aureus skin infections in children. Advice should be sought from local microbiologists.

ANTIFUNGALS (SEE CHAPTER 6)

Indications: Tinea capitis, onychomycosis, cutaneous fungal infections.

Oral azole antifungals (particularly itraconazole) and terbinafine are used in preference to griseofulvin, as they have a broader spectrum of activity and shorter treatment duration. Remember that immunocompromised children are at particular risk of fungal infections. Tables 38.1 and 38.2 provide detailed information regarding age, formulation, appropriate dosages and licensing information.

TABLE 38.1

Formulation and Licensing Information for Oral Antifungals in Children

Generic Name	Formulation	Information
Fluconazole	Capsules 50 mg, 150 mg, 200 mg Oral suspension 50 mg/5 mL, 200 mg/5 mL	Unlicensed for superficial fungal infections in children
Itraconazole	Capsules 100 mg Oral liquid sugar-free 50 mg/5 mL	Unlicensed in children (age range unspecified by manufacturers)
Griseofulvin	Tablets 125 mg, 500 mg Oral spray 10 mg/g	Licensed in children
Terbinafine	Tablets 250 mg	Unlicensed in children

Tinea capitis is predominantly a complaint of pre-adolescent children; infants are affected less commonly. Oral therapy is usually required in order to eradicate the organism, alleviating disease symptoms quickly and safely and to reduce transmission to others. The choice of drug will vary according to the causative organism, but as fungal culture may take up to 1 month, it is reasonable to start therapy immediately. Although griseofulvin is the only drug licensed for the treatment of tinea capitis in children in the UK, newer antifungal agents are gaining popularity, due to their greater cost-effectiveness and safety. In the UK, Trichophyton tonsurans is reported to account for 50–90% of dermatophyte scalp isolates, whereas in Europe Microsporum canis remains the most commonly involved organism.

Griseofulvin is more effective against Microsporum species than Trichophyton species, and the latter may require prolonged therapy. The suspension is more palatable for children but has become expensive and may be difficult to source. Terbinafine has much higher efficacy against Trichophyton species than Microsporum species and may be considered the treatment of choice for T. tonsurans infection. Itraconazole is active against both Microsporum and Trichophyton species and is widely used in many European countries. It is not licensed in children under the age of 12 years in the UK. A liquid formulation exists.

UK guidelines suggest the use of terbinafine or griseofulvin as first-line therapy, dependent on the organism suspected/isolated, with itraconazole used as second-line therapy.

Fluconazole is licensed for use in the treatment of candidiasis in children of all ages and exists in an orange-flavoured liquid formulation. The antifungal medications and dosage regimens suggested for use in children are outlined in Table 38.2.

Onychomycosis is less common in children than in adults. The dominant causative agents in this age group are T. rubrum, T. mentagrophytes and Candida species (in immunosuppressed children). Griseofulvin is no longer recommended for paediatric onychomycosis due to the long treatment duration and lack of efficacy. Daily terbinafine and daily or pulsed itraconazole have been shown to be well-tolerated in paediatric populations, with faster response and higher cure rates than in adults due to the faster growth of the nail plate in children.

Pityriasis versicolor may affect older children and usually responds to topical therapy. If required, it may be treated with oral itraconazole or fluconazole.

Widespread or intractable superficial candidiasis may require systemic therapy. Fluconazole is licensed for use in mucosal and invasive Candida infection in children of all ages. As stated above, itraconazole is not licensed for use in children under 12 years.

ANTIHISTAMINES

Indications: Urticaria, dermographism, pruritus in atopic eczema and allergic rhinitis.

If possible prescribe sugar- and colour-free oral solutions. In practice, higher doses of oral antihistamines than licensed dosages or those recommended in BNFC are often used in chronic urticaria in children, as in adults.

TABLE 38.2

Oral Antifungal Medication and Dosage Regimens for Children

Generic Name	Indication	Oral Dose 12–18 Years	Oral Dose <12 Years
Fluconazole	Oropharyngeal candidiasis	50 mg daily for 7–14 days up to 100 mg daily	<2 weeks: 3–6 mg/kg on day 1, then 3 mg/kg every 72 hours 2–4 weeks: 3–6 mg/kg on day 1, then 3 mg/kg every 48 hours 1 month–11 years: 3–6 mg/kg on day 1, then 3 mg/kg for 7–14 days (max 100 mg)
	Tinea corporis, tinea cruris, tinea pedis, tinea manuum		1 month–17 years: 3 mg/kg (max 50 mg) daily for 2–4 weeks (maximum duration 6 weeks)
	Tinea capitis		1–17 years: 6 mg/kg (maximum 300 mg) daily for 2–4 weeks
Itraconazole	Oropharyngeal candidiasis	100 mg once daily for 15 days	1 month–11 years: 3–5 mg/kg once daily (maximum 100 mg daily)
	Tinea corporis, tinea cruris, tinea pedis, tinea manuum	Either 100 mg once daily for 15 days in tinea corporis and tinea cruris, and 30 days for tinea pedis and tinea manuum, or 200 mg twice daily for 7 days	1 month–11 years: 3–5 mg/kg (maximum 100 mg) daily for 15 days for tinea corporis and tinea cruris and 30 days for tinea pedis and tinea manuum
	Onychomycosis	>50 kg 200 mg daily for 3 months or pulsed 200 mg x2/day for 1 week out of 4; 2 courses fingernails, 3 courses toenails	1–11 years; 5 mg/kg daily (maximum 200 mg) pulsed for 1 week out of 4; 2 pulses fingernails, 3 courses toenails
	Pityriasis versicolor	200 mg once daily for 7 days	1 month–1 years: 3–5 mg/kg once daily (maximum 200 mg) for 7 days
	Tinea capitis		1–17 years: 3–5 mg/kg (maximum 200 mg) daily for 2–6 weeks
Griseofulvin	Tinea capitis	500 mg per day increase to 1g daily in single or divided doses if needed for 6–8 weeks	1 month–11 years: 15–20 mg/kg/d (max per dose 1 g) in single or divided dose for 6–8 weeks
Terbinafine	Tinea capitis	>40 kg: 250 mg/d for 2–4 weeks	<20 kg: 62.5 mg/day for 4 weeks 20–39 kg: 125 mg/day for 4 weeks >40 kg: 250 mg/day for 4 weeks
	Onychomycosis	Above dose for 6 weeks for fingernails and 12 weeks for toenails	Above dose for 6 weeks for fingernails and 12 weeks for toenails

ANTIVIRALS (SEE CHAPTER 8)

Indications: Herpes simplex infection, varicella zoster infection, eczema herpeticum, an acute disseminated herpes simplex virus (HSV) infection in children with atopic eczema. It is often associated with systemic symptoms and should be treated with oral antiviral medication.

Aciclovir (acyclovir) is active against HSV. Tablets and suspension are not licensed in children.

- Tablets: 200 mg, 400 mg and 800 mg.
- Dispersible tablets: 200 mg, 400 mg and 800 mg.
- Suspension: 200 mg/5 mL and 400 mg/5 mL.
- Child 1 month–2 years: 100 mg 5 times daily for 5 days.

- Child 2–18 years: 200 mg 5 times daily for 5 days.
- May need higher doses for immunocompromised +/– varicella zoster/herpes zoster infection.

ANTIMALARIALS (SEE CHAPTER 7)

Indications: Hydroxychloroquine is used for connective tissue disease, lupus erythematosus, some photodermatoses and porphyria cutanea tarda in childhood at a dose of 5–6.5 mg/kg (max 400 mg) once daily.

Biological Drugs Used for Skin Disease in Children and Young People

Biologic medication is recommended as an option for treating moderate to severe plaque psoriasis, atopic eczema and hidradenitis suppurativa in children and young people if:

- Total Psoriasis Area and Severity Index (PASI) is >10.
- Psoriasis has not responded to at least 1 suitable standard systemic therapy, e.g. ciclosporin, methotrexate or phototherapy, or these are contraindicated or not tolerated.
- Atopic eczema (AE) has not responded to at least 1 suitable systemic immunosuppressant or these are not suitable.
- Hidradenitis suppurativa (HS) has not responded to conventional systemic therapy.

See Table 38.3 for NICE guidance on when to assess for adequate response:

- Psoriasis: PASI 75 (75% reduction in PASI score) since start of treatment.
- AE: At least EASI 50 (50% reduction in EASI score) from start of treatment and at least 4 point reduction in CDLQI.
- HS: A reduction of 25% or more in total abscess and inflammatory nodule count and no increase in abscesses and draining fistulas.

TABLE 38.3
Paediatric and Adolescent Biologic Medication

Medication	Age	Dosing Regime	NICE Timelines for Evaluating Response to Therapy	Indication
Anti-TNF				
Etanercept subcutaneous injection	6 years and above	0.8 mg/kg weekly Maximum weekly dose of 50 mg	12 weeks	Psoriasis
Adalimumab subcutaneous injection	4 years and above	0.8 mg/kg or 15 kg–<30 kg = 20 mg >30 kg = 40 mg *Loading dose*: W0, W1 *Maintenance dose*: Fortnightly thereafter	16 weeks	Psoriasis
	12 years and above	>30 kg: *Loading dose*: 80 mg with 40 mg after 1 week *Maintenance dose*: 40 mg fortnightly increased to 40 mg once weekly or 80 mg every 2 weeks if needed	12 weeks	Hidradenitis suppurativa

(Continued)

TABLE 38.3 *(Continued)*

Paediatric and Adolescent Biologic Medication

Medication	Age	Dosing Regime	NICE Timelines for Evaluating Response to Therapy	Indication
IL12/1L 23 Inhibitor				
Ustekinumab subcutaneous injection	6 years and above	<60 kg = 0.75 mg/kg 60–<100 kg = 45 mg >100 kg = 90 mg *Loading dose*: W0, W4 *Maintenance dose*: W16 and 12 weekly thereafter	16 weeks	Psoriasis
IL17A Inhibitor				
Secukinumab subcutaneous injection	6 years and above	<25 kg = 75 mg 25–<50 kg = 75 mg >50 kg = 150 mg but can increase to 300 mg *Loading dose*: W0, 1, 2, 3, 4 *Maintenance dose*: Monthly thereafter	12 weeks (NICE guidance)	Psoriasis
Ixekizumab subcutaneous injection	6 years and above	25 kg–50 kg: *Loading dose*: W0 – 80 mg *Maintenance dose*: 40 mg 4 weekly thereafter >50 kg: *Loading dose*: W0 – 160 mg *Maintenance dose*: 80 mg 4 weekly thereafter	Not yet NICE approved in paediatric population	Psoriasis
IL4/IL 13 Inhibitor				
Dupilumab subcutaneous injection	6–11 years (*Prefilled syringe device only licensed*)	15 kg–<60 kg = 300 mg *Loading dose*: D1 and D15 *Maintenance dose*: Then every 4 weeks thereafter; can increase to 200 mg fortnightly >60 kg: *Loading dose*: W0 (x2 300 mg injections) *Maintenance dose*: W2 and fortnightly thereafter	16 weeks	Atopic eczema
	12–18 years	<60 kg = initial dose of 400 mg then 200 mg fortnightly >60 kg = initial dose of 600 mg then 300 mg fortnightly	16 weeks	Atopic eczema
Janus Kinase 1 Inhibitors				
Abrocitinib oral tablet	12 years and above	100 mg OD; can increase to 200 mg	16 weeks	Atopic eczema
Upaticitinib modified release oral tablet	12 years and above	>30 kg = 15 mg OD	16 weeks	Atopic eczema

Pre-biologic investigations are as per adults:

- FBC, U&Es, LFTs, VZV, Hepatitis, TB and HIV screen, ANA, ENA, CXR, CRP or ESR, pregnancy test if appropriate.

CORTICOSTEROIDS (SEE CHAPTER 15)

Indications: Severe atopic eczema, connective tissue disease, systemic lupus erythematosus, immunobullous skin disease, severe urticaria.

Prednisolone has predominantly glucocorticoid activity and is the corticosteroid most commonly used orally in children with severe atopic dermatitis. There are concerns regarding their potential to suppress growth due to the suppressive action of glucocorticoids on the hypothalamic–pituitary–adrenal axis. This suppression is greatest and most prolonged when the drugs are given at night and least when given in a single dose in the morning.

Alternate-day dosing may reduce growth suppression but can have reduced therapeutic effectiveness against the disease being treated. Prednisolone dosage should be taken with food in the morning as it can affect sleep and may cause hyperactivity in children.

Courses of oral corticosteroids for skin diseases in children are usually prednisolone 1–2 mg/kg in total and should be intermittent and if for regaining control, e.g. of atopic eczema, try and limit higher doses for 1–2 weeks and then reduce slowly over 2–4 weeks rather than stopping suddenly. Prolonged courses increase susceptibility to infections and severity of infections. Clinical presentations of infections may also be atypical or exacerbated.

ISOTRETINOIN (SEE CHAPTER 22)

Although unlicensed in children under 12 years old, isotretinoin has been safely used in infantile acne and in younger children. Capsule contents are light-sensitive and insoluble in water. The author recommends mixing with a fatty food such as peanut butter on toast in the dark. Severe infantile acne should be managed by those with special expertise in paediatric dermatology.

- 1 month–2 years: 0.2 mg/kg daily.
- Child 2–12 years: 0.2–0.5 mg/kg increased if necessary to 1 mg/kg.
- Child 12–18 years: 0.5 mg/kg daily increased if necessary to 1 mg/kg.

IMMUNOSUPPRESSIVE/IMMUNOMODULATORY THERAPY

Indications: Severe atopic eczema, psoriasis, immunobullous disease.

Before beginning systemic immunosuppressive medications in children, it should be established if the child has had chickenpox. If in doubt, the varicella zoster virus (VZV) serology should be checked. Children who are not immune to VZV are at risk of severe chickenpox when taking immunosuppressive therapy, including prolonged corticosteroids. If possible arrange varicella zoster immunisation before treatment (2 injections 4–8 weeks apart). If the child is exposed to chickenpox, advice should be sought from the local microbiology department regarding post-exposure treatment. If the child is confirmed to have chickenpox infection or shingles, they will need urgent specialist care and treatment.

Pre-treatment blood tests advised before starting immunosuppressant/immunomodulatory therapy in children:

- FBC.
- U&Es.
- LFTs.
- Fasting lipids.

- VZV serology.
- CRP.
- TPMT (for Azathioprine).
- TB, hepatitis, HIV screening and CXR if indicated from history.

Note PIIINP not useful in children/young people as raised levels seen due to growth.

Immunizations with live vaccines such as polio and rubella should be avoided while children are taking systemic immunomodulatory, biologic and immunosuppressive drugs, as the immunizations may not be effective.

Most immunosuppressive agents, although commonly used, are not licensed for use in the treatment of skin disease in children, including ciclosporin (not licensed under 16 years), methotrexate and mycophenolate mofetil.

Methotrexate:
- Often used as a first-line systemic agent for atopic eczema and psoriasis.
- Available as oral solution, tablet and subcutaneous injection.
- Give ONCE weekly and if fatigue/nausea occurs give on Fridays to allow weekend recovery.
- 0.1 mg/kg test dose followed by 0.4 mg/kg maintenance dose (maximum dose 25 mg/week).
- Folic acid 1 mg/day, 6 days per week (not on methotrexate day) or 5 mg twice per week can be given to reduce side effects.
- Consider a switch to subcutaneous methotrexate if there is significant nausea/poor efficacy.
- Methotrexate tablets: 2.5 mg (10 mg tablets are available but best avoided in children to reduce drug dosage errors).
- Methotrexate oral solution: 2 mg/mL.
- Methotrexate subcutaneous injection: Available between 7.5 mg to 25 mg in 2.5 mg increasing increments to be used ONCE weekly.

SPECIAL POINT: VITAMIN D SUPPLEMENTATION

Children may have asymptomatic vitamin D deficiency. Furthermore, studies have suggested that there may be an inverse relationship between the severity of atopic dermatitis and vitamin D levels, with vitamin D supplementation leading to a decrease in severity of disease. Therefore, in children with difficult and severe eczema check levels if appropriate.

Simple nutritional vitamin D deficiency can be prevented by oral supplementation with ergocalciferol (calciferol or vitamin D2) or cholecalciferol (vitamin D3) daily, using multivitamin drops or preparations of vitamin A and D.

With acknowledgment to Maria Akinde, Clinical Nurse Specialist, Paediatric Dermatology, St John's Institute of Dermatology, Guy's and St Thomas' Hospitals NHS Foundation Trust for the tables in the chapter.

FURTHER READING

Gupta A, Venkataraman M, Shear N, et al. Onychomycosis in children: Review on treatment and management strategies. J Dermatolog Treat. 2022; 33(3):1213–24.

Irvine A, Jones A, Beattie P, et al. A randomised controlled trial assessing the effectiveness, safety and cost-effectiveness of methotrexate versus ciclosporin in the treatment of severe atopic eczema in children: The TREatment of severe atopic eczema trial (TREAT). Br J Dermatol. 2018 Dec; 179(6):1297–1306.

Menter A, Cordoro K, Davis D, et al. Joint American Academy of Dermatology: National Psoriasis Foundation guidelines of care for the management and treatment of psoriasis in paediatric patients. J Am Acad Dermatol. 2020 Jan; 82(1):161–201.

Simpson E, Paller A, Siegried E, et al. Efficacy and safety of dupilumab in adolescent with uncontrolled moderate to severe atopic dermatitis: A phase 3 randomized clinical trial. JAMA. 2020; 156:44–56.

Smith C, Yiu Z, Bale B, et al. BAD guidelines for biologic therapy for psoriasis 2020: A rapid update. Br J Dermatol. 2020; 183:628–37.

Wollneberg A, Barbarot S, Bieber T, et al. Consensus-based European guidelines for treatment of atopic eczema in adults and children: Part I. J Eur Acad Dermatol Venereol. 2018 May; 32(5):657–682.

39 Systemic Therapy and Kidney Disease

Phil Mason

Many drugs and their metabolites are renally excreted and accumulate in patients with chronic kidney disease (CKD), which may lead to increased toxicity and side effects. Kidney function decreases with age, so otherwise healthy older patients may have unrecognized CKD. It is therefore important to identify such patients in order to modify the dose or dosing frequency. This has become easier with universal reporting of an estimated glomerular filtration rate (eGFR) alongside the creatinine measurement.

Other renal factors may be relevant, in particular heavy proteinuria, hypoalbulinaemia and marked salt and water retention, which may change drug pharmacokinetics (and pharmacodynamics). However, these rarely have a significant effect on drug dosing.

IDENTIFICATION OF PATIENTS WITH IMPAIRED RENAL FUNCTION

Table 39.1 indicates the prevalence of different degrees of CKD. Renal function declines with age so that, for example, approximately 25% of men and approximately 50% of women over the age of 75 years have an eGFR of less than 60 mL/min (CKD3). Although most of these will not progress to more severe CKD (especially in the absence of proteinuria), the reduced GFR will affect drug elimination.

Actual measured GFR (mGFR) using either radioactive isotopes or iohexol is time-consuming, expensive and neither practical nor necessary in clinical practice. A creatinine clearance is a reliable surrogate of actual GFR but requires an accurately collected 24-hour urine sample and blood creatinine, making it unsuitable as a routine measurement. However, the GFR may be estimated by a variety of formulae based on the serum creatinine, which is dependent on renal function but also on muscle mass and dietary meat intake, and can be affected by concurrent medication (Table 39.2). The method of estimating renal function reported by all laboratories now uses the formula developed by the Modification of Diet in Renal Disease Study Group (MDRD), which estimates the GFR based on the patient's age, sex, racial background and creatinine (Table 39.3). It generally underestimates GFR when renal function is near normal (>50 mL/min), but these patients tend not to need dose modification. Most laboratories now use the modified CKD-EPI formula, which gives a result closer to the mGFR.

It should be remembered that any estimate of GFR is only valid for stable patients without an acute illness.

DOSAGES FOR PATIENTS WITH CKD

Drug dose modification is rarely required until the eGFR falls below 60 mL/min (CKD3), and most renally excreted drugs only need adjustment below 30 mL/min (CKD4 and 5). Many drug Summaries of Product Characteristics (SPCs) and the British National Formulary (BNF) recommend dose modifications based on the Cockcroft–Gault formula, but the eGFR is a reasonable surrogate for this.

Before prescribing any drug in patients with CKD, the dosage should be checked in the BNF. The Renal Drug Handbook provides comprehensive dose recommendation for virtually all available drugs and also indicates whether they are removed by different dialysis modalities. Pharmacists and renal units are also available for advice.

DOI: 10.1201/9781003016786-39

TABLE 39.1

Prevalence of Different Stages of Chronic Kidney Disease, 2015–16

Stage	GFR (mL/min/1.73 m²)	Prevalence in the United States
1 (normal function but proteinuria)	>90	4.7%
2	60–89	3.4%
3	30–59	5.8%
4	15–29	0.24%
5	<15 (or dialysis/transplant)	0.2%

Note: Although the data are from the United States, the prevalence is similar in other developed countries.

Source: From K/DOQI-NHANES III study.

Abbreviation: GFR, glomerular filtration rate.

TABLE 39.2

Factors Affecting Creatinine Levels

GFR

Muscle mass

Dietary meat intake

Hydration status

Drugs – direct, e.g. trimethoprim, cimetidine (interfere with renal tubular secretion of creatinine)

NB: Creatinine increased (so eGFR reduced) but mGFR unaltered

Drugs – indirect, e.g. diuretics, which affect hydration status

Drugs which do affect GFR, e.g. NSAIDs or via interstitial nephritis, e.g. PPIs

Abbreviations: GFR, glomerular filtration rate; NSAID, non-steroidal anti-inflammatory drug; PPI, proton pump inhibitor.

TABLE 39.3

Formulae for Calculating Estimates of Kidney Function: The Cockcroft–Gault Formula Estimates a Calculated Creatinine Clearance and the Modification of Diet in Renal Disease (MDRD) and CKD-EPI Estimate GFR

Cockcroft–Gault

$$Crcl = \frac{(140 - age) \times wt \ (kg) \times 1.23\male (1.04\female)}{creatinine \ (\mu mol/L)}$$

MDRD

eGFR = $32788 \times (creatinine, \mu mol/L)^{-1.154} \times age^{-0.203}$
[× 1.212 if black] [× 0.742 if female]

CKD-EPI

eGFR = $141 \times min(S_{cr}/\kappa, 1)^{\alpha} \times max(S_{cr}/\kappa, 1)^{-1.209} \times 0.993^{Age} \times 1.018$ [if female] × 1.159 [if African American]

S_{cr} is serum creatinine in $\mu mol/L$, κ is 61.9 for females and 79.6 for males, α is –0.329 for females and –0.411 for males, min indicates the minimum of S_{cr}/κ or 1, and max indicates the maximum of S_{cr}/κ or 1

Abbreviation: eGFR, estimated glomerular filtration rate.

NEPHROTOXIC DRUGS

Some drugs have predictable dose-related effects on kidney function (but often of variable magnitude in different patients). These include, for example, the calcineurin inhibitors tacrolimus and ciclosporin (cyclosporine), non-steroidal anti-inflammatory drugs (NSAIDs) and aminoglycosides. Other drugs may have idiosyncratic effects, for instance, drugs causing acute interstitial nephritis. Currently, proton pump inhibitors are the most common culprits, but others include antibiotics, mesalazine, allopurinol and diuretics. However, it is important to remember these reactions are actually very rare.

DRUGS COMMONLY USED IN DERMATOLOGY

This is not an exhaustive list, and for patients with CKD, it is important that the correct dose of every prescribed drug be checked.

- Hydroxychloroquine and chloroquine: These drugs and their metabolites are renally excreted, so dose reduction is required and consideration should be given to limiting the duration of treatment. They also increase levels of ciclosporin.
- Mepacrine: No dose reduction is necessary, but renal function should be monitored, as idiosyncratic renal failure may develop.
- Antibiotics: Most antibiotics do not need dose reduction, but tetracycline should be avoided, although doxycycline, minocycline and lymecycline are safe. The macrolides are safe, but erythromycin doses need to be reduced in dialysis patients and those with CKD5. They also inhibit cytochrome P450 (CYP450) 3A4 and increase calcineurin inhibitor levels.
- Retinoids: Isotretinoin and acitretin are safe above a GFR of 10–15 mL/min, but at lower levels (and for patients on dialysis), the situation is unclear and careful titration with monitoring is advised. They are reported to cause glomerulonephritis and vasculitis, but this is very rare.
- Antiproliferative drugs: Azathioprine and mycophenolate do not need dose reduction, but cyclophosphamide and especially methotrexate do. Methotrexate is best avoided with eGFR <20 mL/min.
- Biologics: In general, no dose modifications are necessary, but the SPCs usually advise caution.
- Triazole antifungals: No dose reduction is required in CKD, but they are potent CYP3A4 inhibitors and so drug interactions are common.
- Calcineurin inhibitors (tacrolimus and ciclosporin): There is no doubt that these drugs are nephrotoxic. Patients with non-renal solid organ transplants have a high incidence of developing CKD4–5 (6–21%) at 5 years post-transplant, with an estimated overall incidence of renal failure requiring dialysis or transplantation of 1–1.5% per annum. Renal impairment is also a recognized complication of their use in psoriasis. Higher levels are associated with a higher incidence of CKD, and, although some dermatological data suggest that monitoring levels is not necessary, especially when used at doses of 5 mg/kg or less, some patients will have high levels even at these doses and a proportion of these will develop CKD. Monitoring of levels should be considered, especially in those at risk, soon after commencement, and regular creatinine measurements should be made for the duration of treatment. It is important to warn the patient of potential interactions with drugs (so that anyone prescribing is aware that the patient is on these drugs), foods and over-the-counter preparations (e.g. grapefruit juice and St John's wort), which may increase drug levels. Any decline in renal function should be investigated by referral to a nephrologist, and a biopsy will usually be performed to determine the cause.
- Topical agents: Generally, topical medications can be used in patients with CKD, although caution is required with topical NSAIDs, especially if used frequently and on large areas of skin.

DRUG PRESCRIPTION IN DIALYSIS AND TRANSPLANT PATIENTS

Dialysis patients should be considered to have an eGFR <10%, but it should also be determined if the drug is removed by dialysis, and some drugs are best administered at the end of a dialysis session. It is best to liaise with the renal team involved before prescribing for this group of patients.

Transplant patients often have a degree of CKD, but the main concern is drug interactions that may affect levels of immunosuppressive drugs. Again, it is best to liaise with the transplant team or transplant pharmacists.

FURTHER READING

Ashley C, Dunleavy A. *The Renal Drug Handbook*. 5th Ed. CRC Press, 2018.

Ellis CN, Fradin MS, Messana JM, et al. Cyclosporine for plaque-type psoriasis. Results of a multidose, double-blind trial. N Engl J Med. 1991;324:277–84.

Feutren G, Abeywickrama K, Friend D, von Graffenried B. Renal function and blood pressure in psoriatic patients treated with cyclosporin A. Br J Dermatol. 1990;122(Suppl. 36):57–69.

Ojo AO, Held PJ, Port FK, et al. Chronic renal failure after transplantation of a nonrenal organ. N Engl J Med. 2003;349:931–40.

40 Systemic Therapy and Liver Disease

Maria Bashyam and Shahid A. Khan

INTRODUCTION

Liver disease is increasing worldwide. Most liver disease is preventable, but it is frequently identified too late. Specific dermatological conditions such as psoriasis are associated with an increased incidence of non-alcoholic fatty liver disease. Therefore, the assessment of hepatic function is essential before starting any potentially hepatotoxic drug. Pre-existing liver disease can usually be identified from the clinical history, examination, routine liver function tests (LFTs) and non-invasive assessments of liver fibrosis. Any abnormality requires further investigation to determine the underlying cause and the extent of pre-existing liver damage (fibrosis). This will allow an informed decision to be made regarding the safety of a particular drug Most systemic dermatological medications are safe if regularly monitored. For those known to be hepatotoxic, LFTs should be checked before commencement, with referral to a hepatologist for further investigations if abnormalities are detected, and at regular intervals during their use. Hepatitis B and C virus infection remain highly prevalent globally and screening should be undertaken before starting drugs with immunosuppressant actions.

Most drugs can be used in patients with chronic liver disease, but specific consideration should be given to dosing and monitoring. Systemic drugs that are recognized to cause hepatotoxicity should be discontinued if LFTs increase to be more that 2–3 times the upper limit of normal. Patients with pre-existing liver disease and high-risk cases should be managed jointly with a hepatologist.

ASSESSMENT OF LIVER FUNCTION

- Clinical history: Alcohol consumption, illicit drug use, medication (including over the counter and herbal remedies), metabolic syndrome risk factors and family history of liver disease.
- Clinical examination: Stigmata of chronic liver disease (for example jaundice, spider naevi, hepatomegaly and splenomegaly or ascites).
- Liver function tests
  - Aminotransferases: The enzymes aspartate aminotransferase (AST) and alanine aminotransferase (ALT) are present in hepatocytes and leak into the blood when there is hepatocyte damage/inflammation.
  - Alkaline phosphatase (ALP): Elevations in ALP occur due to cholestasis (i.e. failure of bile secretion or drainage) secondary to intra- or extrahepatic causes. A raised ALP without gamma-glutamyl transferase (GGT) should raise suspicion of bone disease, and specific ALP isoenzymes can be measured if required. ALP levels are raised in pregnancy due to production of the placental isoenzyme, and the normal range is higher in children.
  - Gamma glutamyl transferase (GGT): Elevations in GGT occur in diseases of the liver and biliary system. Causes include excessive alcohol consumption, cholestasis (intra- or extrahepatic) and various medications.
  - Bilirubin: Bilirubin is produced from the breakdown of erythrocytes in the liver and reticuloendothelial system. Bilirubin is conjugated with glucuronic acid in the liver

DOI: 10.1201/9781003016786-40

and excreted in the bile. Rises in unconjugated bilirubin are derived from extrahepatic erythrocyte breakdown (haemolysis) or defects in conjugation, such as in Gilbert's syndrome. A rise in conjugated bilirubin indicates hepatic disease and can be due to hepatocyte damage, cholestasis or synthetic liver failure.

DIAGNOSIS

It is not possible, on clinical grounds, to differentiate hepatitis B from hepatitis caused by other viral agents. Hence, laboratory confirmation of the diagnosis is essential. A number of blood tests are available to diagnose and monitor people with hepatitis B. They can be used to distinguish acute and chronic infections.

Laboratory diagnosis of hepatitis B infection focuses on the detection of the hepatitis B surface antigen (HBsAg). WHO recommends that all blood donations be tested for hepatitis B to ensure blood safety and avoid accidental transmission to people who receive blood products.

- Acute HBV infection is characterized by the presence of HBsAg and the acute immunoglobulin M (lgM) antibody to the core antigen, hepatitis B core antibody (HBcAb). During the initial phase of infection, patients are also seropositive for the hepatitis B e antigen (HBeAg). HBeAg is usually a marker of high levels of replication of the virus. The presence of HBeAg indicates that the blood and body fluids of the infected individual are highly infectious.
- Chronic infection is characterized by the persistence of HBsAg for at least 6 months (with or without concurrent HBeAg). Persistence of HBsAg is the principal marker of risk for developing chronic liver disease and liver cancer (hepatocellular carcinoma) later in life.
- Albumin is synthesized in the liver, and thus a falling serum albumin level may indicate synthetic liver failure.
- Prothrombin time (PT) is a marker of hepatic synthetic function due to the short half-life of prothrombin. The PT may be prolonged in acute liver injury and chronic liver disease (cirrhosis).
- Ultrasound scan is a non-invasive, safe and inexpensive investigation that should be undertaken in all patients with suspected liver disease. It allows identification of parenchymal disease, fatty liver, biliary obstruction, portal hypertension, vascular pathology and liver lesions. If abnormalities of liver function are detected, specialist advice from a hepatologist is essential before starting a potentially hepatotoxic drug to ensure the appropriate choice and dose of drug and adequate monitoring.
- Transient elastography (FibroScan) is a rapid, immediate, cheap, non-invasive, reproducible and validated test that uses ultrasound to measure liver stiffness gauged in kilopascals (kPa) as a marker of fibrosis. It may help limit the need for biopsies, with the latter being reserved for patients whose score is suggestive of moderate fibrosis (i.e. >7.1 kPa) or where clinical suspicion/concern exists.
- Hepatitis virus infection screening for hepatitis B virus (HBV) and hepatitis C virus (HCV) should be carried out before starting high-dose prednisolone, immunosuppressive therapy and psoriasis biological therapy. If hepatitis virus serology indicates possible infection, further advice should be obtained from a hepatologist.
- HBV serology screening tests focus on the identification of the viral surface antigen (HBSAg), which is the first serological marker of acute infection that persists in those with chronic infection. Acute infection is also characterised by presence of the immunoglobulin M (IgM) antibody to the core antigen and seropositivity to the e antigen (HBeAg). The presence of HBeAg indicates that body fluids and blood are highly infectious. Persistence of HBSAg for more than 6 months is a marker of risk for chronic liver disease and hepatocellular carcinoma.

TABLE 40.1

Hepatitis B Virus (HBV) Blood Tests and Their Interpretation

Test	Interpretation of Positive Result
Hepatitis B surface antigen (HBsAg)	Acute or chronic infection with HBV
Hepatitis B surface antibody	Successful response to HBV vaccine or recovery from acute HBV infection
Hepatitis B core antibody (HBcAb)	Past or present infection depending on the above test results
Hepatitis B e antigen (HBeAg)	HBV infection – high infectivity

- HBV surface antibody positivity indicates former infection or immunisation. An antibody to the HBV core antigen may occur in past or present infection according to other serological findings (see Table 40.1). Monitoring of the serum HBV DNA level is also valuable in assessing liver disease activity, treatment and differentiating other aetiologies of hepatitis in HBSAg carriers.
- HCV infection is diagnosed by screening for anti-HCV antibodies, which indicate exposure to the virus followed by a nucleic acid test for HCV RNA to assess ongoing infection and viral load. A new HCV infection is usually asymptomatic, and uncleared infection often remains asymptomatic until symptoms of serious liver damage develop. Direct-acting oral antivirals for 12–24 weeks can cure most cases.

PRESCRIBING IN PATIENTS WITH LIVER DISEASE

Prescribing systemic dermatological treatment in patients with pre-existing liver disease can present challenges, as many of these drugs can cause liver damage. The following factors should be considered:

- Is there an alternative, effective, non-hepatotoxic drug?
- How severe is the underlying liver disease? Does the patient have pre-existing hepatic fibrosis/cirrhosis?
- Could the liver disease be treated/controlled before drug therapy?
- What is the effect of the drug on liver function? Does the drug have the potential to worsen pre-existing liver disease? Is it a dose-dependent or idiosyncratic effect?
- What is the effect of liver disease on drug metabolism and dosage?
- How will the effect of the drug on liver function be monitored?

MONITORING

More than 1,000 drugs have been reported to cause liver injury, with manifestations ranging from asymptomatic elevations in liver enzymes to fulminant hepatic failure resulting in death or requiring liver transplantation. Drug-induced liver injury (DILI) is the most commonly cited reason for withdrawal of an approved drug. The National Institutes of Health (NIH) has a searchable database of drugs, herbs and supplements associated with DILI.

Any prescriber must be vigilant in identifying DILI, as early drug discontinuation can limit its severity. Hepatitic reactions (hepatocyte inflammation) are usually associated with a rise in transaminases, and cholestatic drug reactions are usually associated with a rise in ALP and GGT levels (which can be associated with pruritus), though biochemical features often overlap.

As a general guide, patients commenced on a drug with an established risk of idiosyncratic DILI should undergo monitoring of LFTs every 4 weeks for 3 months and then every 3 months thereafter. If the LFTs rise to more than 2–3 times the upper limit of normal, then the drug should be discontinued and LFTs closely monitored to document resolution. A liver specialist can advise if and when a liver biopsy is indicated.

Re-exposure to a drug implicated in DILI is generally not advisable, even at a reduced dose, as it may lead to a rapid and more severe relapse of DILI. In special circumstances, a re-challenge may be warranted, with close monitoring of LFTs if the drug is considered essential. This should be done under co-management of a liver specialist.

SPECIFIC DRUGS

Anti-TNFs

Anti-TNFs can be associated with a variety of liver function abnormalities. TNF alpha is a key cytokine in the host immune reactions against HBV infection, and due to the risk of HBV reactivation, all patients should be screened for HBV before starting anti-TNF treatment (see Table 40.1). If they are HBV-core antibody-positive, with a negative HBSAg (resolved HBV), they should be treated prophylactically with tenofovir or entecavir concurrently. If they are HBVSAg-positive, this suggests ongoing/chronic HBV infection and advice from a hepatologist should be sought. Careful monitoring of liver function tests and HBV serology should be maintained during treatment and for at least 6 months after.

Adalimumab

Adalimumab can cause an increase in ALP in 5% and, less commonly, hepatic necrosis in <5% of cases. It can also cause a mild and transient elevation in transaminases, rarely requiring dose modification. In 1–3.5% of cases, the ALT can rise to more than 3 × ULN, requiring cessation of the drug. It can also cause autoimmune hepatitis with development of liver autoantibodies: Anti-nuclear antibodies (ANA), smooth muscle antibodies (SMA) and double-stranded DNA antibodies (dsDNA). (See Infliximab.)

Certolizumab Pegol

Certolizumab can be associated with a transient and mild increase in the ALT. Certolizumab is a newer medication, so not as much data is available concerning other patterns of injury, but it is feasible that it could also induce autoantibodies mimicking autoimmune hepatitis that require corticosteroid treatment.

Etanercept

Etanercept can cause minimal asymptomatic ALT elevations which do not require dose adjustments. In approximately <1%, etanercept can cause liver autoantibody induction and cause exacerbation or induction of autoimmune hepatitis, which is usually responsive to corticosteroid treatment. It is not clear whether patients who react to etanercept can tolerate another anti-TNF agent.

Infliximab

Infliximab has been-well described as causing DILI, with a range of dysfunctions that usually resolve when it its discontinued. Transaminitis is usually early in onset after 2–5 doses. Raised enzymes may be transient or progressive, necessitating discontinuation (usually when 3–5 × ULN).

This can also progress to jaundice. These abnormalities normally resolve 4–12 weeks after discontinuation. Affected patients can usually tolerate etanercept.

Infliximab commonly causes induction of autoantibodies: ANA, SMA and dsDNA. This is rarely associated with a clinical autoimmune lupus- or autoimmune hepatitis-like syndrome, and it usually resolves on drug withdrawal. Infliximab can also cause a usually self-limiting cholestatic DILI from 4 days to 24 weeks after starting treatment.

ANTI-IL 12/23 BIOLOGICAL THERAPY

Ustekinumab has been associated with a low rate of mild-to moderate serum enzyme elevations during therapy, which were self-limiting and resolved with ongoing therapy. There appears to be no significant risk of idiosyncratic, clinically apparent liver injury. However, it has immunomodulatory activity and has been associated with reactivation of HBV in susceptible patients, so baseline screening is advised and liaison with hepatology if positive.

ANTI-IL 17 BIOLOGICS

There is a paucity of data about the risk of HBV reactivation with non-TNF–targeted biologics. However, as the TH17/IL-17 axis is thought to play a role in elimination of HBV, its inhibition may increase the risk of HBV reactivation and this has been observed in clinical practice. Antiviral prophylaxis is indicated in those with chronic HBV infection and resolved HBV if their baseline viral load is positive.

ANTIBIOTICS

Flucloxacillin is reported to cause severe hepatotoxicity in approximately 1 in 13,000 patients. This risk is increased at higher doses and for treatment longer than 14 days. Liver dysfunction can occur any time between 1 week and 2 months after starting therapy and up to 6 weeks after stopping. Deranged LFTs typically show a mixed cholestatic and hepatitic profile, with cholestasis and a mixed inflammatory infiltrate on histology. The course of cholestatic hepatitis from flucloxacillin is often prolonged, with persistently abnormal LFTs for over 6 months in 10–30% of cases. These are associated with loss of smaller bile ducts and periportal inflammation, which may progress to biliary cirrhosis and liver failure.

Tetracyclines may also be hepatotoxic, causing jaundice and acute fatty infiltration. Minocycline is associated with two distinct forms of liver injury: An acute hepatitis-like syndrome typically arising within 1–3 months of starting therapy and chronic hepatitis, usually with autoimmune features, which follows long-term therapy. In both forms, hypersensitivity features may be present with rash, fever and eosinophilia. The liver injury is usually self-limiting with prompt drug discontinuation, but if treatment is continued inadvertently, progressive liver fibrosis and cirrhosis may develop.

Sulphonamides have been recognised to cause liver damage since their development as antimicrobial agents. Most cases occur within 2–4 weeks, although the onset may be delayed several months. Hepatocellular injury with marked increases in transaminases is often accompanied by hypersensitivity features (rash and eosinophilia). Recovery may take several months.

ANTIFUNGALS

- Ketoconazole: This is the most hepatotoxic oral azole antifungal drug, due to its extensive metabolism within the liver. Mild asymptomatic and transient elevations (<2 times the upper limit of normal) of transaminases have been estimated to occur in up to 20% of patients, with clinically apparent hepatotoxicity in approximately 1 in 2,000–15,000 users. The presentation is usually with acute hepatitis within 1–6 months of starting the drug.

Recovery usually occurs after drug discontinuation, but acute fulminant hepatic failure requiring transplantation has been reported, so it is no longer indicated for treatment of skin disease in Europe.

- Itraconazole: This has been reported to cause asymptomatic rises in LFTs in 1–5% of patients. Biochemically, the abnormalities are typically cholestatic, but hepatitic or mixed pictures can occur. LFTs generally return to normal within 3 months of discontinuing treatment. Reports of serious hepatotoxicity are extremely rare.
- Fluconazole: Transient mild-to-moderate elevations of serum aminotransferases occur in up to 5% of patients treated with fluconazole. The severity of liver injury ranges from transient asymptomatic enzyme elevations in the majority of cases to clinically apparent hepatitis and acute fatal liver failure in a very small number of cases. The liver injury is typically hepatocellular, occurs within the first few weeks of therapy and can be associated with a rash, fever and eosinophilia. Complete resolution can take up to 4 months following drug withdrawal.
- With all the azoles, there are little data regarding cross-reactivity, and extreme caution should be applied when exposing patients who have had hepatotoxicity to other agents in the same class.
- Terbinafine: This has very rarely been associated with liver dysfunction. Liver injury usually arises within the first 6 weeks of therapy. In a surveillance study including over 25,000 patients, there were only two reports of symptomatic cholestatic liver injury. Asymptomatic elevations in hepatic enzymes were recorded in less than 1% of cases for abnormal liver function tests which usually require no action and less than 0.5% of cases that require cessation, and these normalized within 3–6 months of discontinuation.

Azathioprine

Azathioprine (AZA) has been associated with several forms of hepatotoxicity. Mild transient and asymptomatic rises in serum aminotransferase levels are common during the first 3 months of therapy and resolve rapidly with dose reduction or discontinuation. Acute cholestatic injury may occur within the first year of therapy, and longer-term AZA may cause chronic hepatic damage with nodular regenerative hyperplasia and portal hypertension. Baseline and regular assessment of liver function are therefore required throughout treatment.

Liver function tests alongside other monitoring tests, such as full blood count, should be performed at 1–2-weekly intervals for the first month and/or until a steady dose is achieved. After a stable dose has been established and the initial blood tests are okay, monitoring with blood tests every 2–3 months is sufficient. Additional monitoring with thiopurine metabolites can be helpful. Measurement of therapeutic 6TGN metabolites help guide dose adjustments, whereas 6MMPN levels correlate to the likelihood of hepatotoxicity.

Corticosteroids

Corticosteroids can have major effects on the liver, particularly with long-term or high-dose therapy. Particular caution is needed in patients with pre-existing liver disease.

Corticosteroid therapy can cause steatohepatitis, especially when given in high doses for prolonged periods. Biochemical features include elevated transaminases, and liver histology demonstrates steatosis, hepatocyte ballooning and an inflammatory infiltrate. These findings are usually reversible on dose reduction or discontinuation. Pre-existing non-alcoholic steatohepatitis (NASH) may be aggravated due to a combination of weight gain, insulin resistance and altered lipid metabolism. Prolonged therapy increases the risk of fibrosis and cirrhosis. Dose minimization and alternative drugs should be considered, with monitoring for liver fibrosis in those on long-term treatment.

In patients who are HBV core antibody-positive, high-dose steroids (e.g. prednisolone 60 mg daily or higher) can cause reactivation of viral infection, resulting in acute hepatitis and acute liver failure. Such patients should be closely monitored with 1–3 monthly blood tests and started on antivirals if there is any sign of reactivation. In patients with chronic HBV (i.e. HBV surface antigen-positive), oral corticosteroids are not contraindicated, but advice should be sought from a hepatologist as these drugs may increase the viral load. Abnormal LFTs do not usually develop during treatment due to immunosuppressive effects, but on drug withdrawal, acute hepatitis may occur, which may aggravate underlying liver damage and on rare instances, precipitate acute liver failure.

In patients with HCV infection, corticosteroid therapy can lead to a rise in hepatitis C viral load, which may ultimately accelerate the progression to hepatic fibrosis, so close collaboration with a hepatologist is advised to ensure appropriate monitoring.

CICLOSPORIN

Ciclosporin does not have specific dose adjustments in severe liver disease, but it is largely metabolized by the liver. Levels should be closely monitored and dose adjustments made accordingly in those with severe liver dysfunction.

DAPSONE

Dapsone can cause acute hepatitis and cholestatic jaundice. The onset is usually sudden and associated with fever and a rash (DRESS) followed by jaundice, and it occurs within a few days or weeks of starting treatment. Eosinophilia is commonly seen. In rare instances, dapsone DILI has led to acute liver failure; however, most cases resolve within 2–4 weeks of drug discontinuation.

DUPILUMAB

Dupilumab is a fully recombinant monoclonal antibody directed against the alpha subunit of the IL-4 receptor, it also acts against the IL-13 alpha subunit. It is not known to have any primary hepatotoxicity. Its safety in patients with underlying HBV infection is not known. IL-4 is an anti-inflammatory cytokine, and the alpha subunit has been reported to promote liver regeneration and to regulate fibrosis so there are theoretical risks associated with inhibition of this cytokine. Concomitant antiviral therapy may be indicated with close monitoring of LFTs and HBV status under the guidance of hepatology.

DIMETHYL FUMARATE

Dimethyl fumarate is an anti-inflammatory immunomodulator. It has been associated with mild-to-moderate, transient elevation of serum enzymes in approximately 25% of cases. These are usually asymptomatic and settle with continued use. The elevated liver function blood tests are usually transient and do not require medication cessation. Discontinuation is only needed in less than 1% of cases where the abnormalities do not resolve. Acute hepatitis has been reported that resolved on stopping treatment with no chronic injury or liver failure. Dose-dependent increases in liver enzymes have been reported in patients taking baricitinib. If DILI is suspected, treatment should be interrupted until this diagnosis is excluded.

METHOTREXATE

Short-term low-to-moderate dose treatment with methotrexate (MTX) causes mild, self-limiting elevation in the serum transaminases in about 15–50% of patients. About 5% of patients develop more significantly elevated liver enzymes that usually normalize rapidly with dose reduction or drug discontinuation. Folic acid supplementation has been shown to be protective against this effect and is routinely prescribed in conjunction with methotrexate.

Long-term MTX therapy is associated with the development of dose-dependent hepatic fibrosis, and this drug is therefore contraindicated in those with underlying chronic liver disease, except in exceptional circumstances. The risk and rate of progression to fibrosis or cirrhosis is increased in patients with a heavy alcohol intake, those with diabetes, obesity, renal failure, age >60 years and concomitant use of other potentially hepatotoxic drugs. These factors are therefore considered to be relative contraindications to MTX therapy. Nowadays, a pre-treatment liver biopsy to assess the degree of fibrosis is only recommended in patients who are suspected clinically, biochemically or radiologically to be at risk of or to have underlying liver disease. If fibrosis is confirmed, then methotrexate is best avoided and an alternative therapy considered.

Significant fibrosis can occur in the context of entirely normal LFTs, which are therefore unreliable in isolation for drug monitoring. A significant fibrosis risk is associated with a cumulative dose of MTX exceeding 3.5–4 g with no hepatotoxic risk factors and after every 1–1.5 g in those with risk factors for hepatotoxicity. Historically, due to the dose-dependent risk of hepatic fibrosis, guidelines recommended liver biopsy before starting therapy and after a cumulative dose of 1, 3 and 8 grams. However, although liver biopsy remains the gold standard for assessment of fibrosis, it carries a significant risk of morbidity and is subject to sampling error and is therefore no longer routinely recommended.

Monitoring the blood level of the aminoterminal peptide of type III pro-collagen (PIIINP) (a serological marker of hepatic fibrosis) can be used to screen for liver fibrosis and to reduce the need for routine liver biopsies.

Over the last decade, other additional, non-invasive methods to assess for baseline hepatic fibrosis and to monitor for worsening fibrosis have also become widely available. These are usually radiological or serological and depend on local availability.

Transient elastography can be helpful as a non-invasive measure of fibrosis (see Assessment of Liver Function). Additional serological tests include the Enhanced Liver Fibrosis (ELF) panel, which consists of three markers of fibrosis: Hyaluronic acid, PIIINP and tissue inhibitor of matrix metalloproteinase. A score of >9.8 correlates to a high risk of fibrosis, warranting input from hepatology.

At present, a combination of transient elastography in conjunction with serological tests is likely to provide the ideal method and can be helpful for monitoring of hepatic fibrosis and guiding the need for liver biopsy in patients with psoriasis on methotrexate.

Long-term, low-dose MTX therapy has also been implicated in rare instances to cause reactivation of HBV in patients who are HBV core antibody-positive. However, the majority of the patients were also receiving concomitant corticosteroids (see Corticosteroids). These cases have, however, led to recommendations that baseline screening for the HBV surface antigen and HBV core antibody should be carried out before starting MTX and, if positive, consideration given to prophylaxis with antiviral agents.

As with AZA, LFTs alongside other monitoring bloods should be performed more regularly at 1–2-weekly intervals for the first month and/or until a steady dose is achieved; thereafter, 2–3-monthly bloods can be used for monitoring.

RETINOIDS

- Acitretin: Mild abnormalities in LFTs occur in up to one-third of patients taking acitretin; however, only 1–5% of patients have abnormalities greater than 3 times the upper limit of normal and require drug discontinuation. Clinically, apparent liver injury due to acitretin is rare, but several cases have been reported. The time of onset is wide, ranging from 1 week to 9 months after starting therapy. The biochemical profile is typically of raised transaminases, but cholestatic hepatitis has been reported with rare instances of DRESS. The vast majority of cases resolve on drug discontinuation.

- Bexarotene: Elevated aminotransferase levels occur in about 5% of patients. In most cases, abnormalities are mild and transient, but severe and even fatal hepatotoxicity has been reported, especially at high doses.
- Isotretinoin: Modest increases in serum aminotransferases occur in up to 15% of patients taking isotretinoin, but fewer than 1% of patients have abnormalities greater than 3 times the upper limit of normal. Clinically, apparent liver injury is exceedingly rare. Mild serum aminotransferase elevation is often self-limiting and may resolve without drug discontinuation.
- Alitretinoin: Has also been associated with transient and reversible elevations of serum aminotransferases. All oral retinoids are contraindicated in patients with severely impaired liver function.

With acknowledgements to Jo Puleston and Julian Teare, authors of this chapter in the 1st edition; and Rachel Westbrook and Mark Thursz, authors in the 2nd edition.

FURTHER READING

Akiyama S, Cotter TG, Sakuraba A. Risk of hepatitis B virus reactivation in patients with autoimmune disease undergoing non-tumor necrosis factor-targeted biologics. World J Gastroenterol. 2021;27:2312–24.

Day JW, Rosenberg WM. The enhanced liver fibrosis (ELF) test in diagnosis and management of liver fibrosis. BJHM. 2018;79(12):694–9.

LiverTox: Clinical and Research Information on Drug-Induced Liver Injury [Internet]. Bethesda (MD): National Institute of Diabetes and Digestive and Kidney Diseases; 2012. Available from: https://www.ncbi.nlm.nih.gov/books/NBK547852/.

Loomba R, Liang J. Hepatitis B reactivation associated with immune suppressive and biologic modifier therapies: Current concepts, management strategies, and future directions. Gastroenterology. 2017;152:1297–309.

Menter A, Gelfand JM, Conor C et al. Joint American Academy of Dermatology–National Psoriasis Foundation guidelines of care for the management of psoriasis with systemic nonbiologic therapies. J Am Acad Dermatol. 2020;82:1445–86.

41 Systemic Therapy in Older People

Sarita Singh, Rosanna Fox and Manuraj Singh

INTRODUCTION

Advances in medical science have contributed to a worldwide increase in life expectancy. The World Health Organization predicts that the global population of people aged over 60 will reach 2 billion by 2050. There will be an inevitable increase in the burden of dermatological disease, yet there has been little research on skin disease in older people. Aging is associated with various adverse physiological changes in the skin that render it more susceptible to disease. Skin problems in older people present therapeutic and logistic challenges compounded by problems such as insomnia, dementia, poor eyesight and hearing, comorbidities and polypharmacy. Furthermore, the psychosocial consequences of skin disease in this population impact other family members and carers. Prescribing systemic medications, especially in frail older people, requires careful consideration to minimise adverse effects and maximise therapeutic benefit. This chapter provides an overview of the general principles and considerations when prescribing systemic therapy in older people.

GENERAL PRINCIPLES

POLYPHARMACY

Older patients often take multiple medications due to comorbidities. Commonly prescribed drugs include hypnotics, diuretics, antiparkinsonian drugs, antihypertensives, psychotropics and non-steroidal anti-inflammatory drugs (NSAIDs). These increase the risk of potentially harmful drug interactions and reduced adherence.

PHYSIOLOGICAL CHANGES

Physiological changes associated with older age affect drug pharmacokinetics and pharmacodynamics, increasing the risk of toxicity. Age-related decline in renal function often necessitates dose reductions of renally eliminated drugs. Pharmacokinetics (drug absorption, distribution, metabolism and excretion), mostly related to renal excretion, are important, but pharmacodynamics (drug action on its target), related to the biochemical and physiologic effects of prescribed drugs, are also commonly altered in older patients.

The risk of adverse drug reactions. including cutaneous adverse reactions, is increased in patients over 65. Where possible, skin disease in older people should be managed with topical therapy. However, it is important that patients are not denied effective treatment for dermatoses associated with significant physical and psychosocial morbidity and/or potential mortality.

STOPP AND START

STOPP and START are evidence-based criteria that were proposed in 2008 to review and rationalize medication regimes in older people. These have been shown, in randomized controlled trials, to reduce adverse drug reactions and increase drug appropriateness. STOPP stands for "Screening Tool of Older Persons' potentially inappropriate Prescriptions"; these criteria aim to reduce the incidence of adverse events from potentially inappropriate prescribing and polypharmacy. START stands for "Screening Tool to Alert to Right Treatment"; these criteria are used to avoid omission of indicated and appropriate medicines in older patients with specific conditions.

Individual criteria exist for specific organ systems, such as cardiovascular and musculoskeletal systems, but not as yet for skin disease. An example of a STOPP criteria for prescribing in musculoskeletal disorders that is relevant to dermatological practice is: "NSAID with a history of a peptic ulcer disease or gastrointestinal bleeding, unless with concurrent histamine H2 receptor antagonist or proton pump inhibitor, or misoprostol." Similarly, an example of a START criteria relevant to dermatological practice is: "Bisphosphonates in patients taking maintenance corticosteroid therapy." It is likely that these criteria will require modification and refinement with time as the therapeutic evidence base changes. However, these are helpful tools that can act as a framework for safer therapeutic withdrawal and addition in dermatological prescribing in older people.

Frailty

'Frailty' refers to the syndrome of impaired homeostasis and decline in physiological reserves that results in an increased vulnerability to decompensation in response to low-level stressor events. It is not limited to older people, though the incidence of frailty in those >85 years is about 25–50%. Five 'frailty syndromes' are described by the British Geriatric Society: Falls, delirium, immobility, incontinence and susceptibility to medication side effects. Identifying patients with frailty/those at risk of frailty, is important for holistic patient management and to reduce the risk of exacerbating morbidity via drug side effects in high-risk individuals. Extra care is required when prescribing for patients identified as severely frail and those at high risk of becoming so.

In the UK, the most common frailty scoring systems are the Clinical Frailty Scale (CFS) and the electronic Frailty Index (eFI). The CFS allocates patients a score from 1 (very fit) to 9 (terminally ill) using mobility, fitness and independence factors. It is used as a prognostic and care planning tool, but it is only validated for use in those over 65. The eFI is based on Rockwood's Canadian frailty index and uses a 'cumulative deficit' model to identify and grade frailty severity using patient records. Thirty-six deficits are described and broadly divided into:

1. Disease state, e.g. diabetes, stroke and atrial fibrillation.
2. Signs and symptoms, e.g. polypharmacy, falls and incontinence.
3. Disability, e.g. visual impairment, hearing loss and requirement for care.
4. Abnormal laboratory markers, e.g. anaemia and haematinic deficiency.

The total cumulative deficit is calculated by number of deficits recorded, divided by the total number of deficits considered (e.g. 9 deficits would equate to a score of 0.25 = 9/36). Patients are risk-stratified into: Fit (eFI <0.12), mild frailty (eFI 0.12–0.24), moderate frailty (eFI 0.25–0.36) or severe frailty (eFI >0.36).

The CFS and eFI provide frameworks for identifying and stratifying patients who are at higher risk of harm from medication and can be used to achieve safer and more appropriate prescribing of systemic therapy in older patients with skin disease.

Medication Formulation

It is important to consider the formulation of medication, especially in frail older patients who may have difficulty swallowing tablets or capsules when liquid formulations can be very useful. Patients should be informed of the need to take medication with sufficient water and not to leave tablets in the mouth or take when lying supine, due to the risk of oral and oesophageal ulceration, respectively, with certain drugs.

Drug Toxicity

Older patients are particularly susceptible to pharmacokinetic changes, predominantly associated with increased drug tissue concentration due to age-related decline in renal function. Furthermore, when older patients become acutely unwell, particularly if dehydrated, drug levels can increase rapidly. For drugs with a narrow therapeutic index, this can lead to rapid onset of toxicity and adverse effects. For example, an older patient on a stable dose of methotrexate may develop bone marrow suppression when suffering from an acute gastrointestinal infection, due to dehydration and acute kidney injury.

General Principles Checklist

1. Always consider whether systemic therapy is absolutely necessary.
2. Use a frailty scoring system for all patients over 65 to identify potentially inappropriate prescribing and minimize patient risk.
3. Prescribe the lowest dose that is effective and increase dosage slowly as necessary, with careful monitoring of full blood count (FBC), renal and liver function.
4. If possible, make sure that relevant vaccinations are up-to-date (such as the seasonal flu, COVID-19, pneumococcal and shingles vaccinations) before starting any immunosuppressive drug.
5. Do not deny patients effective medication solely on the basis of age.
6. Regular medication reviews are critical to ensure patient adherence and reduce polypharmacy (and the associated increased risk of adverse drug reactions).

PRESCRIBING PRINCIPLES FOR COMMON SKIN CONDITIONS IN OLDER PEOPLE

The most common indications for systemic dermatological therapy in older people are severe psoriasis or eczema, intractable idiopathic pruritus and bullous pemphigoid.

Pruritus

Pruritus is the most common skin complaint in older people. The prevalence increases with age, affecting more than half of people over 65 years every week. Generalized pruritus is often multifactorial and is compounded by problems faced by many older people. These include insomnia (which increases time available for scratching), boredom and loneliness, bereavement, dementia or memory loss, financial difficulties, chronic health issues and polypharmacy. Xerosis (dry skin) is the leading cause of generalized pruritus in older people. Generalized itch without rash may also indicate systemic disease, such as haematological disorders, nutritional deficiencies, renal dysfunction and cholestatic liver disease.

Drug-induced pruritus should also be considered. Opioids, chloroquine, angiotensin-converting enzyme inhibitors and statins are commonly cited pruritogenic agents, but many systemic drugs and topical agents can cause pruritus. An itch can take several weeks to months to develop. The underlying aetiologies are unclear, but possibilities include deposition of the drug or its metabolites in the skin, cholestatic hepatic injury, phototoxicity, xerosis or neurologic mechanisms. Drug-induced pruritus does not always resolve promptly following discontinuation and may persist for many months or even years. In some patients, no underlying cause is identified ('idiopathic' pruritus).

Management of generalized pruritus is challenging. Any underlying cause should be rectified. The patient's ability to comply with therapy should be considered, and simple topical regimes should be used whenever possible to facilitate adherence. In severe or recalcitrant pruritus, systemic therapy may include non-sedating antihistamines, selective serotonin reuptake inhibitors, tricyclic antidepressants, oral steroids, opioid antagonists, thalidomide or biologic therapies.

Psoriasis

Topical medication should be used as first-line treatment in older people. Narrowband ultraviolet B (UVB) phototherapy may be considered, but it is unsuited to those with poor mobility or at high risk of falls. Systemic therapy such as ciclosporin, methotrexate and acitretin should be reserved for severe/recalcitrant disease and carefully monitored.

Eczema

Intensive topical therapy should be used first-line. A short course of oral corticosteroids may be necessary, but older patients are at increased risk of adverse effects, such as gastric irritation and loss of bone mineral density. Initiation of oral corticosteroids often requires co-prescription of medications for bone and gastric protection, increasing polypharmacy. In addition, underlying conditions, such as diabetes, cardiac disease and psychiatric conditions, may be exacerbated by systemic corticosteroids. Other systemic agents, including ciclosporin and JAK inhibitors, should be reserved for severe, recalcitrant disease. Narrowband UVB phototherapy can be considered as above.

Bullous Pemphigoid

Initial treatment should include topical corticosteroids and an oral tetracycline. If widespread and/or severe, oral corticosteroids are usually required with introduction of a steroid-sparing immunosuppressant, such as mycophenolate mofetil or azathioprine. Dose adjustments may be necessary due to renal impairment.

MONITORING OF SYSTEMIC THERAPY

Immunosuppressive drugs such as azathioprine, methotrexate and mycophenolate mofetil are more likely to cause bone marrow suppression and subsequent infection in older patients, so close monitoring of the FBC is essential. Sun protection advice is important, especially in fair-skinned individuals on long-term immunosuppressive therapy.

COMMONLY PRESCRIBED DRUGS – CONSIDERATIONS IN OLDER PATIENTS

Methotrexate

Methotrexate is almost entirely eliminated by the kidneys, so special attention should be paid to renal function. Nephrotoxic effects of NSAIDs should be considered. Patients with reduced renal function are at increased risk of haematological and liver toxicity. Folic acid should be prescribed, as older people are at increased risk of folate deficiency.

Mycophenolate Mofetil

Mycophenolate mofetil (MMF) is generally considered a good choice as a steroid-sparing drug in older patients. Haematological and biochemical monitoring are necessary, as immuno- and myelosuppression are more common in this population. Older people are at increased risk of gastrointestinal haemorrhage and pulmonary oedema with MMF, and it should be used with particular care in those with frailty.

Antibiotics

In addition to dose adjustment for renal impairment, it is also important to consider the increased risk of cutaneous ADRs (beta-lactams, cephalosporins, fluroquinolones and sulphonamides are the main culprits). In frail, underweight patients (typically <45 kg), dose reduction is required. Patients should be informed about the importance of taking certain drugs, such as doxycycline and clindamycin, with plenty of water and while upright to reduce the risk of oesophageal injury.

RENAL FUNCTION – CONSIDERATIONS

The age-related decline in renal function necessitates dose reduction for many drugs. Stage III chronic kidney disease occurs in approximately 15–30% of patients aged over 65, so renal impairment should be especially considered in this age group. Serum creatinine is a poor marker of renal function in older people due to reduced muscle mass, so a normal serum creatinine can be falsely reassuring. GFR estimation and creatinine clearance should therefore be used in older patients, especially when taking drugs with potential nephrotoxicity. (See Chapter 39.)

HEPATIC FUNCTION – CONSIDERATIONS

In contrast to renal function, hepatic function remains fairly stable in older age, with no abnormalities in routine liver blood tests unless there is underlying liver disease. However, there is a fall in hepatic blood flow, liver volume and hepatocyte function with age, with declining drug clearance and cytochrome P450 activity. This can decrease drug metabolism, increase the risk of hepatotoxicity and lead to toxic serum concentrations. Older patients are at increased risk of drug-induced liver injury (DILI), so drugs with known hepatotoxic effects should only be prescribed when necessary and with regular blood monitoring.

SUMMARY

In conclusion, the complex interactions between polypharmacy, comorbidities, altered pharmacodynamics and even modest changes in pharmacokinetics in older people necessitate an approach to prescribing of 'start low and go slow.' Older patients are more sensitive to the effects of drug therapy, and thus adverse reactions for a specified dose generally increase with age. Consider renal impairment in all older patients and ensure appropriate dose adjustment. Treatment regimens should be made as simple as possible to aid compliance, and frailty should be considered as a risk factor for adverse effects of systemic therapy in any patient over the age of 65.

FURTHER READING

Cullinan S, O'Mahony D, O'Sullivan D, et al. Use of a frailty index to identify potentially inappropriate prescribing and adverse drug reaction risks in older patients. Age Ageing. 2016;45:115–20.
Flammiger A, Maibach H. Drug dosage in the elderly: Dermatological drugs. Drugs Aging. 2006;23:203–15.
O'Mahony D, O'Sullivan D, Byrne S, et al. STOPP/START criteria for potentially inappropriate prescribing in older people: Version 2. Age Ageing. 2015;44:213–8.
Rockwood K, Theou O. Using the clinical frailty scale in allocating scarce health care resources. Can. Geriatric J. 2020;23:254–59.
Singh S, Georgiadou D. Pruritus in the elderly population. Dermatol Pract. 2020;26(1):4–10.

Index

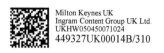

Milton Keynes UK
Ingram Content Group UK Ltd.
UKHW050450071024
449327UK00014B/310